Critical Care for Potential Liver Transplant Candidates

Dmitri Bezinover · Fuat Saner
Editors

Critical Care for Potential Liver Transplant Candidates

Springer

Editors
Dmitri Bezinover
Anesthesiology and Perioperative Medicine
Penn State Hershey Medical Center
Hershey, PA
USA

Fuat Saner
General, Visceral and Transplant Surgery
University of Duisburg-Essen
Essen
Germany

ISBN 978-3-319-92933-0 ISBN 978-3-319-92934-7 (eBook)
https://doi.org/10.1007/978-3-319-92934-7

Library of Congress Control Number: 2018962551

This Springer imprint is published by the registered company Springer Nature Switzerland AG
The registered company address is: Gewerbestrasse 11, 6330 Cham, Switzerland

Foreword

Since its introduction to clinical practice in 1963, liver transplantation has become *the* treatment for both acute and chronic end-stage liver failure as well as for liver-dependent metabolic diseases. By any measure, the improvements seen in this therapeutic option have been spectacular. Even its founding father, Thomas E. Starzl, could not have foreseen how commonplace this procedure would become such that as of today more than 400,000 liver transplantations have been performed worldwide. In the Western world, most transplantations are performed using grafts from deceased donors. However, in the Eastern world, the procedure, instead, relies almost entirely on grafts from live donors.

According to a statement from the 1983 NIH Consensus Conference, transplantation may be a promising alternative to current therapy in the management of a variety of serious liver diseases in their late phase. This would be true for both children and adults. In addition, the conference report not only defined ten absolute and five relative contraindications to transplantation but also outlined the characteristics of the ideal recipient. However, if we were to follow these recommendations today, not a single patient would receive a transplant. Improvements in surgical techniques in both donor and recipient as well as in anaesthesia and peri-operative care have nearly eliminated all but one (active, non-hepatic-related sepsis) of these contraindications. Early survival rates (in the 20% range) pale in comparison to today's rates, which approach 90%. Long-term outcomes, however, have remained almost unchanged. This is due to the fact that many patients with functioning grafts die from cardiovascular, renal, and infectious diseases and also as a result of de novo tumor formation. Most of these complications are either directly or indirectly linked to life-long immunosuppression. This will be the focus, no doubt, of intense research in the next few years.

The spectacular progress made in recent years has, however, caused a serious problem. Liver transplantation, in some ways, has become a victim of its own success. The increasing number of referrals to transplant centers around the world has resulted in an ever-widening gap between the number of potential recipients and the number of available grafts. This gap is steadily increasing, resulting in an increase in mortality while patients wait for a life-saving transplant (up to 30%). This is because, with increasing experience, transplant teams are selecting more and more patients with severe comorbidities. Unfortunately, many of these patients succumb to their comorbidities while on the wait-list. Care of these potential recipients is very labor-intensive and care of these newly transplanted patients is carried out in a context of high risk. This situation is complicated further by the development of surgical variants of the procedure (e.g., split and living donor liver transplantation) and the frequent use of *extended criteria* grafts in order to offer transplantation to as many patients as possible. As a result of these developments, experienced transplant physicians may have the impression that we have returned to the high morbidity and mortality experienced in the adolescent phase of transplantation (1964–1990). The dedicated professionals in transplant centers continue to pave the way for a new generation of transplant caregivers. This new generation of transplant teams has expanded their interest, expertise, and influence in areas specifically related to managing hepatic encephalopathy, infectious diseases, cardiovascular, renal, and mechanical ventilatory support, as well as in the growing fields of combined transplantation and transplant oncology. The transplant team most familiar with each individual patient must be intimately involved in all decisions regarding patient care, including listing and, even more importantly, delisting.

This book, *Critical Care for Potential Liver Transplant Candidates*, is a timely addition to the literature. An international group of highly respected transplant clinicians outline the diagnosis and management of a wide variety of cardiopulmonary, renal, coagulation, infectious, and electrolyte disturbances seen in liver transplant recipients. Current knowledge and areas of uncertainty in need of research specific to these patients are discussed.

The editors of this book, Dmitri Bezinover from Penn State University, Penn State School of Medicine, USA, and Fuat Saner from Essen University Hospital, Germany, should be congratulated for bringing together a group of world experts to prepare this book. It should be on the desk of all clinicians involved in the care of liver transplant patients.

Jan Lerut
Past President of ESOT and ILTS and
Past Director of the Starzl Abdominal Transplant Unit
Université catholique de Louvain,
Brussels, Belgium

Contents

Chapter 1
Cardiac Evaluation and Management

Christopher Wray and James Y. Findlay

Introduction

Liver transplantation constitutes a significant cardiovascular challenge. It involves undertaking a major surgical procedure on a patient with an already altered cardiovascular status during which there is the potential for large and rapid volume shifts, changes in cardiac loading and vascular compliance, and alterations in electrolytes. Pre-existing cardiac conditions may increase the risk of perioperative morbidity and mortality. Additionally, cardiac conditions can influence post-transplant long-term survival. The pretransplant cardiac evaluation is thus a critical part of the evaluation process, with the goal of identifying conditions that can affect the transplant outcome in both the immediate perioperative period and the longer term. Identification of conditions allows pretransplant interventions, as indicated, to be undertaken, perioperative management to be optimized, and postoperative follow-up to be planned. An increased risk of both perioperative and long-term mortality associated with cardiac conditions can also play a significant part in the determination of transplant candidacy.

C. Wray
Liver Transplant Division, Department of Anesthesiology and Perioperative Medicine, Ronald Reagan UCLA Medical Center, Los Angeles, CA, USA

J. Y. Findlay (✉)
Solid Organ Transplant Anesthesia, Department of Anesthesiology and Perioperative Medicine, Mayo Clinic, Rochester, MN, USA
e-mail: Findlay.james@mayo.edu

D. Bezinover, F. Saner (eds.), *Critical Care for Potential Liver Transplant Candidates*,
https://doi.org/10.1007/978-3-319-92934-7_1

Coronary Artery Disease

Interest in underlying cardiovascular disease in liver transplant (LT) patients has increased in the past two decades. Recognition of the impact of cardiovascular disease on post-transplant outcomes has driven research and the publication of consensus documents regarding preoperative cardiac evaluation in LT candidates [1, 2]. Although postoperative survival has continued to improve during this time, major demographic shifts in LT candidates have occurred. Reflecting the general population, LT candidates are aging. More than 20% of LT candidates in the United States are now aged 65 years or older [3]. Cardiovascular disease is highly associated with aging, as are many conditions that impact cardiac risk. End-stage liver disease (ESLD) patterns are changing in LT candidates as well. New antiviral treatment regimens for hepatitis C virus (HCV) infection and the emergence of non-alcoholic fatty liver disease (NAFLD) as a major cause of cirrhosis are likely to play a role in determining future LT candidate populations. Older patients with comorbidities including cardiovascular disease may be excluded from LT candidacy. Likewise, in intensive care unit (ICU) LT patients with a severe manifestation of ESLD, underlying cardiovascular disease may impart additional perioperative risk. Although a number of cardiovascular conditions are of concern in adult LT candidates, coronary artery disease (CAD) is the primary focus of pretransplant cardiac assessment.

Importance

The negative impact of CAD on post-LT survival was initially reported in patients in the 1990s and early 2000s. These series demonstrated inferior outcomes in single-center cohorts with CAD [4–6]. Recent studies have shown that cardiovascular morbidity and mortality are common in the post-transplant period, although direct causation from underlying CAD is difficult to determine in retrospective analyses. Cardiac events were one of the most common etiologies of early postoperative mortality in a large OPTN database analysis of LT patients in the United States over a 10-year period [7]. In another large database series from the United Kingdom over a 13-year period, cardiac disease was the fourth most common cause of postoperative mortality after 1 year, responsible for 8.7% of deaths [8]. Postoperative immunosuppression contributes to the development of hypertension, hyperlipidemia, diabetes, and renal dysfunction, which may enhance the progression of underlying CAD. The cure for ESLD is also associated with significant metabolic changes that can lead to CAD. In a single-center series, 30% of LT recipients with a diagnosis of post-transplant metabolic syndrome suffered cardiovascular complications compared to 6% of patients without that diagnosis [9]. In the last 15 years, significant attention has focused on the detection and management of CAD in LT patients. The expansion of upper age limits for LT candidacy and the aging of the general population have further driven this interest. Compared to the corresponding period for most non-cardiac surgical procedures, the perioperative period in LT is associated with prolonged hemodynamic and metabolic instability and the potential for a hypercoagulable state. Underlying obstructive CAD in this setting may increase the likelihood for plaque rupture and/or a mismatch between coronary supply and demand.

There is wide variance in the prevalence of CAD reported in LT candidates [10]. Differences in patient populations, diagnostic methods, and categorizations of CAD severity contribute to this variability. Most studies have been conducted with a single-center cohort and a relatively small sample size. Overall, recent studies suggest that the prevalence of CAD in LT candidates is at least equal to that of the general population (the reported rate of CAD in the general US population aged 45–64 years in 2015 was 6.1%) [1, 11]. In older LT candidates and in those with traditional CAD risk factors, CAD prevalence may be much higher [12]. Patients with a diagnosis of NAFLD have a higher likelihood of CAD compared to the general population, with prevalence rates reported as ranging from 7.4 to 21.6% [13, 14]. The prevalence of CAD is likely to increase in LT candidates as the population ages and the rates of CAD risk factors increase. The emergence of NAFLD is likely to have a major impact on the cardiovascular risk of LT candidates as well. According to 2016 UNOS data, HCV infection is no longer the leading indication for LT in the United States, which is likely to represent an increased number of LTs for the diagnosis of NAFLD [15].

Screening

Screening for asymptomatic CAD has become an essential part of the preoperative selection process for adult LT candidates. However, preoperative cardiac evaluation of LT patients is challenging. Currently, there is no standard for the preoperative CAD evaluation of LT candidates, and randomized prospective studies investigating preoperative paradigms are lacking for this population. Even though the majority of LT programs use the guidelines of the American Association for the Study of Liver Diseases (AASLD), there are wide variations in practice between centers. Candidates may remain listed for long periods of time prior to an organ offer, and CAD may progress during the interim. Progression of cirrhosis resulting in severe manifestations of ESLD may necessitate an urgent cardiac reevaluation prior to transplant. The urgency of surgery, the continued mismatch between organ supply and demand, and the need for programs to maintain acceptable outcomes distinguish LT from other non-cardiac surgeries.

History, Risk Factors, Cardiac Symptoms, and Functional Capacity

Current ACC/AHA guidelines recommend a stepwise process for the preoperative cardiac evaluation of non-cardiac surgical patients that relies on determining functional status and analyzing key risk factors. An indication for noninvasive ischemia testing is based on this approach in most clinical situations [16].

A known history of previous CAD in an LT candidate requires an updated cardiology evaluation prior to listing. However, the frequency of reevaluation over an extended listing period has yet to be precisely defined. As the ESLD population ages, more patients are likely to have traditional CAD risk factors. CAD risk factor analysis is important for LT candidates, as having more than one pretransplant risk factor has been shown to correlate with the risk of significant CAD [17].

Diagnosis of occult CAD on the basis of a history of cardiac symptoms is problematic in LT candidates. A variety of cardiovascular conditions that may produce cardiac symptomatology are prevalent in this population. The presence of cardiac dysfunction due to cirrhosis, a syndrome termed cirrhotic cardiomyopathy (CCM), may be responsible for many cardiac symptoms. In critically ill transplant candidates, underlying renal failure due to hepatorenal syndrome (HRS) may contribute to volume overload and symptoms of diastolic heart failure. Etiologies of systolic failure such as alcoholic cardiomyopathy may produce symptoms of congestive heart failure. Deconditioned ESLD patients are usually unable to exercise to the point of producing ischemic symptoms. Finally, asymptomatic myocardial ischemia and silent myocardial infarction (MI) are common in candidates with longstanding diabetes.

Determining the functional capacity of LT candidates is also challenging. ESLD contributes to deconditioning, malnutrition, sarcopenia, renal failure, and pulmonary complications. These factors collectively impact exercise tolerance and mobility. Critically ill ICU LT candidates may have a prolonged history of immobility that prevents an accurate assessment of their functional status.

Noninvasive Ischemia Testing

Based on the known prevalence of underlying CAD and the difficulty of applying current American College of Cardiology (ACC)/American Heart Association (AHA) guidelines for noninvasive ischemia testing to LT candidates, most centers perform comprehensive noninvasive testing on a large proportion of adult LT candidates. There is a significant body of research focused on evaluating a variety of noninvasive methods in LT candidates. In general, most studies have been performed with small, single-center cohorts, and results vary across studies due to differences in study methods, patient characteristics, and outcome measurements. In particular, a comparison of noninvasive results with coronary angiography, the current standard for determining a diagnosis of CAD, was not performed in many of the studies. Although comprehensive noninvasive testing is common in most centers, there are concerns regarding efficacy, cost, and logistics [1]. Nevertheless, important information on the utility of noninvasive methods for the detection of asymptomatic CAD in LT candidates has emerged.

Resting Electrocardiogram (EKG)

A preoperative resting 12-lead EKG is necessary prior to listing adult LT candidates. Although occult obstructive CAD may be present despite a normal resting EKG, the presence of Q waves, left bundle branch block, frequent premature ventricular contractions (PVCs), and repolarization abnormalities associated with silent myocardial ischemia provide valuable diagnostic information that can direct further CAD evaluation. In addition, EKG manifestations of CCM such as prolongation of the QT interval, bradycardia due to chronotropic dysfunction, and arrhythmias such as atrial fibrillation (AF) are especially important to consider in documenting the condition of critically ill patients with advanced ESLD [18].

Stress Echocardiography

Pharmacologic stress echocardiography with dobutamine (DSE) has been extensively evaluated in LT candidates. The use of exercise echocardiography is limited by poor functional capacity in many patients with cirrhosis and has rarely been studied. Although an early single-center study demonstrated a strong positive predictive value (PPV) for the detection of obstructive CAD, further studies have shown significant variability in both the sensitivity and specificity of DSE for the prediction of underlying obstructive CAD compared to coronary angiography [19–22]. Incomplete and non-diagnostic studies are common with DSE in LT candidates due to failure to reach the target heart rate, and beta blockade for portal hypertension and chronotropic dysfunction from CCM may be implicated [22]. In LT candidates with an underlying vasodilatory state, tests may be terminated early due to cardiac symptoms, dysrhythmia, or hypotension. Despite the inaccuracy of DSE for predicting underlying obstructive CAD, the test appears to have value for identifying patients at low risk for postoperative cardiac events. In an analysis of seven studies in which DSE was employed for the preoperative screening of LT candidates, the reported specificities and negative predictive values for perioperative and long-term postoperative cardiac events were very good [23]. These findings suggest that a normal DSE predicts a low likelihood of perioperative cardiac events, especially in candidates with few CAD risk factors. Many centers use DSE as the initial CAD screening test in pretransplant paradigms. However, as the sensitivity of DSE for detecting obstructive CAD in LT candidates is poor compared to the general population, candidates at high risk for underlying CAD may be referred for coronary angiography regardless of DSE results.

Nuclear Myocardial Perfusion Imaging

Stress myocardial perfusion scintigraphy or single photon emission contrast tomography (SPECT) has been studied in LT cohorts as well. A number of studies have shown wide variability in both sensitivity and specificity for the detection of obstructive CAD with SPECT in LT candidates [24–26]. The results of one study showed that SPECT had the same accuracy as risk factor analysis for the detection of severe CAD in a cohort of LT candidates [26]. The vasodilatory state associated with ESLD may have an impact on the efficacy of SPECT in LT candidates.

Cardiac Contrast Tomography/Coronary CT Angiography

Cardiac contrast tomography (CT) scanning for quantifying the calcium burden present in coronary arteries has been described as a viable screening method for CAD in a cohort of low-risk LT candidates [27]. Cardiac CT has advantages in LT candidates, as diagnostic accuracy is not affected by exercise capacity, vasodilatory state, or heart rate. Likewise, coronary CT angiography, an alternative to invasive coronary angiography, provides detailed imaging of coronary anatomy, and has been described as a viable screening test in a cohort of low- and medium-risk LT candidates [28].

Cardiopulmonary Fitness Evaluation

Functional cardiovascular testing including the assessment of metabolic equivalents (METs) that patients are able to attain may be employed in the preoperative testing paradigm for non-cardiac surgery. Functional testing for the preoperative assessment of LT candidates has been studied. Both the 6-min walk distance test and the cardiopulmonary exercise test (CPET) have been assessed in LT candidates, and a limited cardiopulmonary reserve has been shown to correlate with worse post-transplant survival using either method [10]. It should be noted that in many LT candidates, especially in those with critical illness, functional cardiac testing is not likely to be applicable.

Coronary Angiography

Coronary angiography allows for the definitive diagnosis of the severity and distribution of CAD, regardless of its functional impact. Angiography is invasive and associated with risks that may be increased in LT candidates. Studies have demonstrated the safety of angiography in patients with cirrhosis, although with only small samples [29, 30]. Vascular injuries and transfusion are more common with angiography in ESLD patients compared to patients without cirrhosis [30]. Upper extremity arterial access for coronary angiography has become standard at many centers and has been shown to be safe and effective in a cohort of ESLD patients [31].

Recommendations

Two recently published documents provide recommendations for the preoperative evaluation of CAD in LT candidates, although these two documents differ in terms of some specific details [1, 2]. According to a consensus document from the American Heart Association (AHA) and the American College of Cardiology Foundation (ACCF), noninvasive stress testing should be considered regardless of functional status based on the presence of three or more CAD risk factors. These risk factors include an age of greater than 60 years, a history of tobacco use, hypertension, hyperlipidemia, left-ventricular hypertrophy, diabetes, and a history of known cardiovascular disease. This document also includes the recommendation that each center identify a cardiology consultant for the preoperative evaluation of LT candidates [1]. In an AASLD and American Society of Transplantation (AST) practice guideline included in the document, both an assessment of cardiac risk factors and stress echocardiography as an initial CAD screening test are recommended. Also recommended are the use of coronary angiography as indicated by the clinical situation and consideration for cardiac revascularization in LT candidates with significant CAD [2].

Many centers use screening paradigms that include compulsory noninvasive testing, aggressive coronary angiography for positive or non-diagnostic stress test results, and direct coronary angiography for high-risk candidates regardless of stress test results. Although angiography allows for standardized grading of CAD lesions, the severity of CAD that may be of significance during the perioperative period of LT has not been defined. Fractional flow reserve (FFR), a method for determining the functional significance of a flow-limiting coronary lesion, has become the standard for assessing the need for revascularization in intermediate coronary lesions [32]. FFR is likely to have a significant role in determining the need for preoperative revascularization of discrete coronary lesions in LT candidates.

Management of CAD in LT Candidates

There is no consensus regarding management strategies for LT candidates with significant CAD. Furthermore, the extent of CAD that excludes candidates from LT has not been defined. Current ACC/AHA guidelines do not recommend revascularization for asymptomatic CAD prior to elective non-cardiac surgery [16]. However, LT surgery is unique compared to other elective non-cardiac surgeries. Severe hemodynamic, metabolic, and hemostatic changes occur during the perioperative period and may persist in critically ill patients for many days during the postoperative period. The impact of underlying obstructive CAD in relation to LT may adversely impact outcomes to a greater extent compared to routine elective surgery. In addition, organs are a scarce and precious resource. Centers are usually unwilling to risk early mortality from a cardiovascular complication in a patient with severe underlying CAD without performing pretransplant revascularization, although this practice has not been validated in randomized studies. Unlike in the non-transplant surgical population, significant logistical, ethical, and practical issues prevent the design and implementation of a properly powered, randomized study comparing medical management to pretransplant revascularization in an LT population.

In many centers, obstructive CAD identified on pretransplant angiography is treated using percutaneous coronary intervention (PCI). In LT candidates, especially in those with high MELD scores and a likelihood of undergoing LT in the near future, PCI with a bare metal stent (BMS) is the favored approach as the duration of antiplatelet therapy is shorter with BMS. In general, listing for LT is usually delayed for 4 weeks following BMS placement per recent guidelines; however, listing dilemmas may occur after revascularization in patients with decompensated liver disease [33]. Centers must balance the risk of stent thrombosis against the risk of delaying transplant in high-MELD candidates with an escalating risk of mortality from progressive ESLD without LT. Furthermore, the timing of the withdrawal of antiplatelet therapy may need to be addressed, adding to the complexity of treating these patients. Difficult listing decisions for LT candidates with CAD including for those with a history of recent revascularization require close communication between all clinicians involved in the care of these patients.

Cardiac surgical revascularization prior to LT may be undertaken in candidates with multi-vessel disease not amenable to PCI. However, a very high rate of mortality is well recognized in patients with advanced cirrhosis following cardiac surgery [34]. Off-pump coronary artery bypass grafting (CABG) is a less invasive revascularization option and may be considered in appropriate LT candidates. There are reports of improved outcomes in off-pump surgery compared to conventional CABG in patients with cirrhosis; however, each of these studies included only a small number of patients [35, 36]. Combined CABG-LT surgeries have been performed successfully in LT candidates with multi-vessel CAD; however, experience is limited to case reports and small, single-center series [37].

Prior to listing for LT, all candidates should be maintained on long-term lifestyle and dietary modifications to limit the development and progression of CAD. Medical therapies may be considered in patients with risk factors or with a proven diagnosis of CAD [16]. Per ACC/ACCF recommendations, chronic condition medical management of CAD in LT candidates should be directed by a cardiologist [1]. Statin therapy has been shown to decrease perioperative cardiac events and mortality in non-transplant surgical patients, and its use is reasonable in high-risk patients including LT candidates [16]. In non-LT surgical populations, there is mixed evidence for the benefit of perioperative beta blockade, and it is not recommended to initiate beta blockade at the time of surgery in patients not previously receiving beta-blockers [16]. The impact of perioperative beta blockade has been evaluated in LT patients. In a single-center series of LT patients, perioperative beta blockade was protective against both early mortality and a composite of nonfatal myocardial infarction (MI) and early mortality [6]. In another single-center study on LT patients, intraoperative hemodynamic data and postoperative outcomes were compared between patients who had received preoperative beta blockade and patients who had not received this treatment. Intraoperative hemodynamic parameters such as heart rate and cardiac index were lower in the group that received beta-blockers; however, there were no differences in outcome data between the groups, including in regard to early mortality [38]. Many LT candidates may receive chronic beta blockade therapy for the management of portal hypertension. It is reasonable to maintain perioperative beta blockade in these patients, although the risk of bradycardia during the perioperative period should be considered.

Outcomes in LT Candidates with CAD

As previously mentioned, there are no prospective randomized controlled studies that include a comparison between revascularization and medical therapy in LT patients with CAD. Retrospective series, mostly in single-center cohorts, have provided outcome data for LT patients with documented CAD. Of particular interest are studies conducted within the past 15 years. These studies report outcomes in patients who received transplants in the current MELD score organ allocation era in the United States (after 2002). Current CAD management strategies including PCI with post-intervention antiplatelet therapy were routine during this time period as well.

In a recent single-center study of LT candidates over a 10-year period, coronary angiography rates and postoperative LT outcomes were evaluated. During the study period, the pretransplant cardiac evaluation policy evolved from a general cardiology consultation to a dedicated LT cardiology service based on a paradigm that included standard indications for angiography. The authors found that rates of coronary angiography and PCI increased over the study period. Postoperative MI and unadjusted 1-year mortality decreased during the study period as well. Interestingly, the majority of postoperative MI patients from the early period of the study did not undergo preoperative angiography, and more than half of the patients who underwent preoperative PCI had normal stress tests. The authors concluded that a lower threshold for performing pretransplant coronary angiography may impact post-transplant outcomes [39]. Based on the study methodology, the impact of coronary angiography and pretransplant coronary revascularization cannot be directly correlated with a survival benefit. However, the results are compelling.

In three recent studies, post-transplant outcomes in LT patients with documented CAD are evaluated. In a single-center study of 87 LT patients who underwent pretransplant angiography, 29 patients were found to have angiographically proven obstructive CAD, of whom 22 underwent pretransplant revascularization. Post-transplant outcomes in this cohort were compared to those of control groups from the same institution. There was no significant difference in survival between the patients with CAD and either the patients with no CAD on angiogram or the control group patients. The authors concluded that post-LT survival is not dependent on the severity of underlying CAD or the number of coronary arteries involved [40]. In another single-center study of 386 LT patients over a 4-year period, postoperative survival was compared with national UNOS data. The single-center cohort included patients with a diagnosis of CAD. Postoperative survival was similar between the studied group and the national database group, and survival was similar regardless of the severity of CAD or the preoperative cardiovascular risk index [41]. Finally, in a multi-center study of 630 LT patients who had undergone pretransplant angiography, 151 patients with obstructive CAD were identified. These patients underwent treatment per the discretion of each center. In total, 80 patients underwent pretransplant interventions; 46 patients received coronary stents; and 32 patients underwent CABG. Seventy-one patients were managed medically prior to LT. There was no difference in adjusted mortality between the groups with and without obstructive CAD. The authors concluded that when current CAD management is used, patients with proven obstructive CAD can safely undergo LT provided they are otherwise appropriate candidates [42].

Based on the above evidence, LT in patients with appropriately treated CAD using current practices appears to be justified. However, given that cardiac disease is a leading cause of late post-LT mortality, further studies examining the impact of underlying CAD on long-term outcomes are required. In addition, the current UNOS national database for LT does not archive information on cardiac risk factors or cardiac outcomes. Individual centers must maintain their own databases of LT populations with cardiac diseases. Collecting sufficient data on LT patients with underlying CAD is challenging, as the overall volume of transplants performed on patients with obstructive CAD is relatively low, despite the recent increase in the prevalence of CAD.

CAD Management in LT ICU Patients

There are no studies directly addressing the impact of CAD on critically ill LT patients in the ICU setting. Most ICU LT candidates have high MELD scores, generally considered a score of 35 or higher. These patients have a high prevalence of renal failure requiring renal replacement therapy, mechanical ventilation, hemodynamic instability requiring vasopressor infusions, and treatment of coagulopathy. In the MELD allocation era, high-MELD patients are prioritized for receiving an LT given that their risk of mortality is acute. LT outcomes based on MELD score have been studied with mixed results; overall, however, the preoperative MELD score is not a highly accurate predictor of post-LT survival [43–45]. The impact of underlying cardiac disease on post-LT outcomes in high-MELD patients has been studied.

In a single-center study, post-LT outcomes were analyzed in 169 LT recipients with MELD scores of 40 or greater over an 8-year period. Early (3 months) mortality was 22%. An analysis of the pretransplant risk factors in survivors and in the group with early mortality demonstrated that chronic morbidities, sepsis, and cardiac conditions strongly predicted post-LT mortality in this high-MELD cohort. Severe CAD (defined as 70% stenosis of a coronary artery or a history of revascularization), a history of MI, and wall motion abnormalities on stress testing were included in the cardiac predictors of early mortality [46]. This study provides evidence that underlying CAD has a significant impact on critically ill, high-MELD LT candidates.

Evaluating ICU patients for CAD can be challenging. Functional status cannot be determined. Cardiac symptoms may be masked or absent. Logistics for performing noninvasive testing are difficult. In some centers, critically ill LT candidates may undergo direct coronary angiography prior to listing to rule out obstructive CAD, especially in patients with hemodynamic instability and with elevated levels of cardiac biomarkers. The threshold for determining exclusionary criteria in high-MELD candidates with underlying CAD is difficult, as each clinical situation is unique. Listing dilemmas are common in critically ill ICU LT candidates, and underlying CAD adds to the complexity of treating these patients. A multidisciplinary team including surgeons, cardiologists, transplant anesthesiologists, hepatologists, and critical care physicians should be included in the preoperative management, evaluation, and determination of candidacy of critically ill patients with CAD.

Structural Heart Disease

Patients presenting for liver transplant evaluation may have known structural heart disease, or it may be discovered on pretransplant screening, particularly on echocardiography. As a general approach, cardiac symptoms should be sought, although in the context of liver failure the interpretation of these may be difficult (e.g., exercise limitation, shortness of breath, or edema). The lesion should be characterized by appropriate measurements of severity, many of which can be obtained by echocardiography. It should be noted that echocardiography is able to detect small degrees of valvular abnormalities; those reported as trivial or mild are rarely of clinical significance. The potential influence of altered physiology during the perioperative period should be considered in making a decision on the suitability of a candidate for transplant. In some circumstances, stress echocardiography may assist in assessing the significance of a cardiac lesion and potential responses to the stresses of transplant surgery. The potential interventions to ameliorate or correct the lesion should also be considered along with the associated risk, particularly if cardiac surgery may be required. The outcome literature regarding patients with structural heart disease undergoing LT is rather scant and generally of low evidential quality. The studies that do exist report the outcome of those patients selected to advance to transplant, which limits the general guidance that can be taken from it. The decision-making process relies on sound clinical judgment and close collaboration between members of the transplant team along with cardiology and cardiac surgery input.

Valvular Heart Disease

Stenotic Lesions

The presence of moderate or severe aortic stenosis has been reported as resulting in a fivefold increase in perioperative mortality and morbidity, with the highest risk reported for patients with severe disease [47]. Data related to LT and this condition are not available, as most programs deny LT to candidates with untreated high-grade stenosis. If pretransplant intervention can be undertaken, this is typically recommended. Operative valve replacement can be considered. However, with increasing severity of liver failure, the high risk of perioperative decompensation and mortality associated with cardiac surgery in ESLD may limit acceptance of this [48]. One approach has been to perform valve replacement and LT in the same procedure, as reported in case reports and small series [49, 50]. However, this approach can be challenging from both an operative management and organizational standpoint. More recently, transcatheter techniques, both valvuloplasty and valve replacement, have become available and have been successfully used prior to LT [51, 52]. In centers with experience in these techniques, these may represent the best bridge to transplant for suitable candidates.

Mitral stenosis causes obstruction of blood flow between the left atrium (LA) and the left ventricle, resulting in LA dilation and elevated pressures in the LA, the pulmonary vasculature, and the right side of the heart. Options for management include surgical and percutaneous techniques, of which the latter have been reported as a bridge to LT [53].

Insufficiency

Trivial or mild valvular regurgitation is a frequent finding on echocardiography and of little significance. Indeed, it may be a normal finding, such as the tricuspid regurgitation used to estimate right-sided systolic pressure. More severe degrees of aortic and mitral regurgitation can lead to left-ventricular volume overload and failure; such patients are poor candidates for LT without correction. A further consideration with left-sided regurgitation is the possibility of it worsening in the post-transplant period as SVR increases [54].

Tricuspid regurgitation (TR), if severe, results in increased right-sided filling pressure, which may compromise blood flow to the transplanted liver. In an evaluation of TR in liver failure, it should be remembered that functional TR can be related to volume status and may show marked improvement with diuresis. TR of any degree greater than mild has been associated with more intraoperative hemodynamic instability and higher per-transplant morbidity and mortality. Yet, how this information should be incorporated into pretransplant risk stratification is unclear [55, 56].

Outflow Tract Obstruction

Left ventricular outflow tract (LVOT) obstruction occurs when a narrowing of the LVOT and high flow result in a pressure gradient causing systolic anterior motion of the mitral valve (SAM) into the LVOT, a resultant obstruction, and a drop in cardiac output and blood pressure. Left-ventricular hyperdynamism and low SVR, as present in ESLD and during LT, are predisposing factors. An inducible LVOT obstruction (not present at rest but present during stress) is a not uncommon finding on DSE performed on LT candidates. Patients who exhibit this have a higher incidence of intraoperative hypotension, but post-LT outcomes are not affected [57]. Intraoperative TEE aids in identifying the occurrence of LVOT obstruction and guiding management with fluid administration, pressor use, and avoidance of hyperdynamism.

LVOT obstruction secondary to a fixed lesion occurs in the more common variant of hypertrophic cardiomyopathy (HCM). Successful LT has been reported in HCM patients with appropriate monitoring and management [58, 59]. While operative myomectomy is the definitive treatment, alcohol septal ablation has been used as a bridge to LT [60].

PFO/ASD

A finding of patent foramen ovale (PFO) is common and has been identified on echocardiography in 25% of adults [61]. Theoretically, PFO could place patients at risk for perioperative morbidity while undergoing LT, particularly embolic events. However, published studies show no increased morbidity or mortality and no influence of PFO size [62, 63]. The findings for atrial septal defect in pediatric patients undergoing LT are similar [64, 65].

Congenital Heart Disease

Fontan Circulation

Correction of congenital heart disease by the Fontan procedure results in a circulation that is prone to the development of liver disease. Such patients present a complex problem: if further heart surgery is contemplated, they are at risk for hepatic decompensation; if LT is considered, the influence of the Fontan physiology on the transplanted liver is uncertain, and experience is limited [66]. Of particular concern is that a CVP adequate to maintain pulmonary blood flow (which is passive in these patients) is required, which may compromise liver blood flow. Yet, successful combined heart liver transplantation has been reported [67].

Other Congenital Defects

A large variety of congenital cardiac defects may be identified in LT candidates, uncorrected or corrected. In some pediatric candidates, the cardiac defects may be part of the syndrome with liver failure (e.g., Alagille syndrome). In each case, the particular lesions and how these could influence both the transplant procedure and the postoperative course should be considered in concert with appropriate expert consultation.

Cirrhotic Cardiomyopathy

Cirrhotic cardiomyopathy (CCM) is a cardiac dysfunction occurring in patients with cirrhosis. Although there is no universally accepted definition, a proposed working definition describes it as characterized by impaired contractile responsiveness to stress and/or altered diastolic relaxation with electrophysiological abnormalities in the absence of other known cardiac disease [68]. A constellation of alterations in cardiovascular receptor function, molecular mediators, cardiac membrane function, and autonomic function have been described in cirrhotic patients and are believed to contribute to the development of CCM [68, 69]. Investigative findings include systolic dysfunction (low resting EF), blunted systolic response to stress, diastolic dysfunction, and electrophysiological abnormalities including prolonged QT [68–71]. Reversal of clinical abnormalities post-LT has been described [71]. Assessing the significance of CCM in the LT population is problematic. There is no definitive test for CCM. Systolic dysfunction is masked in ESLD by the associated vasodilation, and there is no standardized test for blunted cardiac responsiveness. Diastolic dysfunction is common in LT candidates, being found in 43% in one study [72]. Diastolic dysfunction is not associated with the severity of liver disease; however, it is associated with volume status, particularly in the presence of ascites and with other factors described in a non-ESLD population such as increased age [72–74]. Studies in which the influence of diastolic dysfunction on outcomes in both cirrhotic patients and post-LT patients are evaluated present conflicting conclusions. Diastolic dysfunction has been reported as not associated with worsened outcomes [73, 75], as associated with worse outcomes but not as an independent factor [76], and as independently associated with increased graft failure and mortality [77]. The later study also showed a "dose effect" with worse outcomes for higher grades of diastolic dysfunction. Further, diastolic dysfunction has been associated with increased hemodynamic instability during LT [78]. At this point, the importance of identifying CCM in LT candidates is unclear, as is the relationship between CCM and diastolic dysfunction, and between the latter and the outcomes.

Arrhythmia

Severe arrhythmias may impact the LT patient population in the preoperative, intraoperative, and postoperative phases. Pre-existing arrhythmia in an LT candidate requires a complete cardiology evaluation. In certain cases, definitive therapy may be warranted prior to listing. The presence of an unstable arrhythmia may impact the candidacy of a patient and should be addressed prior to proceeding with LT. In the perioperative period, a severe arrhythmia may adversely impact the LT patient. Underlying CCM, electrolyte and acid base abnormalities, chronic cardiac conditions, and hemodynamic instability may all contribute to the development of an arrhythmia and worsen the clinical course. An arrhythmia may develop during critical intraoperative events, particularly at reperfusion of the new graft. Severely ill ICU LT patients may be at higher risk for an arrhythmia secondary to a prolonged high-catecholamine state and multi-organ dysfunction. In all cases, a new severe arrhythmia in an LT patient requires prompt cardiology evaluation and treatment.

Ventricular Arrhythmias

The prevalence of ventricular arrhythmias has rarely been studied in LT patients, and sudden cardiac death is seldom reported in cirrhosis patients. Despite this, the underlying presence of CCM may create conditions in the myocardium that enable the development of a ventricular arrhythmia. QT prolongation is a common feature of CCM, occurring in half of all patients with cirrhosis [79]. In ESLD patients, toxins accumulate in the central circulation and act on cardiac myocytes, resulting in cellular changes that manifest as a prolonged QT interval [80]. The increased sympathetic state in CCM may contribute to the development of QT prolongation as well [81]. It is well known that QT prolongation may induce a fatal ventricular arrhythmia, particularly torsades de pointes. In addition to a prolonged QT interval, underlying ventricular dysfunction may further contribute to the development of a ventricular arrhythmia. The presence of alcoholic cardiomyopathy (CM), the most common form of dilated CM in cirrhosis, may further contribute, particularly in the late stages of heart failure. Underlying CAD, valvular disease, and right-ventricular (RV) failure from severe portopulmonary hypertension (PPH) may lead to ventricular arrhythmias in LT patients as well.

The perioperative period during LT increases the likelihood for a ventricular arrhythmia in patients with QT prolongation. The hemodynamic stress of surgery, electrolyte and acid-base derangements, and medications that further prolong the QT interval may all have an impact. The acute physiologic changes associated with reperfusion of the graft, including postreperfusion syndrome, create the highest risk for ventricular arrhythmias during the perioperative period. Central venous access procedures and pulmonary artery catheterization may predispose to ventricular ectopy. In critically ill ICU patients with multi-organ disease, a ventricular arrhythmia may impact the clinical course in both the preoperative and postoperative periods. Ventricular ectopy may signify a severe underlying cardiac condition such as left-ventricular (LV) failure, myocardial ischemia, MI, or acute right-ventricular (RV) failure. In the postoperative period, LV failure from stress-induced CM (takotsubo CM) may present with ventricular irritability. Regardless of the phase of LT, prompt recognition and treatment of an unstable arrhythmia using advanced cardiac life support (ACLS) treatments including cardioversion are indicated. In the operating room, some centers may place defibrillator patches as part of a standard institutional protocol in all patients prior to surgery. In all cases of ventricular arrhythmia, cardiology consultation is warranted for the diagnosis of underlying cardiac conditions and further management. Patients with a history of ventricular arrhythmia or those with the onset of ventricular arrhythmia in the preoperative period require a comprehensive cardiology evaluation, and LT candidacy may be impacted.

Despite a large number of publications documenting cardiac events in the perioperative and postoperative periods in LT populations, few provide information on ventricular arrhythmia. Most studies are retrospective reports from single centers, and the methodology may not differentiate between the types of arrhythmia; some report only atrial fibrillation. A ventricular arrhythmia may be a manifestation of another cardiac condition, particularly heart failure and MI. Nevertheless, there are case reports of ventricular arrhythmias including torsade de pointes complicating LT [82–84]. In a prospective series of 105 patients who received an LT, 37% developed significant ventricular ectopy during pulmonary artery catheterization (defined as 3 or more premature ventricular beats); 4 patients developed a sustained ventricular arrhythmia [85]. In a single-center series that reported cardiac events in LT patients, there were 12 intraoperative arrhythmias resulting in 2 intraoperative deaths, although the types of arrhythmia were not specified [86]. Many studies have documented arrhythmias in the early postoperative period in LT patients; however, few have specifically documented ventricular arrhythmias. In one single-center report, arrhythmia was one of the most common postoperative cardiac complications; however the majority of arrhythmias were atrial fibrillation [87]. In another single-center series that reported 70 early postoperative cardiac events, 24 atrial arrhythmias and 2 ventricular tachycardia events were documented [88]. In all phases of LT, the anesthesiologist should be vigilant regarding the early diagnosis and prompt treatment of ventricular arrhythmias. A preoperative EKG is necessary, and the QT interval should be assessed. Medications that prolong the QT interval should be avoided if possible. Cardiology consultation is advisable for the further management of LT patients with a ventricular arrhythmia.

Atrial Fibrillation

Based on reports documenting the frequent occurrence of atrial fibrillation (AF) during the perioperative period in LT patients, a number of recent studies specifically investigating AF in LT populations have been published. AF appears to be much more common than ventricular arrhythmia in LT patients. AF is the most common dysrhythmia in adults, and its prevalence increases with age due to cardiac structural and electrophysiologic changes [89]. AF is associated with significant morbidity and mortality, including stroke and heart failure. In the perioperative period, the onset of AF can significantly impact hemodynamic stability due to loss of the atrial contribution to stroke volume. A rapid ventricular response (RVR) can further impact hemodynamic stability. AF is categorized as paroxysmal, recurrent, and chronic persistent. The evaluation and treatment of AF have been well studied and are beyond the scope of this chapter [89].

AF has been investigated in LT patients in all phases of the perioperative period. In a single-center series of 717 consecutive LTs, 32 patients (4.5%) had documented AF on EKG prior to surgery. Compared to an age-matched control group, patients with AF had more adverse cardiovascular events during the intraoperative phase and more AF-related postoperative events. However, overall graft and patient survival was similar between the groups [90]. In another single-center series of 757 LT patients, 19 (2.5%) had documented preoperative AF. Compared to the non-AF patients, the patients with AF had lower 30-day (84 vs. 97%) and 1-year (68 versus 90%) survival [91]. The impact of postoperative AF was studied in a large single-center series of LT patients. In 1,387 consecutive LT patients, the prevalence of postoperative AF within 30 days of surgery was 7.4%. Patients with postoperative AF were older, had a higher MELD score, and were more likely to require preoperative intubation, dialysis, and vasopressors. Crude mortality and graft failure were significantly higher in patients with postoperative AF, as were the incidence of postoperative renal failure and the duration of hospitalization. Multivariate analysis demonstrated that postoperative AF is an independent predictor for mortality. Interestingly, postoperative AF correlated closely with MELD score: nearly a third of patients with MELD scores of 32 or higher developed AF. These findings suggest that the development of postoperative AF is highly associated with underlying severe ESLD, multi-organ disease, and severe CCM [92].

The prevalence and adverse impact of AF in surgical populations are well documented [93]. The presence of AF in any phase of the perioperative period may impact outcomes in LT as well. It is advisable for patients with documented preoperative AF to undergo a cardiology evaluation. In patients with chronic AF, decisions regarding medical therapy and anticoagulation management may increase the complexity of care during the perioperative period. The onset of acute AF with RVR during LT may significantly impact hemodynamics, and appropriate management may include cardioversion and cardiology consultation. Unstable AF in the preoperative and intraoperative phases may impact LT candidacy. Postoperative AF is an important risk factor for mortality and morbidity in LT patients. AF with RVR may precipitate tachycardia-induced LV failure. Postoperative LT patients with underlying CCM and baseline hemodynamic instability may be at a particularly elevated risk. Management of new onset AF in the postoperative period should include cardiology consultation.

Bradyarrhythmias

The underlying state of CCM in LT patients creates the potential for bradycardia and dysrhythmia related to a low heart rate, despite the hyperdynamic circulation of cirrhosis. Chronotropic dysfunction is a recognized feature of CCM. Abnormal heart rate responses to pharmacologic and physiologic stimulation are common in patients with ESLD [94]. Chronotropic incompetence during DSE is a common reason for incomplete test results. In one series, 49% of LT candidates did not achieve the target heart rate during DSE [22]. Chronotropic incompetence in cirrhosis is thought to occur due to many factors, including beta-receptor downregulation, reduced baroreflex responses, and autonomic neuropathy [22, 79]. Reduced heart rate variability has been documented in cirrhotic patients [95]. In addition, many LT candidates receive chronic beta-blockade therapy for portal hypertension, further contributing to the potential for low heart rate responses.

Bradyarrhythmias in the perioperative period in LT patients have received little research attention. Nevertheless, bradycardia is regularly encountered during LT, particularly at reperfusion. The release of pooled venous blood from the lower half of the body after opening of the vena cava clamps results in the rapid return of cold, acidotic blood to the heart. Bradycardic responses at reperfusion are common, although most are self-limited. In rare cases, heart block or asystole requiring resuscitation may occur. A reduction in heart rate may also occur with postreperfusion syndrome (PRS) and may further exacerbate bradycardia in the early neohepatic phase of LT [96]. Severe bradyarrhythmias including heart block have been reported in all phases of LT, including in the preoperative and postoperative settings [97]. Bradycardia may be exacerbated by pharmacologic agents, particularly beta-blockers. Cardiology evaluation is warranted in the preoperative and postoperative setting, especially with cases of high-grade atrioventricular block. Successful LT in patients with permanent and temporary pacemakers has been reported [97].

Key Points

1. Pre-existing cardiac conditions in liver transplant candidates may adversely impact post-transplant outcomes and may affect transplant candidacy. Cardiovascular events are an important cause of peri- and post-transplant morbidity and mortality.
2. Coronary artery disease is the most important cardiovascular condition in liver transplant candidates. Screening for asymptomatic ischemic heart disease is an essential part of the preoperative selection process.
3. Published guidelines recommend non-invasive ischemia testing in candidates at risk for coronary artery disease. Although there is no consensus regarding management strategies, coronary angiography and revascularization of obstructive lesions have important roles.
4. Structural and valvular cardiac disease may impact transplant candidacy. Preoperative echocardiography is indicated to identify major cardiac conditions such as dilated cardiomyopathy and aortic stenosis.
5. Cirrhotic cardiomyopathy, a constellation of cardiovascular changes associated with advanced liver disease, may contribute to the perioperative cardiovascular risk in liver transplant patients.

References

1. Lentine K, Costa S, Weir M, Robb J, Fleisher L, Kasiske B, et al. Cardiac disease evaluation and management among kidney and liver transplantation candidates: a scientific statement from the American Heart Association and the American College of Cardiology Foundation. Circulation. 2012;126(5):617–63.
2. Martin P, DiMartini A, Feng S, Brown R, Fallon M. Evaluation for liver transplantation in adults: 2013 practice guideline by the American Association for the Study of Liver Diseases and the American Society of Transplantation. Hepatology. 2014;59(3):1144–65.
3. https://optn.transplant.hrsa.gov/data/view-data-reports/national-data/#. Accessed 4/31/17.
4. Plotkin J, Scott V, Pinna A, Dobsch B, De Wolf A, Kang Y. Morbidity and mortality in patients with coronary artery disease undergoing orthotopic liver transplantation. Liver Transpl Surg. 1996;2(6):426–30.
5. Diedrich D, Findlay J, Harrison B, Rosen C. Influence of coronary artery disease on outcomes after liver transplantation. Transplant Proc. 2008;40(10):3554–7.
6. Safadi A, Homsi M, Maskoun W, Lane K, Singh I, Sawada S, et al. Perioperative risk predictors of cardiac outcomes in patients undergoing liver transplantation surgery. Circulation. 2009;120(13):1189–94.
7. VanWagner L, Lapin B, Levitsky J, Wilkins J, Abecassis M, Skaro A, et al. High early cardiovascular mortality after liver transplantation. Liver Transpl. 2014;20(11):1306–16.
8. Gelson W, Hoare M, Dawwas M, Vowler S, Gibbs P, Alexander G. The pattern of late mortality in liver transplant recipients in the United Kingdom. Transplantation. 2011;91(11):1240–4.
9. Laryea M, Watt K, Molinari M, Walsh M, McAlister V, Marotta P, et al. Metabolic syndrome in liver transplant recipients: prevalence and association with major vascular events. Liver Transpl. 2007;13(8):1109–14.
10. Hogan B, Gonsalkorala E, Heneghan M. Evaluation of coronary artery disease in potential liver transplant recipients. Liver Transpl. 2017;23(3):386–95.
11. https://ftp.cdc.gov/pub/Health_Statistics/NCHS/NHIS/SHS/2015_SHS_Table_A-1.pdf. Accessed 5/1/17.
12. Tiukinhoy-Laing S, Rossi J, Bayram M, De Luca L, Gafoor S, Blei A, et al. Cardiac hemodynamic and coronary angiographic characteristics of patients being evaluated for liver transplantation. Am J Cardiol. 2006;98(2):178–81.
13. Kadayifci A, Tan V, Ursell P, Merriman R, Bass N. Clinical and pathologic risk factors for atherosclerosis in cirrhosis: a comparison between NASH-related cirrhosis and cirrhosis due to other aetiologies. J Hepatol. 2008;49(4):595–9.
14. Gologorsky E, Pretto E, Fukazawa K. Coronary artery disease and its risk factors in patients presenting for liver transplantation. J Clin Anesth. 2013;25(8):618–23.
15. Kim W, Lake J, Smith J, Skeans M, Schladt D, et al. OPTN/SRTR 2015 annual data report: liver. Am J Transplant. 2017;17(Suppl 1):174–251.
16. Fleisher L, Fleischmann K, Auerbach A, Barnason S, Beckman J, et al. ACC/AHA guideline on perioperative cardiovascular evaluation and management of patients undergoing noncardiac surgery: executive summary: A report of the American College of Cardiology/American Heart Association Task Force on Practice Guidelines. Circulation. 2014;130:2215–45.
17. Patel S, Kiefer T, Ahmed A, Ali Z, Tremmel J, et al. Comparison of the frequency of coronary artery disease in alcohol-related versus non-alcohol-related endstage liver disease. Am J Cardiol. 2011;108:1552–5.
18. Moller S, Bernardi M. Interactions of the heart and the liver. Eur Heart J. 2013;34:2804–11.
19. Plotkin J, Benitez R, Kuo P, Njoku M, Ridge L, et al. Dobutamine stress echocardiography for preoperative cardiac risk stratification in patients undergoing orthotopic liver transplantation. Liver Transpl Surg. 1998;4:253–7.
20. Snipelisky D, Levy M, Shapiro B. Utility of dobutamine stress echocardiography as part of the pre-liver transplant evaluation: an evaluation of its efficacy. Clin Cardiol. 2014;37:468–72.

21. Harinstein M, Flaherty J, Ansari A, Robin J, Davidson C, et al. Predictive value of dobutamine stress echocardiography for coronary artery disease detection in liver transplant candidates. Am J Transplant. 2008;8:1523–8.
22. Singhal A, Mukerji A, Thomaides A, Karachristos A, Maloo M, et al. Chronotropic incompetence on dobutamine stress echocardiography in candidates for a liver transplant. Exp Clin Transplant. 2013;11:546–53.
23. Nguyen P, Plotkin J, Fishbein T, Lauren J, Satoskar R, et al. Dobutamine stress echocardiography in patients undergoing orthotopic liver transplantation: a pooled analysis of accuracy, perioperative and long term cardiovascular prognosis. Int J Cardiovasc Imaging. 2013;29(8):1741–8.
24. Aydinalp A, Bal U, Atar I, Urtan C, Yildirir A, et al. Value of stress myocardial perfusion scanning in diagnosis of severe coronary artery disease in liver transplantation candidates. Transplant Proc. 2009;41(9):3757–60.
25. Senzolo M, Bassanello M, Graziotto A, Zucchetta P, Cillo U, et al. Microvascular autonomic dysfunction may justify false-positive stress myocardial perfusion imaging in patients with liver cirrhosis undergoing liver transplantation. Transplant Proc. 2008;40(6):1916–7.
26. Bhutani S, Tobis J, Gevorgyan R, Sinha A, Suh W, et al. Accuracy of stress myocardial perfusion imaging to diagnose coronary artery disease in end stage liver disease patients. Am J Cardiol. 2013;111(7):1057–61.
27. Kemmer N, Case J, Chandna S, Neff G. The role of coronary calcium score in the risk assessment of liver transplant candidates. Transplant Proc. 2014;46(1):230–3.
28. Poulin M, Chan E, Doukky R. Coronary computed tomographic angiography in the evaluation of liver transplant candidates. Angiology. 2015;66(9):803–10.
29. Pillarisetti J, Patel P, Duthuluru S, Roberts J, Chen W, et al. Cardiac catheterization in patients with end-stage liver disease: safety and outcomes. Catheterization Cardiovasc Intervent. 2011;77(1):45–8.
30. Sharma M, Yong C, Majure D, Zellner C, Roberts J, et al. Safety of cardiac catheterization in patients with end-stage liver disease awaiting liver transplantation. Am J Cardiol. 2009;103(5):742–6.
31. Jacobs E, Singh V, Damluji A, Shah N, Warsch J, et al. Safety of transradial cardiac catheterization in patients with end-stage liver disease. Catheterization Cardiovasc Intervent. 2014;83(3):360–6.
32. Shantouf R, Mehra A. Coronary fractional flow reserve. Am J Roentgenol. 2015;204(3):261–5.
33. Levine G, Bates E, Bittl J, Brindis R, Fihn S, et al. ACC/AHA guideline focused update on duration of dual antiplatelet therapy in patients with coronary artery disease. J Am Coll Cardiol. 2016;68(10):1082–115.
34. Shaheen A, Kaplan G, Hubbard J, Myers R. Morbidity and mortality following coronary artery bypass graft surgery in patients with cirrhosis: a population-based study. Liver Int. 2009;29(8):1141–51.
35. Filsoufi F, Salzberg S, Rahmanian P, Schiano T, Elsiesy H, et al. Early and late outcome of cardiac surgery in patients with liver cirrhosis. Liver Transpl. 2007;13(7):990–5.
36. Hayashida N, Shoujima T, Teshima H, Yokokura Y, Takagi K, et al. Clinical outcome after cardiac operations in patients with cirrhosis. Ann Thorac Surg. 2004;77(2):500–5.
37. Giakoustidis A, Cherian T, Antoniadis N, Giakoustidis D. Combined cardiac surgery and liver transplantation: three decades of worldwide results. J Gastrointestin Liver Dis. 2011;20(4):415–21.
38. Milan Z, Taylor C, Armstrong D, Davies P, Roberts S, et al. Does preoperative Beta-blocker use influence intraoperative hemodynamic profile and post-operative course of liver transplantation? Transplant Proc. 2016;48(1):111–5.
39. Maddur H, Bourdillon P, Liangpunsakul S, Joseph Tector A, Fridell A, et al. Role of cardiac catheterization and percutaneous coronary intervention in the preoperative assessment and management of patients before orthotopic liver transplantation. Liver Transpl. 2014;20(6):664–72.

40. Satapathy S, Vanatta J, Helmick R, Flowers A, Kedia S, et al. Outcome of liver transplant recipients with Revascularized coronary artery disease: a comparative analysis with and without cardiovascular risk factors. Transplantation. 2017;101(4):793–803.
41. Skaro A, Gallon L, Lyuksemburg V, Jay C, Ladner D, et al. The impact of coronary artery disease on outcomes after liver transplantation. J Cardiovasc Med (Hagerstown). 2016;17(12):875–85.
42. Wray C, Scovotti J, Tobis J, Niemann C, Planinsic R, et al. Liver transplantation outcome in patients with angiographically proven coronary artery disease: a multi-institutional study. Am J Transplant. 2013;13(1):184–91.
43. Alexopoulos S, Matsuoka L, Cho Y, Thomas E, Sheikh M, et al. Outcomes after liver transplantation in patients achieving a model for end-stage liver disease score of 40 or higher. Transplantation. 2013;95(3):507–12.
44. Kaltenborn A, Hartmann C, Salinas R, Ramackers W, Kleine M, et al. Risk factors for short- and long-term mortality in liver transplant recipients with MELD score >/=30. Ann Transplant. 2015;20:59–69.
45. Onaca N, Levy M, Sanchez E, Chinnakotia S, Fasola C, et al. A correlation between the pretransplantation MELD score and mortality in the first two years after liver transplantation. Liver Transpl. 2003;9(3):117–23.
46. Petrowsky H, Rana A, Kaldas F, Sharma A, Hong J, et al. Liver transplantation in highest acuity recipients: identifying factors to avoid futility. Ann Surg. 2014;259(6):1186–94.
47. Kertai MD, Bountioukos M, Boersma E, Bax JJ, Thomson IR, Sozzi F, et al. Aortic stenosis: an underestimated risk factor for perioperative complications in patients undergoing noncardiac surgery. Am J Med. 2004;116(1):8–13.
48. Thielmann M, Mechmet A, Neuhauser M, Wendt D, Tossios P, Canbay A, et al. Risk prediction and outcomes in patients with liver cirrhosis undergoing open-heart surgery. Eur J Cardiothorac Surg. 2010;38(5):592–9.
49. Eckhoff DE, Frenette L, Sellers MT, McGuire BM, Contreras JL, Bynon JS, et al. Combined cardiac surgery and liver transplantation. Liver Transpl. 2001;7(1):60–1.
50. Parker BM, Mayes JT, Henderson JM, Savage RM. Combined aortic valve replacement and orthotopic liver transplantation. J Cardiothorac Vasc Anesth. 2001;15(4):474–6.
51. Kalarickal P, Liu Q, Rathor R, Ishag S, Kerr T, Kangrga I. Balloon aortic valvuloplasty as a bridge to liver transplantation in patients with severe aortic stenosis: a case series. Transplant Proc. 2014;46(10):3492–5.
52. Silvestre OM, Bacal F, Ramos DS, Tarasoutchi F, Acorsi TD, Fernandes F, et al. Transcatheter aortic valve implantation as rescue therapy for liver transplant candidates with aortic valve stenosis. Liver Transpl. 2014;20(10):1277–9.
53. Moreno R, Delcan JL, Garcia E, Villacastin J, Ortega A, Perez E. Emergent mitral percutaneous valvuloplasty before emergent liver transplantation. Catheter Cardiovasc Diagn. 1997;41(2):229–30.
54. Navasa M, Feu F, Garcia-Pagan JC, Jimenez W, Llach J, Rimola A, et al. Hemodynamic and humoral changes after liver transplantation in patients with cirrhosis. Hepatology. 1993;17(3):355–60.
55. Alper I, Ulukaya S, Demir F, Kilic M. Effects of cardiac valve dysfunction on perioperative management of liver transplantation. Transplant Proc. 2009;41(5):1722–6.
56. Kia L, Shah SJ, Wang E, Sharma D, Selvaraj S, Medina C, et al. Role of pretransplant echocardiographic evaluation in predicting outcomes following liver transplantation. Am J Transplant. 2013;13(9):2395–401.
57. Maraj S, Jacobs LE, Maraj R, Contreras R, Rerkpattanapipat P, Malik TA, et al. Inducible left ventricular outflow tract gradient during dobutamine stress echocardiography: an association with intraoperative hypotension but not a contraindication to liver transplantation. Echocardiography. 2004;21(8):681–5.
58. Harley ID, Jones EF, Liu G, McCall PR, McNicol PL. Orthotopic liver transplantation in two patients with hypertrophic obstructive cardiomyopathy. Br J Anaesth. 1996;77(5):675–7.

59. Hensley N, Dietrich J, Nyhan D, Mitter N, Yee MS, Brady M. Hypertrophic cardiomyopathy: a review. Anesth Analg. 2015;120(3):554–69.
60. Paramesh AS, Fairchild RB, Quinn TM, Leya F, George M, Van Thiel DH. Amelioration of hypertrophic cardiomyopathy using nonsurgical septal ablation in a cirrhotic patient prior to liver transplantation. Liver Transpl. 2005;11(2):236–8.
61. Meissner I, Whisnant JP, Khandheria BK, Spittell PC, O'Fallon WM, Pascoe RD, et al. Prevalence of potential risk factors for stroke assessed by transesophageal echocardiography and carotid ultrasonography: the SPARC study. Stroke Prevent: Assessment Risk Commun Mayo Clin Proc. 1999;74(9):862–9.
62. Alba AC, Verocai Flaman F, Granton J, Delgado DH. Patent foramen ovale does not have a negative impact on early outcomes in patients undergoing liver transplantation. Clin Transpl. 2011;25(1):151–5.
63. Werlang ME, Palmer WC, Boyd EA, Cangemi DJ, Harnois DM, Taner CB, et al. Patent foramen ovale in liver transplant recipients does not negatively impact short-term outcomes. Clin Transpl. 2016;30(1):26–32.
64. Concejero A, Chen CL, Liang CD, Wang CC, Wang SH, Lin CC, et al. Atrial septal defect in end-stage liver disease children before and after liver transplantation. Surgery. 2008;143(2):271–7.
65. Tam NL, Concejero AM, Liang CD. Fate of atrial septal defect in children with end-stage liver disease undergoing living donor liver transplantation. Transplant Proc. 2008;40(8):2510–1.
66. Asrani SK, Asrani NS, Freese DK, Phillips SD, Warnes CA, Heimbach J, et al. Congenital heart disease and the liver. Hepatology. 2012;56(3):1160–9.
67. D'Souza BA, Fuller S, Gleason LP, Hornsby N, Wald J, Krok K, et al. Single-center outcomes of combined heart and liver transplantation in the failing Fontan. Clin Transpl. 2017;31(3)
68. Moller S, Henriksen JH. Cardiovascular complications of cirrhosis. Gut. 2008;57(2):268–78.
69. Zardi EM, Abbate A, Zardi DM, Dobrina A, Margiotta D, Van Tassell BW, et al. Cirrhotic cardiomyopathy. J Am Coll Cardiol. 2010;56(7):539–49.
70. Rahman S, Mallett SV. Cirrhotic cardiomyopathy: implications for the perioperative management of liver transplant patients. World J Hepatol. 2015;7(3):507–20.
71. Torregrosa M, Aguade S, Dos L, Segura R, Gonzalez A, Evangelista A, et al. Cardiac alterations in cirrhosis: reversibility after liver transplantation. J Hepatol. 2005;42(1):68–74.
72. Raevens S, De Pauw M, Geerts A, Berrevoet F, Rogiers X, Troisi RI, et al. Prevalence and outcome of diastolic dysfunction in liver transplantation recipients. Acta Cardiol. 2014;69(3):273–80.
73. Merli M, Calicchia A, Ruffa A, Pellicori P, Riggio O, Giusto M, et al. Cardiac dysfunction in cirrhosis is not associated with the severity of liver disease. Eur J Intern Med. 2013;24(2):172–6.
74. Pozzi M, Carugo S, Boari G, Pecci V, de Ceglia S, Maggiolini S, et al. Evidence of functional and structural cardiac abnormalities in cirrhotic patients with and without ascites. Hepatology. 1997;26(5):1131–7.
75. Sampaio F, Pimenta J, Bettencourt N, Fontes-Carvalho R, Silva AP, Valente J, et al. Systolic dysfunction and diastolic dysfunction do not influence medium-term prognosis in patients with cirrhosis. Eur J Intern Med. 2014;25(3):241–6.
76. Alexopoulou A, Papatheodoridis G, Pouriki S, Chrysohoou C, Raftopoulos L, Stefanadis C, et al. Diastolic myocardial dysfunction does not affect survival in patients with cirrhosis. Transpl Int. 2012;25(11):1174–81.
77. Mittal C, Qureshi W, Singla S, Ahmad U, Huang MA. Pre-transplant left ventricular diastolic dysfunction is associated with post transplant acute graft rejection and graft failure. Dig Dis Sci. 2014;59(3):674–80.
78. Escobar B, Taura P, Martinez-Palli G, Fondevila C, Balust J, Beltran J, et al. Stroke volume response to liver graft reperfusion stress in cirrhotic patients. World J Surg. 2014;38(4):927–35.
79. Moller S, Henriksen J. Cirrhotic cardiomyopathy. J Hepatol. 2010;53(1):179–90.
80. Trevisani F, Merli M, Savelli F, Valeriono V, Zambruni A, et al. QT interval in patients with non-cirrhotic portal hypertension and in cirrhotic patients treated with transjugular intrahepatic porto-systemic shunt. J Hepatol. 2003;38(3):461–7.

81. Bernardi M, Maggioli C, Dibra V, Zaccherini G. QT interval prolongation in liver cirrhosis: innocent bystander or serious threat. Expert Rev Gastroenterol Hepatol. 2012;6(1):57–66.
82. Chung E, Jeon Y, Kim H, Lee K, Lee J, et al. Torsade de pointes in liver transplantation recipient after induction of general anesthesia: a case report. Korean J Anesthesiol. 2014;66(1):80–4.
83. Kim M, Kim N, Park J, Nam S. Ventricular arrhythmia in patients with prolonged QT interval during liver transplantation: two cases report. Korean J Anesthesiol. 2014;67(6):416–20.
84. Chin J, Park J, Kim S, Kim S, Kong Y, et al. Torsades de pointes triggered by severe diastolic hypotension with low hematocrit in the Neohepatic stage of liver transplantation: a case report. Transplant Proc. 2010;42(5):1959–62.
85. Gwak M, Kim J, Kim G, Choi S, Ahn H, et al. Incidence of severe ventricular arrhythmias during pulmonary artery catheterization in liver allograft recipients. Liver Transpl. 2007;13(10):1451–4.
86. Eleid M, Hurst T, Vargas H, Rakela J, Mulligan D, et al. Short-term cardiac and noncardiac mortality following liver transplantation. J Transplant. 2010;7:Article ID 910165. https://doi.org/10.1155/2010/910165.
87. Nicolau-Raducu R, Gitman M, Ganier D, Loss G, Cohen A, et al. Adverse cardiac events after orthotopic liver transplantation: a cross-sectional study in 389 consecutive patients. Liver Transpl. 2015;21(1):13–21.
88. Josefsson A, Fu M, Björnsson E, Kalaitzakis E. Prevalence of pre-transplant electrocardiographic abnormalities and post-transplant cardiac events in patients with liver cirrhosis. Bio Med Central Gastroenterol. 2014;14:65. https://doi.org/10.1186/1471-230X-14-65. 11 pages
89. January C, Wann L, Alpert J, Calkins H, Cigarroa J, et al. 2014 AHA/ACC/HRS guideline for the management of patients with atrial fibrillation a report of the American College of Cardiology/American Heart Association task force on practice guidelines and the Heart Rhythm Society. Circulation. 2014;130(23):e199–267.
90. Bargehr J, Trejo-Gutierrez J, Patel T, Rosser B, Aranda-Michel J, et al. Preexisting atrial fibrillation and cardiac complications after liver transplantation. Liver Transpl. 2015;21(3):314–20.
91. Vannucci A, Rathor R, Vachharajani N, Chapman W, Kangrga I. Atrial fibrillation in patients undergoing liver transplantation-a single-center experience. Transplant Proceed. 2014;46(5):1432–7.
92. Xia V, Worapot A, Huang S, Dhillon A, Gudzenko V, et al. Postoperative atrial fibrillation in liver transplantation. Am J Transplant. 2015;15(3):687–94.
93. Vallurupalli S, Shanbhag A, Mehta J. Controversies in postoperative atrial fibrillation after noncardiothoracic surgery: clinical and research implications. Clin Cardiol. 2017;40(5):329–32.
94. Fede G, Privitera G, Tomaselli T, Spadaro L, Purrello F. Cardiovascular dysfunction in patients with liver cirrhosis. Ann Gastroenterol. 2015;28(1):31–40.
95. Ates F, Topal E, Kosar F, Karincaoglu M, Yildirim B, et al. The relationship of heart rate variability with severity and prognosis of cirrhosis. Dig Dis Sci. 2006;51(9):1614–8.
96. Siniscalchi A, Gamberini L, Laici C, Bardi T, Ercolani G, et al. Post reperfusion syndrome during liver transplantation: from pathophysiology to therapy and preventive strategies. World J Gastroenterol. 2016;22(4):1551–69.
97. Kobayashi T, Sato Y, Yamamoto S, Oya H, Takeishi T, et al. Temporary cardiac pacing for fatal arrhythmia in living-donor liver transplantation: three case reports. Transplant Proc. 2008;40(8):2818–20.

Chapter 2
Pulmonary Evaluation of Liver Transplant Candidates

Hilary M. DuBrock and Michael J. Krowka

Introduction

Pulmonary diseases are frequently encountered comorbidities in liver transplant (LT) candidates. Pulmonary disease can develop as a complication of liver disease or in association with risk factors such as smoking that are common in patients with end-stage liver disease. A systematic and comprehensive pretransplant pulmonary evaluation of LT candidates is necessary in order to recognize and treat conditions that are associated with increased perioperative and long-term morbidity and mortality. Some pulmonary complications of liver disease also have significant implications for prioritizing organ allocation according to the current Model for End-Stage Liver Disease (MELD) exception policy. This chapter will provide an overview of the pulmonary preoperative evaluation of LT candidates with an emphasis on the perioperative evaluation and management of pulmonary vascular complications of liver disease, hepatopulmonary syndrome (HPS), and portopulmonary hypertension (POPH).

An Overview of Pulmonary Diseases that Affect Liver Transplant Candidates

Hepatopulmonary Syndrome (HPS)

Diagnosis

HPS is characterized by the following triad (Table 2.1):

H. M. DuBrock (✉) · M. J. Krowka
Mayo Clinic, Rochester, MN, USA
e-mail: dubrock.hilary@mayo.edu

D. Bezinover, F. Saner (eds.), *Critical Care for Potential Liver Transplant Candidates*,
https://doi.org/10.1007/978-3-319-92934-7_2

Table 2.1 Diagnostic criteria for hepatopulmonary syndrome and portopulmonary hypertension

	HPS	POPH
Diagnostic testing[a]	1. Room air upright arterial blood gas 2. Contrast-enhanced transthoracic echocardiogram	1. Right-heart catheterization
Diagnostic criteria	1. IPVD as detected by CE-TTE 2. A-a gradient > 15 mmHg (or > 20 mmHg if age > 64 years) 3. Liver disease	1. mPAP > 25 mmHg 2. PVR > 3 Wood units (240 dynes•s•cm^{-5}) 3. PAWP < 15 mmHg 4. Portal hypertension

A-a alveolar-arterial, *CE-TTE* contrast-enhanced transthoracic echocardiogram, *IPVD* intrapulmonary vasodilatation, *mPAP* mean pulmonary arterial pressure, *PAWP* pulmonary arterial wedge pressure, *PVR* pulmonary vascular resistance

[a]In addition to appropriate workup for other causes of hypoxemia in patients with suspected HPS and appropriate workup for other causes of pulmonary hypertension in patients with suspected POPH

Table 2.2 Classification of disease severity in hepatopulmonary syndrome

Disease severity	A-a gradient	PaO2
Mild	≥ 15 mmHg or > 20 mmHg if age > 64	≥ 80 mmHg
Moderate		60–79 mmHg
Severe		50–59 mmHg
Very severe		< 50 mmHg

A-a alveolar-arterial, *PaO2* partial pressure of oxygen in arterial blood

1. Abnormal arterial oxygenation [defined as an Alveolar-arterial (A-a) oxygen gradient ≥ 15 mmHg (or > 20 mmHg if age > 64) on room air arterial blood gas]
2. Intrapulmonary vascular dilatation (IPVD), detected by contrast-enhanced transthoracic echocardiogram
3. Advanced liver disease

HPS can be classified as mild, moderate, severe, or very severe based on the level of hypoxemia. Mild HPS is defined by a PaO2 > 80 mmHg, moderate HPS by a PaO2 of 60–80 mmHg, severe HPS by a PaO2 of 50–59 mmHg, and very severe HPS by a PaO2 < 50 mmHg (measurements performed on room air) [1] (Table 2.2).

Epidemiology

HPS develops in 4–32% of LT candidates [1]. HPS is not associated with age, sex, or liver disease severity or etiology [2]. Compared to LT candidates without HPS, patients who develop HPS are less likely to have a history of smoking [2]. Genetic predisposition may also be important in disease epidemiology. Multi-center case-control studies have identified an association between HPS and alterations in genes involved in the regulation of angiogenesis [3].

Pathophysiology

HPS typically develops in the setting of portal hypertension and cirrhosis but can also develop in acute or chronic hepatitis, acute liver failure, and vascular abnormalities that limit hepatic blood flow to the lungs, such as cavopulmonary shunts and congenital portosystemic shunts [1]. Dilatation of capillary and precapillary pulmonary blood vessels results in hypoxemia via a ventilation-perfusion (V-Q) mismatch, anatomic shunting, and diffusion limitation. The pathophysiology of HPS has not yet been elucidated, but clinical studies and animal models suggest that vasoactive mediators of inflammation, vasodilatation, and angiogenesis, such as tumor necrosis factor alpha, nitric oxide, endothelin-1, and vascular endothelial growth factor, may play a role in disease pathogenesis [1].

Portopulmonary Hypertension

Diagnosis

Portopulmonary hypertension is a clinical and hemodynamic diagnosis. It is defined as the presence of pulmonary arterial hypertension (PAH) in the setting of portal hypertension without an alternative cause of pulmonary hypertension [1] (Table 2.1). PAH is further defined as an elevated mean pulmonary arterial pressure (mPAP) > 25 mmHg in the setting of an elevated pulmonary vascular resistance (PVR) > 3 Wood units and a normal pulmonary arterial wedge pressure (PAWP) < 15 mmHg. Right-heart catheterization and thorough exclusion of alternative causes of pulmonary hypertension, such as chronic thromboembolic pulmonary hypertension, sleep-disordered breathing, diastolic dysfunction, and significant obstructive or restrictive lung disease, are required for diagnosis. It is important to distinguish the hemodynamic profile of POPH from other frequently encountered causes of an elevated mean pulmonary arterial pressure in patients with liver disease, such as a hyperdynamic cardiac output and an elevated wedge pressure (Fig. 2.1), as accurate diagnosis has significant implications for management. POPH severity is further classified by mPAP as mild, moderate, or severe (Table 2.3). Lastly, although a PVR of 3 Wood units is used as a threshold in the diagnostic criteria, it should be noted that a

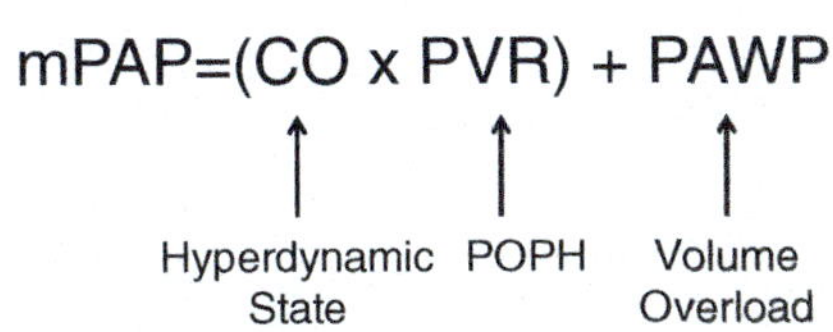

Fig. 2.1 Mean pulmonary arterial pressure (mPAP) can be elevated due to elevated cardiac output (CO) related to hyperdynamic circulation, elevated pulmonary vascular resistance (PVR) related to pulmonary vasoconstriction and obstruction to arterial flow, or elevated pulmonary arterial wedge pressure (PAWP) related to volume overload

PVR between 2 and 3 Wood units in the setting of a hyperdynamic cardiac output may be abnormal and associated with adverse post-transplant outcomes [4].

Epidemiology

Approximately 5–6% of patients evaluated for LT meet the criteria for POPH [5, 6]. Similar to HPS, POPH is not associated with liver disease severity. Female sex and autoimmune hepatitis are independent clinical risk factors for POPH [7]. Genetic variations in estrogen signaling have been identified in patients with POPH, suggesting a genetic predisposition [8]. Table 2.4 summarizes and compares the clinical features of HPS and POPH.

Table 2.3 Classification of disease severity in portopulmonary hypertension

Disease severity	PVR	mPAP
Mild	> 3 Wood units	25–34
Moderate		35–44
Severe		≥ 45

mPAP mean pulmonary arterial pressure, *PVR* pulmonary vascular resistance

Table 2.4 Clinical features of hepatopulmonary syndrome and portopulmonary hypertension

	HPS	POPH
Signs and symptoms	Dyspnea, fatigue, platypnea, orthodeoxia, clubbing, cyanosis, spider angiomas	Dyspnea, fatigue, prominent P2, jugular venous distension, tricuspid regurgitation murmur, lower extremity edema
Prevalence in liver transplant candidates	4–32%	5–6%
Clinical risk factors	History of never smoking	Female gender, autoimmune liver disease
Associated with liver disease severity	No	No
Oxygenation	Mild to severe hypoxemia	Normal or mild hypoxemia
PFT abnormalities	Reduced DLCO	Reduced DLCO
CE-TTE	Intrapulmonary vasodilatation (IPVD)	Elevated right-ventricular systolic pressure ± right-ventricular dilation or dysfunction; concomitant IPVD is not uncommon
Treatment	Supportive	PAH-targeted therapy
Improves with transplant	Yes	Often, in selected patients

DLCO diffusion capacity for carbon monoxide, *IPVD* intrapulmonary vasodilatation, *P2* pulmonic component of the second heart sounds, *PAH* pulmonary arterial hypertension, *PFT* pulmonary function test

Pathophysiology

Similar to other forms of PAH, POPH is characterized by vasoconstriction, vascular remodeling, and obstruction to arterial flow. The pathophysiology of POPH is unknown. Estrogen signaling and a higher prevalence of spontaneous portosystemic shunts have been associated with the presence of POPH [8, 9]. Circulating mediators of inflammation and vasoconstriction, such as macrophage migration inhibitory factor and endothelin-1, have also been implicated in disease pathogenesis [1, 10].

Other: Hepatic Hydrothorax, Chronic Obstructive Pulmonary Disease, Alpha-1 Antitrypsin Deficiency, Interstitial Lung Disease, Obstructive Sleep Apnea, Hereditary Hemorrhagic Telangiectasia, and Pulmonary Nodules

Although this chapter focuses on pulmonary vascular complications of liver disease, other pulmonary diseases may affect LT consideration as well. These include hepatic hydrothorax, advanced chronic obstructive pulmonary disease (COPD), interstitial lung disease (ILD), pulmonary nodules, and inherited diseases, such as alpha-1 antitrypsin deficiency and hereditary hemorrhagic telangiectasia, which affect both the liver and the lungs.

Hepatic hydrothorax (HH) refers to the accumulation of ascitic fluid within the pleural space. It develops in the setting of ascites due to negative intrathoracic pressure and microscopic holes in the diaphragm, which can lead to the passage of fluid from the abdominal into the thoracic cavity [11]. HH affects 5–12% of patients with advanced liver disease. Treatment involves salt restriction and diuretic therapy. A refractory hydrothorax refers to persistent symptomatic pleural effusion despite sodium restriction to < 2 grams per day and high-dose diuretic therapy or the need for repeated thoracentesis [11]. Although thoracentesis and paracentesis can transiently decrease symptoms related to HH, they typically recur if the underlying problems are not addressed. In refractory HH, transjugular intrahepatic portosystemic shunt may also be considered to minimize fluid accumulation. Although HH is not considered an indication for LT, post-transplant outcomes of HH are favorable overall [11]. In one case series of 28 patients, resolution was reported in all patients by the 3-month post-transplant point [12]. As there are alternative treatment approaches and no data to support increased waitlist mortality related to HH, standardized MELD exceptions are not available for patients with HH [11].

Chronic obstructive pulmonary disease or emphysema is diagnosed in ~18% of LT candidates [13] among whom a history of smoking is relatively common. According to multi-center prospective studies, 60% of LT candidates had a history of current or past smoking [13]. Although a diagnosis of COPD does not specifically affect LT listing, it is important to recognize and treat pulmonary comorbidities, such as COPD, in order to ensure pulmonary function optimization prior to LT.

Patients with poorly controlled COPD may require prolonged intubation and/or hospitalization. There are currently no guidelines to define the severity of COPD that would preclude LT. Some patients with severe or very severe COPD may not be appropriate candidates for LT if the prognosis related to their COPD is poor. A prognosis related to COPD using validated scoring systems can be helpful in guiding decisions regarding listing. One easy-to-use prognostic calculator available for COPD is the BODE index [14]. Consisting of body mass index, obstruction severity (FEV1% predicted), dyspnea score, and exercise capacity (6-min walk distance), the index can be used to predict survival in patients with COPD. It should be noted, however, that some components of the BODE index, such as the 6-min walk distance, may be affected by liver disease severity [15].

Alpha-1 antitrypsin (AAT) deficiency can lead to both emphysema and liver disease. AAT deficiency is a rare genetic disease caused by abnormal production of AAT, a serine protease inhibitor. Individuals with two M alleles have normal AAT structure and function and normal circulating levels of AAT. The S and Z alleles are associated with abnormal AAT structure and function [16]. The dysfunctional protein accumulates in the liver, which can lead to cirrhosis. Accumulation in the liver also results in circulating deficiency of AAT, which leads to emphysema. Emphysema is typically panlobular or lower lobe predominant [11]. LT cures cirrhosis and results in normalization of circulating AAT levels. Despite normalization of circulating AAT levels post-transplant, however, FEV1% continues to decline post-transplant in some patients. At this time, decreased lung function related to AAT deficiency is not considered an indication for LT. According to one study, the 1-, 3-, 5-, and 10-year post-LT survival rates were 86%, 83%, 80%, and 72%, respectively, for ZZ patients and 91%, 86%, 79%, and 79%, respectively, for SZ patients [16].

Interstitial lung disease (ILD) refers to a heterogenous group of pulmonary diseases, often characterized by pulmonary fibrosis, that affect the pulmonary parenchyma. ILD typically results in increased lung stiffness, which is associated with reduced total lung capacity and a restrictive defect on PFTs. ILD can develop in numerous settings in the context of liver disease. ILD is correlated with some autoimmune diseases and is associated with primary biliary cirrhosis and autoimmune hepatitis [11]. Concomitant ILD and cryptogenic cirrhosis have also been described in association with telomerase mutations. In addition to cirrhosis and ILD, patients can also present with bone marrow failure [17]. Although ILD can be associated with some liver diseases, it does not typically improve with LT and may continue to progress. In highly selected cases, sequential liver-lung transplant can be considered [11]. Newer antifibrotic drugs are now available for the treatment of some types of ILD to slow disease progression, but are not curative. Similar to COPD, there are no guidelines that define the severity of ILD that would preclude LT, but moderate to severe restriction due to ILD is generally considered a contraindication to LT [11].

Sleep-disordered breathing is common in the general population and may be undiagnosed at the time of initial LT evaluation. Untreated obstructive sleep apnea, which can lead to episodic airway obstruction, oxygen desaturation, and hypercapnia can present distinctive challenges to perioperative management [18]. Screening tests, such as the STOP-BANG Questionnaire, can be a useful tool to identify patients at risk for obstructive sleep apnea [19]. Patients who are at an increased risk should undergo additional testing, such as overnight oximetry or polysomnogram, to evaluate for sleep-disordered breathing. According to the most recent guidelines from the American Society of Anesthesiologists, preoperative initiation of CPAP should be considered in patients with confirmed OSA, especially if OSA is severe [18]. Patients with OSA also need to be monitored closely postoperatively for respiratory compromise, as they are particularly susceptible to respiratory depression from sedatives and opiates [18].

Hereditary hemorrhagic telangiectasia is an autosomal dominant disorder characterized by recurrent epistaxis, cutaneous telangiectasias, and visceral arteriovenous malformations (AVMs). AVMs can affect numerous organs, including the lungs, liver, gastrointestinal tract, and brain. Liver involvement is observed in up to 74% of patients, but no more than 8% are symptomatic [20]. Hepatic AVMs can lead to three distinct complications: high-output heart failure, portal hypertension, and biliary necrosis. All three are considered indications for LT, although there are no standardized MELD exception criteria for HHT as this is a relatively rare indication for LT [11]. Outcomes of LT in the setting of high-output heart failure related to hepatic AVMs are favorable to date [11]. Bevacizumab can also be considered for the treatment of high-output heart failure associated with hepatic AVMs. In these patients, a phase II randomized clinical trial of bevacizumab versus placebo demonstrated reduced cardiac output, improved quality of life, and reduced epistaxis [20]. Successful outcomes with embolization of hepatic AVMs have been described in centers with extensive experience but can also lead to ischemic biliary necrosis. Lastly, pulmonary AVMs occur in 15–50% of patients with HHT and are associated with life-threatening complications, such as stroke, brain abscess, and hemoptysis. All patients with HHT should be screened for the presence of pulmonary AVMs, and coil embolization is recommended in order to prevent complications [21]. Pulmonary hypertension can also develop in a subset of patients with HHT. Similar to patients with cirrhosis, PH can occur by multiple mechanisms, including an elevated PVR, an elevated PAWP, or a hyperdynamic cardiac output. Regardless of mechanism, PH in patients with HHT is associated with a trend toward a lower survival rate than is the case for patients without PH [22].

Pulmonary nodules may be detected on routine preoperative chest imaging. The decision to proceed with LT in the setting of undifferentiated pulmonary nodules is challenging. A biopsy of suspicious or enlarged lesions should be performed prior to transplant for diagnostic purposes. Pulmonary nodules may represent primary lung malignancy or treatable granulomatous infection, which should be treated prior to LT [11]. In patients with hepatocellular carcinoma, pulmonary nodules may represent metastatic disease, which is considered a contraindication to LT. FDG-PET can be helpful in the evaluation of nodules > 10 mm in diameter. A report based on a meta-analysis of 239 cases showed 77% sensitivity and 98% specificity for FDG-PET in identifying pulmonary metastases in the setting of newly diagnosed HCC [23]. A CT scan, however, is preferable for the evaluation of smaller nodules < 8–10 mm in diameter due to the limited resolution of an FDG-PET scan. If pulmonary nodules due to metastatic disease are detected post-transplant, surgical excision can be considered for management [11].

Pulmonary Preoperative Evaluation of Liver Transplant Candidates

History

The preoperative pulmonary evaluation of LT candidates should start with a thorough cardiopulmonary review of symptoms, such as dyspnea, orthopnea, platypnea, cough, sputum production, wheezing, chest pain, and peripheral edema, all of which should be assessed and characterized. As dyspnea can be multifactorial in patients with liver disease (Table 2.5), it is important to define the duration and timing of symptoms as well as modifying factors. For example, when dyspnea occurs as a result of an accumulation of ascites in the abdomen, patients typically report relief of symptoms following large-volume paracentesis. A history of dyspnea associated with a chronic cough, sputum production, or wheezing can provide clues to a concomitant diagnosis of COPD, asthma, or ILD. Patients should also be asked about daytime sleepiness and symptoms of sleep-disordered breathing, such as snoring,

Table 2.5 Differential diagnosis of dyspnea in patients with liver disease

Differential diagnosis of dyspnea in liver disease
Related to liver disease
A. Pulmonary
1. Pulmonary vascular disease
Hepatopulmonary syndrome
Portopulmonary hypertension
2. Pulmonary parenchymal disease
Interstitial lung disease (e.g., associated with primary biliary cirrhosis)
Emphysema (e.g., associated with alpha-1 antitrypsin deficiency)
Atelectasis (related to pleural effusions, ascites, and abdominal distension)
3. Pleural
Hepatic hydrothorax
B. Extrapulmonary
Ascites and abdominal distension
Cirrhotic cardiomyopathy
High-output heart failure
Anemia
Sarcopenia/deconditioning
Unrelated to liver disease
Obstructive lung disease
Restrictive lung disease
Diastolic or systolic heart failure
Other

frequent arousals, or witnessed apneas. In the social history, patients should be asked about their smoking history and occupational exposure, such as asbestos, that may be associated with ILD and may impact pulmonary function. A thorough family history is also important to screen for HHT or AATD.

Physical Examination

Physical examination findings can also provide clues to the diagnosis of pulmonary comorbidities. Reduced oxygen saturation is a nonspecific sign of pulmonary diseases, such as HPS, and should prompt further evaluation. Assessment of the BMI is important to screen for OSA and to determine prognosis related to diseases, such as COPD [14, 19]. Airway and neck examination can also be helpful to assess the risk of sleep-disordered breathing or difficult intubation. On the cardiac examination, a systolic murmur at the left lower sternal border and a loud or prominent pulmonic component of the second heart sound, right-ventricular heave, and jugular venous distension may be signs of pulmonary hypertension. Pulmonary examination may identify adventitious breath sounds, such as crackles, wheezes, or rhonchi, that can be suggestive of pulmonary parenchymal, airway, or pleural diseases, such as ILD, COPD, or HH. Extremities should be assessed for the presence of clubbing or peripheral edema, which can be a sign of HPS or right-heart failure, respectively. Abnormal skin findings that may suggest the presence of pulmonary disease include finger clubbing, cyanosis, and spider angiomata, which are nonspecific but have been described in association with HPS [24].

Laboratory Tests and Studies

Laboratory tests are helpful in the evaluation and management of dyspnea and pulmonary disease. Although not directly related to the pulmonary evaluation, the severity of liver disease as assessed by the MELD score can help determine the urgency of a preoperative assessment and the need for expedited LT evaluation [25]. Measurement of alpha-1 antitrypsin levels and assessment of the alpha-1 antitrypsin phenotype or genotype (for the M, S, or Z alleles) are used to screen for alpha-1 antitrypsin deficiency. In patients with POPH, NT-pro brain natriuretic peptide is a useful prognostic indicator [26]. Arterial blood gas is necessary to diagnose HPS and to classify disease severity. In the setting of IPVD and liver disease, abnormal gas exchange in the absence of an alternative etiology defines the presence of HPS. ABG can also be used to identify hypercapnia and hypoxemia related to other etiologies, such as hypoventilation. HPS is classically associated with orthodeoxia, a decrease in the partial pressure of oxygen in arterial blood (PaO2) of more than 5% or more than 4 mmHg with a change in the patient's position from supine to upright, but this finding is only present in up to 25% of patients [27].

Chest X-rays and an electrocardiogram are typically performed as part of the pre-transplant evaluation to evaluate for cardiopulmonary disease. If initial chest imaging is abnormal, a computed tomography scan can be obtained to further define the pattern of pulmonary parenchymal abnormalities. An electrocardiogram is helpful to evaluate heart rhythm and any evidence of structural heart disease or chamber enlargement.

Pulmonary function tests are important in the preoperative evaluation of LT candidates, particularly if the patient is a smoker and/or has signs or symptoms of pulmonary disease by history or physical examination. PFTs can identify the presence of obstructive or restrictive ventilatory deficits suggestive of COPD or interstitial lung disease, respectively. A reduced diffusion capacity for carbon monoxide in the absence of other abnormalities is suggestive of pulmonary vascular disease, such as HPS or POPH, but can also be reduced in ILD.

The 6-min walk is an important prognostic test for LT candidates. Although non-specific, it quantifies exercise capacity and can be reduced in patients with cardiopulmonary disease, end-stage liver disease, or deconditioning. In LT candidates, a reduced 6-min walk distance < 250 m has also been shown to be associated with worse survival [15].

TTE to assess right-ventricular size and function and estimated right-ventricular systolic pressure is a critical screening test for POPH. It is also used to screen for left-sided heart disease, such as left-ventricular systolic or diastolic dysfunction or significant valvular disease. According to current guidelines, TTE screening should be performed for all LT candidates [28]. The optimal interval for follow-up testing in patients with a normal initial echocardiogram is not clear, but annual testing while on the transplant list seems like a reasonable approach. In various studies, the utility of different RVSP thresholds have been evaluated for prompting further invasive testing with right-heart catheterization. An RVSP greater than 38–50 mmHg or the presence of right-ventricular dilation or dysfunction has been suggested, but trade-offs between sensitivity and specificity exist at different thresholds [1, 29]. The most recent American Association for the Study of Liver Diseases (AASLD) guidelines recommend pursuing right-heart catheterization in patients with an estimated RVSP ≥ 45 mmHg by echocardiogram [28].

In patients with an elevated RVSP or RV dysfunction on echocardiogram, right-heart catheterization should be used to evaluate for POPH. Right-heart catheterization is an invasive (usually outpatient) procedure but is required for the diagnosis of POPH. It is also a critical component of perioperative risk stratification in patients with known pulmonary hypertension and should ideally be performed within 1–3 months of LT. Right-heart catheterization involves introducing a Swan-Ganz catheter into a central vein. Platelet counts should preferably be > 50 k and INR < 1.5. The catheter is then used to measure the mPAP and the PAWP (also referred to as pulmonary capillary wedge pressure). Cardiac output (CO) is measured using either the Fick or thermodilution method, and pulmonary vascular resistance can be calculated based on the following equation: PVR = (mPAP - PAWP)/CO. The difference between the mPAP and PAWP is referred to as the transpulmonary gradient. POPH is diagnosed when the mPAP is > 25 mmHg, the PAWP is < 15 mmHg, and the PVR is > 3 Wood units.

An echocardiogram with contrast enhancement, or a "bubble study," can also be used to evaluate a patient for intracardiac or intrapulmonary shunting. For the contrast study, agitated saline is injected via a peripheral vein. This creates microbubbles of ~10 um in diameter [24]. Normally, these bubbles are visualized in the right atrium and then become trapped in the pulmonary capillaries so are not subsequently visualized in the left atrium. In the setting of intracardiac shunting, bubbles are visualized in the left atrium "early," typically within one to two cardiac cycles, whereas in the setting of IPVD or pulmonary AVMs, microbubbles are visualized in the left heart "late," at three or more cardiac cycles [1].

In patients with possible HPS (liver disease, abnormal gas exchange, and IPVD) in the context of comorbid pulmonary parenchymal disease, a technetium-labeled macroaggregated albumin (^{99m}TcMAA) scan can be helpful in determining whether hypoxemia can be attributed to HPS. Significant shunting or brain uptake > 6% is consistent with HPS, while the absence of significant brain uptake is more consistent with pulmonary parenchymal disease as the primary etiology of hypoxemia [1]. It should be noted, however, that a ^{99m}TcMAA scan does not differentiate between intracardiac and intrapulmonary shunting. However, a transesophageal echocardiogram used to directly visualize the source of microbubbles in the left heart can be useful to distinguish intracardiac from intrapulmonary shunting [1].

Lastly, overnight oximetry is a useful and simple screening test for sleep-disordered breathing [30]. Although not required as part of the routine LT evaluation, it is used to identify patients at risk for sleep-disordered breathing who should be referred for polysomnogram and further sleep evaluation.

Management of Hepatopulmonary Syndrome and Portopulmonary Hypertension

Hepatopulmonary Syndrome

Preoperative Management

Once a diagnosis of HPS is made, management is predominantly supportive. There are no effective medical therapies for HPS. Experimental therapies, such as somatostatin, almitrine, indomethacin, norfloxacin, pentoxifylline, and inhaled L-NAME, have all been studied without showing a consistent benefit [1]. Oral garlic extract has been shown to improve oxygenation in a small randomized controlled trial but has not been evaluated in large multi-center studies [31]. Oxygen saturation should be maintained with the use of supplemental oxygen, which is recommended to maintain oxygen saturation > 89%. However, it should be noted that this recommendation is extrapolated from patients with other lung diseases, and the optimal oxygen saturation in HPS is not known [1]. Chest computed tomography and arterial blood gas on 100% inhaled oxygen demonstrating a $PaO_2 < 300$ mmHg consistent

Table 2.6 Model for end-stage liver disease exception criteria for HPS and POPH

	HPS	POPH
Criteria for initial MELD exception	1. Clinical evidence of portal hypertension 2. Evidence of IPVD by CE-TTE 3. PaO2 < 60 mmHg on room air 4. No significant clinical evidence of underlying primary pulmonary disease	1. Initial mPAP > 35 mmHg 2. Initial PVR > 240 dynes•s•cm^{-5} 3. Posttreatment mPAP < 35 mmHg and PVR < 400 dynes•s•cm^{-5}
Criteria for MELD exception extension	Repeat arterial blood gas with PaO2 < 60 mmHg	Repeat right-heart catheterization with post-treatment mPAP < 35 mmHg and PVR < 400 dynes•s•cm^{-5}

mPAP mean pulmonary arterial pressure, *PaO2* partial pressure of oxygen in arterial blood, *PVR* pulmonary vascular resistance

with shunting can be helpful to identify rare patients with HPS and discrete AVMs who may benefit from pulmonary angiography and coil embolization [1].

As further discussed below, increased mortality is seen in all patients with HPS regardless of oxygenation [2]. Due to the increased mortality associated with HPS, the lack of effective medical therapies and the expected improvement in oxygenation following LT, patients should be referred for early consideration of LT, preferably before the development of severe to very severe hypoxemia. As of 2002, patients with HPS have been eligible to receive a MELD exception if the PaO2 is < 60 mmHg related to HPS without evidence of other clinically significant pulmonary disease (Table 2.6). An initial score of 22 is assigned, and the score increases by 10% mortality equivalent points if repeat arterial blood gas testing continues to demonstrate a PaO2 < 60 mmHg [11]. There are no formal recommendations or guidelines regarding oxygen saturation or PaO2 that would preclude LT. There is no agreement about any particular PaO2 threshold as an absolute contraindication to LT.

Intraoperative Management

Intraoperative management of HPS is also supportive. Most patients with HPS can achieve adequate oxygen saturation with 100% inspired oxygen. There are no defined cutoffs for canceling a case due to severe hypoxemia. Due to orthodeoxia, supine positioning in the operating room may also result in improved oxygenation when compared to upright oxygen saturation or arterial blood gas [1]. Patients are typically intubated and mechanically ventilated with lung-protective tidal volumes (6–8 cc/kg) [1]. Continuous monitoring of mixed venous oxygen saturation (SvO2) in the operating room can help guide decisions to initiate venovenous bypass. If SvO2 decreases to below 65% on vascular exclusion of the liver, venovenous bypass can be considered [1, 32].

Post-transplant and Intensive Care Unit Management

Immediately post-transplant, oxygen saturation typically worsens due to volume overload, atelectasis, hypoventilation, sedation, and/or aspiration [1]. Early extubation should be a goal to minimize infectious complications, such as ventilator-associated pneumonia. Severe post-transplant hypoxemia, defined as the need for 100% inspired oxygen to maintain oxygen saturation ≥ 85%, develops in 6–21% of patients with HPS and is associated with prolonged ICU stays and 45% mortality [33]. A clinical management algorithm was recently proposed based on best available evidence and expert opinion [33]. Options for management of severe post-transplant hypoxemia include Trendelenburg positioning, 100% inspired high-flow oxygen, inhaled vasodilators such as epoprostenol or nitric oxide (to optimize V-Q matching), and intravenous methylene blue (with or without inhaled vasodilators). Intravenous methylene blue is a vasoconstrictor that acts through inhibition of cyclic GMP. It has been used to improve oxygenation in HPS, presumably by vasoconstricting regions of vasodilatation, thus improving V-Q matching [34, 35]. Extracorporeal venovenous membrane oxygenation (ECMO) both pre- and post-LT has also been reported as improving oxygenation in HPS and can be considered as a last resort when other less invasive options have failed [33].

Hypoxemia secondary to HPS almost universally improves following LT, but time to recovery may be related to the severity of pretransplant hypoxemia [24, 36]. Postoperatively, patients are typically followed with pulse oximetry, and discontinuation of supplemental oxygen can be considered when oxygen saturation remains > 88%.

Portopulmonary Hypertension

Preoperative Management

Preoperative evaluation and management of POPH is complex and should be performed at an experienced center familiar with the management of pulmonary arterial hypertension (PAH) and the specific goals of treatment in the setting of LT. POPH, similar to other types of World Health Organization Group 1 PAH, is treated with PAH-targeted therapy. The main goal of PAH therapy is to improve symptoms, quality of life, exercise capacity, and survival. In LT candidates, improvement in pulmonary hemodynamics and RV function in order to facilitate safe LT is an additional treatment goal [37].

There are now more than ten approved medications for the treatment of pulmonary arterial hypertension. PAH-targeted therapy is available in oral, inhaled, subcutaneous, and intravenous administration routes. These medications target three distinct pathways that are involved in the pathogenesis of PAH. Prostacyclin analogues, such as epoprostenol, treprostinil and iloprost, and IP receptor agonists, such as selexipag, target the prostacyclin pathway. Endothelin receptor antagonists, such as bosentan, macitentan, and ambrisentan, target the endothelin-1 pathway. Bosentan has been associated with liver injury and liver failure and requires monthly monitoring based on liver function tests. Ambrisentan and macitentan do not require regular monitoring, but it is recommended that patients have baseline liver function tests with follow-up as clinically indicated. Phosphodiesterase-5 inhibitors, such as tadalafil and sildenafil, and soluble guanylate cyclase stimulators, such as riociguat, target the nitric oxide pathway. A more detailed review of PAH-targeted therapy is beyond the scope of this chapter.

Although these drugs are approved to treat POPH, it should be noted that most studies have not included patients with POPH in prospective clinical trials [37]. Consequently, decisions regarding PAH therapy in POPH are based on clinical experience and retrospective studies. Macitentan, an endothelin receptor antagonist, is the first drug to be prospectively studied specifically in patients with POPH in a randomized double-blind placebo-controlled clinical trial, but the results of this study are not yet available. There is no prospective data showing that one agent or pathway is preferable to another drug or pathway in POPH. Intravenous prostacyclin therapy is often used if patients require expedited LT evaluation or if they present with significant symptoms of syncope, right-heart failure, or dyspnea at rest. Progressive splenomegaly and thrombocytopenia have been reported with intravenous prostacyclin use in POPH [38]. Calcium channel blockers, which are sometimes used in idiopathic PAH, are generally avoided in POPH due to the lack of significant response [1].

PAH therapy is generally effective in POPH. Although subject to publication bias, a recent systematic review reported improved hemodynamics and exercise capacity in patients with POPH with the use of PAH-targeted therapy [39]. In addition to PAH therapy, it is also important to optimize volume status and right-heart filling pressure with the judicious use of diuretic therapy. Similar to HPS, supplemental oxygen should be used to maintain oxygen saturation > 89% in order to minimize pulmonary vasoconstriction.

Although POPH is not considered an indication for LT by itself in the absence of decompensated liver disease, LT can be safely performed in patients with adequately treated POPH and normal RV function. POPH may also improve post-transplant [1]. Since 2006, patients with POPH and an adequate hemodynamic response to PAH therapy (defined as an mPAP < 35 mmHg and PVR < 400 dynes•s•cm^{-5} or 5 Wood units) have been eligible to receive standardized MELD exceptions in order to expedite LT [1] (Table 2.6). These hemodynamic criteria were developed predominantly on the basis of a single-center retrospective study in which patients with untreated POPH with an elevated PVR and an elevated mPAP at the time of transplant were found to have an increased risk of death. Patients with an mPAP < 35 mmHg had 0% mortality, while patients with an mPAP of 35–50 mmHg had a 50% mortality rate, and patients with an mPAP > 50 mmHg had 100% perioperative mortality [40]. An mPAP > 50 mmHg is considered an absolute contraindication to LT. It is not known if patients who have an elevated mPAP between 35 and 50 mmHg due to elevated cardiac output with a normal PVR are also at an increased risk of death, but additional data regarding this clinical dilemma are emerging. A recent report from the Mayo Clinic described similar transplant hospitalization mortality rates in patients with an mPAP > 35 mmHg and normal PVR compared to those with an mPAP < 35 mmHg at the time of transplant. This cohort included four patients with treated POPH [41]. In addition to specific hemodynamic parameters, it is also important to assess RV function in the perioperative risk stratification of patients with POPH. It is not clear how best to define normal RV function, but echocardiographic assessments of RV function are critical. Similar to patients with HPS, patients with approved POPH MELD exceptions receive an initial MELD exception score of 22. Following this, they must undergo repeated right-heart catheterizations in order to demonstrate sustained hemodynamic response and to accrue 10% mortality equivalent points every 3 months.

In moderate to severe POPH, transjugular intrahepatic portosystemic shunts (TIPS) should be avoided due to the decreased ability of the right heart to tolerate the increased preload associated with TIPS [1]. The risks and benefits of prophylactic beta-blockade should also be considered on a case-by-case basis. Discontinuation of beta-blockers should be considered due to worsening cardiac output and exercise capacity in patients with POPH [42]. Lastly, coexistence of HPS and POPH is not uncommon [43]. It is not known whether the combination of these two conditions requires treatment that differs from that given when only POPH is present.

Intraoperative Management

Due to the initiation of appropriate screening as recommended by the American Association for the Study of Liver Diseases [28, 44], identification of POPH in the operating room is now relatively uncommon. Intraoperative and perioperative management of POPH is challenging and should be performed by an experienced multidisciplinary team of clinicians. Prior to abdominal incision, a pulmonary artery catheter should be placed to ensure that pulmonary hemodynamics are satisfactory prior to transplant. For patients with an elevated mPAP, obtaining an accurate PAWP measurement is critical to determine whether the mPAP is elevated due to an elevated PVR, CO, or PAWP (Fig. 2.1). According to the most recent International Liver Transplantation Society guidelines, if mPAP is > 45–50 mmHg before abdominal incision, deferment of LT is advised [1].

Continuous intraoperative and postoperative monitoring with a right-heart catheter is critical due to rapid fluctuations in hemodynamics. Intraoperative TEE can also be helpful in monitoring RV function [1]. During reperfusion, cardiac output can increase considerably, leading to an abrupt increase in pulmonary pressure. In the setting of fixed pulmonary vascular resistance, this can precipitate right-ventricular strain and subsequent failure [45, 46]. PAH-targeted therapy should be continued throughout the perioperative and immediate post-transplant period. Abrupt discontinuation of PAH therapy, particularly in patients on parenteral prostacyclin therapy, can lead to acute right-heart failure and death. In addition to continuing a patient's preoperative PAH-targeted therapy, other treatment options during and after LT include the use of inhaled vasodilators, such as nitric oxide or epoprostenol, intravenous prostacyclin analogues, milrinone, and ECMO [47–49]. Similar to all patients with pulmonary hypertension who undergo noncardiac surgery, it is also advised to avoid hypoxia and hypercapnia. End-tidal carbon dioxide should be maintained close to baseline. Although challenging, it is also important to maintain euvolemia as much as possible in order to maintain right-ventricular preload.

Post-transplant and Intensive Care Unit Management

In the intensive care unit (ICU), continuous hemodynamic monitoring should be continued immediately post-transplant to assist with the management of pulmonary hypertension and to monitor mean pulmonary arterial pressure, PVR, and cardiac output. Similar to intraoperative management, ICU management of POPH requires avoidance of hypoxia, hypercapnia, hypovolemia, and hypotension. In patients who develop right-ventricular failure, inotropes, such as dobutamine or milrinone, may be needed to augment contractility, and vasopressors may be needed to avoid hypotension. Norepinephrine and vasopressin are generally the preferred agents in the setting of pulmonary hypertension.

Post-transplant, PAH therapy should be continued with subsequent consideration of weaning based on symptoms, echocardiogram results, and pulmonary hemodynamics. There are no guidelines regarding weaning PAH therapy post-transplant. Typically, major changes in the immediate post-transplant period are not advised. It can take up to 3–6 months or longer post-transplant to wean or discontinue therapy. Decisions regarding medication adjustments are made on an individual basis in reference to symptoms, side effects, and right-ventricular function.

Prognosis

A diagnosis of HPS is associated with a significantly lower survival rate and poorer quality of life [2]. Patients with HPS have a twofold increased risk of death compared to patients without HPS with similar severity of cirrhosis [2]. In the absence of LT, survival is poor. According to an analysis of the United Network for Organ Sharing database, patients with very severe HPS and a PaO2 < 45 mmHg had increased post-transplant mortality [50]. In some experienced centers, however, HPS severity and a PaO2 < 50 mmHg was not associated with increased post-transplant mortality [51].

Patients with HPS have an excellent post-transplant prognosis. Most patients with HPS have improved oxygenation post-transplant and should be expected to no longer require supplemental oxygen, although this can often take months [1]. Recurrence of HPS is relatively rare and often related to recurrence of the underlying liver disease. Although oxygenation typically improves post-LT, development of post-transplant POPH in patients with antecedent HPS has also been described [52]. Whether this is due to the development of de novo POPH or unmasking of preexistent POPH as the pulmonary vasodilatation associated with HPS improves is not known.

In POPH, 5-year survival without LT or PAH therapy is dismal at 14%, while 1-year survival is 35–46% [53]. Different studies have reported variable survival estimates for patients with POPH. Theoretical reasons for these differences may be due to differences in liver disease severity, POPH disease severity, time period of enrollment, and whether patients underwent LT or were treated with PAH therapy. According to the United States multi-center REVEAL registry, patients with POPH have worse 5-year survival compared to idiopathic and familial PAH (40% vs 64%) despite having lower right-atrial pressure and a higher cardiac index, factors typically associated with a better prognosis [54]. In the United Kingdom, survival rates of 85%, 60%, and 35% at 1, 3, and 5 years, respectively, were recently reported for patients with POPH diagnosed between 2001 and 2010 ($n = 110$) [55]. According to a French study, 5-year survival for patients with POPH was 68% [56]. In this cohort, cardiac index and liver disease severity as assessed by the Child-Pugh score were significant predictors of overall mortality [56]. In patients in the United States with approved POPH MELD exceptions, predictors of waitlist mortality included PVR and liver disease severity as assessed by the initial MELD score. Increased mean pulmonary arterial pressure was not associated with worse survival in these patients [57]. Lastly, the presence of IPVD in patients with POPH is also associated with increased mortality [43].

Unlike for HPS, the post-transplant outcomes of POPH are variable. Both clinical improvement and worsening as well as intraoperative and postoperative death have all been described. There are limited data from which to prognosticate the long-term post-transplant outcomes of POPH or to identify patients who are most likely to benefit from LT. In France, overall survival estimates after LT were 80%, 77%, and 77% at 6 months, 1 year, and 3 years, respectively [4]. In the United States, 1-year post-transplant survival in patients with POPH MELD exceptions was 85% [57, 58]. Compared to non-exception LT candidates, however, patients with POPH had increased post-transplant mortality [58]. According to one single-center study in the United States, graft and patient survival rates post-transplant were 85.7% at a median follow-up of 7.8 years [59]. The United Kingdom recently reported 42.9% mortality (12/28) for patients with POPH during the period from 1992 to 2012, and the majority of deaths (10/12) occurred within 6 months of transplant [60]. A recent study from France also suggested that pulmonary hemodynamics may transiently worsen within the first 6 months post-transplant but then subsequently improve, allowing weaning and discontinuation of PAH therapy [4]. Post-transplant, many patients are able to wean or discontinue therapy. In single-center studies, discontinuation of PAH therapy has been reported in 29–64% of patients with POPH [1].

Summary

In summary, pulmonary disease is common in LT candidates. A systematic and thorough pretransplant pulmonary evaluation of LT candidates is necessary in order to appropriately identify and treat pulmonary comorbidities that affect perioperative and postoperative management.

Key Points

1. A systematic and comprehensive pretransplant pulmonary evaluation of LT candidates is necessary in order to recognize and treat conditions that affect LT candidacy and perioperative management.
2. Hepatopulmonary syndrome is characterized by the clinical triad of intrapulmonary vasodilatation, abnormal arterial oxygenation, and liver disease.
3. Portopulmonary hypertension is a clinical and hemodynamic diagnosis defined by elevated mean pulmonary arterial pressure > 25 mmHg, elevated pulmonary vascular resistance, and normal wedge pressure in the setting of portal hypertension and in the absence of alternative etiologies of pulmonary hypertension.
4. HPS typically improves following LT, while post-transplant outcomes of POPH are variable.

References

1. Krowka MJ, Fallon MB, Kawut SM, Fuhrmann V, Heimbach JK, Ramsay MA, Sitbon O, Sokol RJ. International liver transplant society practice guidelines: diagnosis and Management of Hepatopulmonary Syndrome and Portopulmonary Hypertension. Transplantation. 2016;100:1440–52.
2. Fallon MB, Krowka MJ, Brown RS, Trotter JF, Zacks S, Roberts KE, Shah VH, Kaplowitz N, Forman L, Wille K, Kawut SM. Pulmonary vascular complications of liver disease study G. Impact of hepatopulmonary syndrome on quality of life and survival in liver transplant candidates. Gastroenterology. 2008;135:1168–75.
3. Roberts KE, Kawut SM, Krowka MJ, Brown RS Jr, Trotter JF, Shah V, Peter I, Tighiouart H, Mitra N, Handorf E, Knowles JA, Zacks S, Fallon MB. Pulmonary vascular complications of liver disease study G. Genetic risk factors for hepatopulmonary syndrome in patients with advanced liver disease. Gastroenterology. 2010;139:130–9. e124
4. Savale L, Sattler C, Coilly A, Conti F, Renard S, Francoz C, Bouvaist H, Feray C, Borentain P, Jais X, Montani D, Parent F, O'Connell C, Herve P, Humbert M, Simonneau G, Samuel D, Calmus Y, Duvoux C, Durand F, Duclos-Vallee JC, Sitbon O. Long-term outcome in liver transplantation candidates with portopulmonary hypertension. Hepatology. 2017;65:1683–92.
5. Krowka MJ, Swanson KL, Frantz RP, McGoon MD, Wiesner RH. Portopulmonary hypertension: results from a 10-year screening algorithm. Hepatology. 2006;44:1502–10.
6. Colle IO, Moreau R, Godinho E, Belghiti J, Ettori F, Cohen-Solal A, Mal H, Bernuau J, Marty J, Lebrec D, Valla D, Durand F. Diagnosis of portopulmonary hypertension in candidates for liver transplantation: a prospective study. Hepatology. 2003;37:401–9.
7. Kawut SM, Krowka MJ, Trotter JF, Roberts KE, Benza RL, Badesch DB, Taichman DB, Horn EM, Zacks S, Kaplowitz N, Brown RS Jr, Fallon MB. Pulmonary vascular complications of liver disease study G. Clinical risk factors for portopulmonary hypertension. Hepatology. 2008;48:196–203.
8. Roberts KE, Fallon MB, Krowka MJ, Brown RS, Trotter JF, Peter I, Tighiouart H, Knowles JA, Rabinowitz D, Benza RL, Badesch DB, Taichman DB, Horn EM, Zacks S, Kaplowitz N, Kawut SM. Pulmonary vascular complications of liver disease study G. Genetic risk factors for portopulmonary hypertension in patients with advanced liver disease. Am J Respir Crit Care Med. 2009;179:835–42.

9. Talwalkar JA, Swanson KL, Krowka MJ, Andrews JC, Kamath PS. Prevalence of spontaneous portosystemic shunts in patients with portopulmonary hypertension and effect on treatment. Gastroenterology. 2011;141:1673–9.
10. DuBrock HM, Rodriguez-Lopez JM, LeVarge BL, Curry MP, VanderLaan PA, Zsengeller ZK, Pernicone E, Preston IR, Yu PB, Nikolic I, Xu D, Thadhani RI, Channick RN, Ananth Karumanchi S. Macrophage migration inhibitory factor as a novel biomarker of portopulmonary hypertension. Pulmonary circulation. 2016;6:498–507.
11. Krowka MJ, Wiesner RH, Heimbach JK. Pulmonary contraindications, indications and MELD exceptions for liver transplantation: a contemporary view and look forward. J Hepatol. 2013;59:367–74.
12. Xiol X, Tremosa G, Castellote J, Gornals J, Lama C, Lopez C, Figueras J. Liver transplantation in patients with hepatic hydrothorax. Transplant Int: Off J Eur Soc Organ Transplant. 2005;18:672–5.
13. Rybak D, Fallon MB, Krowka MJ, Brown RS Jr, Reinen J, Stadheim L, Faulk D, Nielsen C, Al-Naamani N, Roberts K, Zacks S, Perry T, Trotter J, Kawut SM. Pulmonary vascular complications of liver disease study G. Risk factors and impact of chronic obstructive pulmonary disease in candidates for liver transplantation. Liver Transplant: Off Publ Am Assoc Study Liver Diseases Inte Liver Transplant Soc. 2008;14:1357–65.
14. Celli BR, Cote CG, Marin JM, Casanova C, Montes de Oca M, Mendez RA, Pinto Plata V, Cabral HJ. The body-mass index, airflow obstruction, dyspnea, and exercise capacity index in chronic obstructive pulmonary disease. N Engl J Med. 2004;350:1005–12.
15. Carey EJ, Steidley DE, Aqel BA, Byrne TJ, Mekeel KL, Rakela J, Vargas HE, Douglas DD. Six-minute walk distance predicts mortality in liver transplant candidates. Liver Transplant: Off Publ Am Assoc Study Liver Diseases Inte Liver Transplant Soc. 2010;16:1373–8.
16. Carey EJ, Iyer VN, Nelson DR, Nguyen JH, Krowka MJ. Outcomes for recipients of liver transplantation for alpha-1-antitrypsin deficiency-related cirrhosis. Liver Transplant: Off Publ Am Assoc Study Liver Diseases Inte Liver Transplant Soc. 2013;19:1370–6.
17. Alder JK, Chen JJ, Lancaster L, Danoff S, Su SC, Cogan JD, Vulto I, Xie M, Qi X, Tuder RM, Phillips JA 3rd, Lansdorp PM, Loyd JE, Armanios MY. Short telomeres are a risk factor for idiopathic pulmonary fibrosis. Proc Natl Acad Sci U S A. 2008;105:13051–6.
18. Corso RM, Gregoretti C, Braghiroli A, Fanfulla F, Insalaco G. Practice guidelines for the perioperative Management of Patients with obstructive sleep apnea: navigating through uncertainty. Anesthesiology. 2014;121:664–5.
19. Chung F, Abdullah HR, Liao P. STOP-Bang questionnaire: a practical approach to screen for obstructive sleep apnea. Chest. 2016;149:631–8.
20. Dupuis-Girod S, Ginon I, Saurin JC, Marion D, Guillot E, Decullier E, Roux A, Carette MF, Gilbert-Dussardier B, Hatron PY, Lacombe P, Lorcerie B, Riviere S, Corre R, Giraud S, Bailly S, Paintaud G, Ternant D, Valette PJ, Plauchu H, Faure F. Bevacizumab in patients with hereditary hemorrhagic telangiectasia and severe hepatic vascular malformations and high cardiac output. JAMA. 2012;307:948–55.
21. Trerotola SO, Pyeritz RE, White RI Jr, Picus D, Miller FJ, Foundation HHT, Centers HHT. 2009 treatment guidelines for hereditary hemorrhagic telangiectasia. J Vasc Interv Radiol. 2010;21:179.
22. Lyle MA, Fenstad ER, McGoon MD, Frantz RP, Krowka MJ, Kane GC, Swanson KL. Pulmonary hypertension in hereditary hemorrhagic telangiectasia. Chest. 2016;149:362–71.
23. Lin CY, Chen JH, Liang JA, Lin CC, Jeng LB, Kao CH. 18F-FDG PET or PET/CT for detecting extrahepatic metastases or recurrent hepatocellular carcinoma: a systematic review and meta-analysis. Eur J Radiol. 2012;81:2417–22.
24. Rodriguez-Roisin R, Krowka MJ. Hepatopulmonary syndrome--a liver-induced lung vascular disorder. N Engl J Med. 2008;358:2378–87.
25. Wiesner RH, McDiarmid SV, Kamath PS, Edwards EB, Malinchoc M, Kremers WK, Krom RA, Kim WR. MELD and PELD: application of survival models to liver allocation. Liver Transplant: Off Publ Am Assoc Study Liver Diseases Inte Liver Transplant Soc. 2001;7:567–80.

26. Benza RL, Miller DP, Gomberg-Maitland M, Frantz RP, Foreman AJ, Coffey CS, Frost A, Barst RJ, Badesch DB, Elliott CG, Liou TG, McGoon MD. Predicting survival in pulmonary arterial hypertension: insights from the registry to evaluate early and long-term pulmonary arterial hypertension disease management (REVEAL). Circulation. 2010;122:164–72.
27. Machicao VI, Balakrishnan M, Fallon MB. Pulmonary complications in chronic liver disease. Hepatology. 2014;59:1627–37.
28. Martin P, DiMartini A, Feng S, Brown R Jr, Fallon M. Evaluation for liver transplantation in adults: 2013 practice guideline by the American Association for the Study of Liver Diseases and the American Society of Transplantation. Hepatology. 2014;59:1144–65.
29. Raevens S, Colle I, Reyntjens K, Geerts A, Berrevoet F, Rogiers X, Troisi RI, Van Vlierberghe H, De Pauw M. Echocardiography for the detection of portopulmonary hypertension in liver transplant candidates: an analysis of cutoff values. Liver Transpl. 2013;19:602–10.
30. Netzer N, Eliasson AH, Netzer C, Kristo DA. Overnight pulse oximetry for sleep-disordered breathing in adults: a review. Chest. 2001;120:625–33.
31. De BK, Dutta D, Pal SK, Gangopadhyay S, Das Baksi S, Pani A. The role of garlic in hepatopulmonary syndrome: a randomized controlled trial. Can J Gastroenterol. 2010;24:183–8.
32. Fauconnet P, Klopfenstein CE, Schiffer E. Hepatopulmonary syndrome: the anaesthetic considerations. Eur J Anaesthesiol. 2013;30:721–30.
33. Nayyar D, Man HS, Granton J, Lilly LB, Gupta S. Proposed management algorithm for severe hypoxemia after liver transplantation in the hepatopulmonary syndrome. Am J Transplant Off J Am Soc Transplant Am Soc Transplant Surg. 2015;15:903–13.
34. Schenk P, Madl C, Rezaie-Majd S, Lehr S, Muller C. Methylene blue improves the hepatopulmonary syndrome. Ann Intern Med. 2000;133:701–6.
35. Roma J, Balbi E, Pacheco-Moreira L, Gonzalez AC, Leal CG, Pousa F, Zynger I, Leite D, Halpern M, Guerra PP, Covelo M, Carius L, Agoglia L, Oliveira A, Enne M. Methylene blue used as a bridge to liver transplantation postoperative recovery: a case report. Transplant Proc. 2010;42:601–4.
36. Taille C, Cadranel J, Bellocq A, Thabut G, Soubrane O, Durand F, Ichai P, Duvoux C, Belghiti J, Calmus Y, Mal H. Liver transplantation for hepatopulmonary syndrome: a ten-year experience in Paris, France. Transplantation. 2003;75:1482–9. discussion 1446-1487
37. DuBrock HM, Channick RN, Krowka MJ. What's new in the treatment of portopulmonary hypertension? Expert Rev Gastroenterol Hepatol. 2015;9:983–92.
38. Findlay JY, Plevak DJ, Krowka MJ, Sack EM, Porayko MK. Progressive splenomegaly after epoprostenol therapy in portopulmonary hypertension. Liver Transpl Surg. 1999;5:362–5.
39. Faisal M, Siddiqi F, Alkaddour A, Bajwa AA, Shujaat A. Effect of PAH specific therapy on pulmonary hemodynamics and six-minute walk distance in portopulmonary hypertension: a systematic review and meta-analysis. Pulmonary medicine. 2014;2014:528783.
40. Krowka MJ, Plevak DJ, Findlay JY, Rosen CB, Wiesner RH, Krom RA. Pulmonary hemodynamics and perioperative cardiopulmonary-related mortality in patients with portopulmonary hypertension undergoing liver transplantation. Liver Transplant: Off Publ Am Assoc Study Liver Diseases Inte Liver Transplant Soc. 2000;6:443–50.
41. DeMartino ES, Cartin-Ceba R, Findlay JY, Heimbach JK, Krowka MJ. Frequency and outcomes of patients with increased mean pulmonary artery pressure at the time of liver transplantation. Transplantation. 2017;101:101–6.
42. Provencher S, Herve P, Jais X, Lebrec D, Humbert M, Simonneau G, Sitbon O. Deleterious effects of beta-blockers on exercise capacity and hemodynamics in patients with portopulmonary hypertension. Gastroenterology. 2006;130:120–6.
43. Fussner LA, Iyer VN, Cartin-Ceba R, Lin G, Watt KD, Krowka MJ. Intrapulmonary vascular dilatations are common in portopulmonary hypertension and may be associated with decreased survival. In: Liver transplantation : official publication of the American Association for the Study of Liver Diseases and the international liver transplantation society, vol. 21; 2015. p. 1355.
44. Murray KF, Carithers RL Jr. AASLD. AASLD practice guidelines: evaluation of the patient for liver transplantation. Hepatology. 2005;41:1407–32.

45. Ramsay M. Portopulmonary hypertension and right heart failure in patients with cirrhosis. Curr Opin Anaesthesiol. 2010;23:145–50.
46. Safdar Z, Bartolome S, Sussman N. Portopulmonary hypertension: an update. Liver Transplant: Off Publ Am Assoc Study Liver Diseases Inte Liver Transplant Soc. 2012;18:881–91.
47. Ramsay MA, Spikes C, East CA, Lynch K, Hein HA, Ramsay KJ, Klintmalm GB. The perioperative management of portopulmonary hypertension with nitric oxide and epoprostenol. Anesthesiology. 1999;90:299–301.
48. Stratta C, Lavezzo B, Ballaris MA, Panio A, Crucitti M, Andruetto P, Fanelli V, Grosso Marra W, Ranieri MV, Salizzoni M. Extracorporeal membrane oxygenation rescue therapy in a case of portopulmonary hypertension during liver transplantation: a case report. Transplant Proc. 2013;45:2774–5.
49. Fukazawa K, Poliac LC, Pretto EA. Rapid assessment and safe management of severe pulmonary hypertension with milrinone during orthotopic liver transplantation. Clin Transpl. 2010;24:515–9.
50. Goldberg DS, Krok K, Batra S, Trotter JF, Kawut SM, Fallon MB. Impact of the hepatopulmonary syndrome MELD exception policy on outcomes of patients after liver transplantation: an analysis of the UNOS database. Gastroenterology. 2014;146:1256–65. e1251
51. Iyer VN, Swanson KL, Cartin-Ceba R, Dierkhising RA, Rosen CB, Heimbach JK, Wiesner RH, Krowka MJ. Hepatopulmonary syndrome: favorable outcomes in the MELD exception era. Hepatology. 2013;57:2427–35.
52. Aucejo F, Miller C, Vogt D, Eghtesad B, Nakagawa S, Stoller JK. Pulmonary hypertension after liver transplantation in patients with antecedent hepatopulmonary syndrome: a report of 2 cases and review of the literature. Liver Transplant: Off Publ Am Assoc Study Liver Diseases Inte Liver Transplant Soc. 2006;12:1278–82.
53. Swanson KL, Wiesner RH, Nyberg SL, Rosen CB, Krowka MJ. Survival in portopulmonary hypertension: Mayo Clinic experience categorized by treatment subgroups. Am J Transplant. 2008;8:2445–53.
54. Krowka MJ, Miller DP, Barst RJ, Taichman D, Dweik RA, Badesch DB, McGoon MD. Portopulmonary hypertension: a report from the US-based REVEAL registry. Chest. 2012;141:906–15.
55. Sithamparanathan S, Nair A, Thirugnanasothy L, Coghlan JG, Condliffe R, Dimopoulos K, Elliot CA, Fisher AJ, Gaine S, Gibbs JSR, Gatzoulis MA, EH C, Howard LS, Johnson M, Kiely DG, Lordan JL, Peacock AJ, Pepke-Zaba J, Schreiber BE, Sheares KKK, Wort SJ, Corris PA. National Pulmonary Hypertension Service Research Collaboration of the united K, Ireland. Survival in portopulmonary hypertension: outcomes of the United Kingdom National Pulmonary Arterial Hypertension Registry. J Heart Lung Transplant. 2017;36:770–9.
56. Le Pavec J, Souza R, Herve P, Lebrec D, Savale L, Tcherakian C, Jais X, Yaici A, Humbert M, Simonneau G, Sitbon O. Portopulmonary hypertension: survival and prognostic factors. Am J Respir Crit Care Med. 2008;178:637–43.
57. DuBrock HM, Goldberg DS, Sussman NL, Bartolome SD, Kadry Z, Salgia RJ, Mulligan DC, Kremers WK, Kawut SM, Krowka MJ, Channick RN. Predictors of waitlist mortality in Portopulmonary hypertension. Transplantation. 2017;101:1609–15.
58. Salgia RJ, Goodrich NP, Simpson H, Merion RM, Sharma P. Outcomes of liver transplantation for Porto-pulmonary hypertension in model for end-stage liver disease era. Dig Dis Sci. 2014;59:1976–82.
59. Khaderi S, Khan R, Safdar Z, Stribling R, Vierling JM, Goss JA, Sussman NL. Long-term follow-up of portopulmonary hypertension patients after liver transplantation. Liver Transpl. 2014;20:724–7.
60. Verma S, Hand F, Armstrong MJ, de Vos M, Thorburn D, Pan T, Klinck J, Westbrook RH, Auzinger G, Bathgate A, Masson S, Holt A, Houlihan DD, Ferguson JW. Portopulmonary hypertension: still an appropriate consideration for liver transplantation? Liver Transpl. 2016;22:1637–42.

Chapter 3
Critical Care for Potential Liver Transplant Candidates: Ventilation

Catherine Paugam-Burtz, Emmanuel Weiss, and Samir Jaber

Introduction

End-stage liver disease or cirrhotic patients may require critical care for numerous reasons related to complications or a worsening of their condition. At the time of admission to the ICU, a small percentage of them are already on the waiting list for liver transplantation (LT) and are naturally considered liver transplant candidates. The larger percentage are not on the list, with some of them not even diagnosed as cirrhotic at this time [1]. However, among this population, a significant proportion will probably be liver transplant candidates for two main reasons [2]. First, if the early prognosis for cirrhotic patients admitted to the ICU has improved over time, the midterm prognosis (6 months) for ICU survivors remains very poor, particularly for patients who did not have access to LT including those who were not eligible for this treatment [3, 4]. Second, a significant number of cirrhotic patients may develop acute-on-chronic hepatic failure associated with organ failure and there is an extremely poor prognosis for nontransplanted patients for whom this is the case [3]. These two circumstances highlight the importance of LT for ICU survivors and even for patients during a stay in the ICU, as LT could offer a very significant survival benefit for these patients [4]. All these potential liver transplant candidates shared a similar feature: mechanical ventilation (MV) is associated with a significantly

C. Paugam-Burtz (✉) · E. Weiss
Department of Anesthesiology and Critical Care Medicine, Hôpital Beaujon, APHP, Clichy, France

Paris Diderot (Paris 7) University, Paris France and Inserm UMR_S1149, Center for Research on Inflammation, Paris, France
e-mail: catherine.paugam@aphp.fr

S. Jaber
Department of Anesthesiology and Critical Care Medicine B (DAR B), Saint-Eloi Hospital, University Teaching Hospital of Montpellier, INSERM U104680, Montpellier, France

D. Bezinover, F. Saner (eds.), *Critical Care for Potential Liver Transplant Candidates*,
https://doi.org/10.1007/978-3-319-92934-7_3

increased risk of hospital mortality [5, 6]. In part, this association is probably related to the selection of the sickest patients with the most pronounced multiorgan failure syndrome. However, even if MV is lifesaving, it has become increasingly obvious that MV per se also has the potential to negatively impact the outcomes of critically ill patients. Tremendous efforts have been made to improve MV settings to limit additional pulmonary insults and improve outcomes. A very large body of evidence related to MV in ICU or intraoperative patients is now available. Liver transplant candidates as end-stage liver disease patients have been excluded from the landmark trials of MV in acute lung injury or acute respiratory distress syndrome (ARDS), but most of the results and practices are probably suitable for these patients.

This chapter will address briefly the reasons for respiratory failure in liver transplant candidates and the management strategies for ventilatory support for these patients with a particular focus on the perioperative pulmonary care around liver transplantation.

Reasons for MV

There are various reasons for critically ill cirrhotic patients to require MV [5, 7]. Endotracheal intubation may have to be performed for airway protection in advanced-grade encephalopathy. Ventilatory support may also be required for hypoxia and respiratory failure caused by numerous reasons: atelectasis from the compressive effects of ascites, underlying chronic pulmonary disease, sepsis, or pneumonia. Muscle wasting and intra-abdominal hypertension increase the work of breathing. Infection is probably a leading cause of acute respiratory failure (ARF) requiring MV. Furthermore, there are various reasons why cirrhotic patients develop ARDS, i.e., as a result of inflammation, aspiration, or bacterial pulmonary or non-pulmonary sepsis.

Mechanical Ventilation in the ICU

When a critically ill cirrhotic patient becomes an LT candidate, pulmonary care should be considered as a continuum pathway from the preoperative to the intra- and post-operative period. Preoperative MV requirement is a predictor of postoperative pulmonary complications, ARDS, and prolonged postoperative MV after LT [8, 9]. Prolonged postoperative MV is associated with pulmonary infections and mortality [10, 11]. Because of this close relationship, everything should be done to optimize MV at each step. Although beyond the scope of this chapter, it is nonetheless important to consider MV as part of a global approach to "pulmonary" care. This is particularly true for hemodynamic resuscitation strategies that may impact respiratory outcomes: excessive fluid resuscitation and fluid overload have a negative impact; preoperative fluid status will also impact the incidence of postoperative acute lung injury [12].

How Can Invasive Mechanical Ventilation be Avoided?

When treatment of ARF is a possibility, the first step is to consider how to avoid endotracheal intubation, which refers to invasive MV. On the other hand, noninvasive ventilation (NIV), which uses a facial mask as an interface between patient and ventilator to deliver positive end-expiratory pressure (PEEP) and pressure support, has become the standard of care for acute decompensation of COPD or ARF related to pulmonary edema. However, in hypoxemic ARF, mainly because of various reasons leading to this condition, the overall benefit of NIV techniques has been difficult to show in this population. However, in well-trained teams with adequate interfaces, NIV could be proposed as a first-line treatment for patients with ARF, as these techniques are associated with a reduction of health-care-associated pneumonia. This point may be of particular interest for cirrhotic patients with immune dysfunction and high susceptibility to infections (see infra). However, NIV should not be applied in cases of encephalopathy because of the risk of aspiration.

High-flow nasal cannula (HFNC) oxygen therapy allows continuous nasal delivery of a high flow of heated and humidified gas. It has recently been proposed as an interesting noninvasive option to treat severe hypoxemic ARF. In a randomized trial with hypoxemic patients mostly with pneumonia, HFNC compared to NIV or conventional oxygen therapy did not improve the primary trial endpoint, i.e., the overall intubation rate, but did reduce mortality in the whole cohort and reduced the need for intubation in the subgroup of the most severe hypoxemic patients [13]. In two recent meta-analyses, compared to the use of conventional oxygen therapy, HFNC showed a decreased intubation rate in patients with ARF. However, when compared to NIV, HFNC may not provide better outcomes. To date, the appropriate use of this technique is yet to be determined [14, 15].

Ventilator Settings in Cases of Invasive Mechanical Ventilation

End-stage liver disease patients requiring MV do not all suffer from ARDS, but acute lung injury is frequent in this population. The beneficial effect of a strategy of lung-protective ventilation combining low-tidal volume and PEEP has been demonstrated, and this strategy should be considered as a standard of care for all patients requiring MV [16, 17].

The tidal volume setting should be guided by the patient's predicted body weight. As in obese patients, this is a matter of concern in cirrhotic patients who may have very large variations in weight related to ascites or edema.

The American Thoracic Society, the European Society of Intensive Care Medicine, and the Society of Critical Care Medicine have recently published clinical practice guidelines for mechanical ventilation in adult patients with ARDS. They state that "for all patients with ARDS, MV using lower-tidal volumes (4–8 ml/kg predicted body weight) and lower inspiratory pressures (plateau pressure: 30 cm H2O) (moderate confidence in effect estimates) is strongly recommended. For patients with severe ARDS, prone positioning for more than 12 h/day (moderate confidence in effect estimates) is strongly recommended. For patients with moderate or severe ARDS, the guidelines strongly recommend against the routine use of high-frequency oscillatory ventilation (high confidence in effect estimates) and conditionally recommend it for higher PEEP (moderate confidence in effect estimates) and recruitment maneuvers (low confidence in effect estimates). Additional evidence is necessary to make a definitive recommendation for or against the use of extracorporeal membrane oxygenation in patients with severe ARDS."

Finally, they add that "Clinicians managing patients with ARDS should personalize decisions for their patients, particularly regarding the conditional recommendations in this guideline" [18]. As stated before, even though the population of liver transplant candidates has not been specifically studied, there is no obvious reason not to follow these recommendations.

Prevention of Ventilator-Associated Pneumonia

Patients with liver cirrhosis have an increased risk of microbial infections and are at high risk of death from sepsis. This is related to numerous conditions such as a complex immune dysfunction or increased bacterial translocation through the intestinal wall because of increased gut permeability, reduced gut motility, and altered gut flora. This increased bacterial translocation and consequent endotoxemia leads to increased bloodstream bacterial infections that cause systemic inflammatory response syndrome, sepsis, multi-organ failure, and death. Additionally, cirrhosis-associated immune dysfunction leads to alterations in both innate and acquired immunity, due to defects in the local immunity of the liver as well as in systemic immunity. This dysfunction combines both increased systemic inflammation and immunodeficiency and is responsible for 30% mortality [19, 20].

This very high susceptibility for infections underlines the importance of the prevention of ventilator-associated pneumonia (VAP) in liver transplant candidates under MV. First, it should be kept in mind that probably the most efficient way to reduce VAP is to reduce the duration of MV. This can be achieved through the application of a bundle of care including adequate use of sedation, systematic evaluation for weaning, and extubation [21].

Choice of sedative agents, depth of sedation, and sedative management can influence the risk for VAP in mechanically ventilated patients [22]. If VAP is used, the minimum dose should be applied using titration, and caution should be paid to overdosing and excessive sedation, which can cause accumulation and delayed recovery even after the resolution of liver function.

Second, multifaceted ventilator bundle components seem to be associated with the reduction of VAP [23, 24]. Bundle components may combine head-of-bed elevation, sedative infusion interruptions, spontaneous breathing trials, daily oral care with chlorhexidine, adequate endotracheal tube cuff pressure (20–30 mmHg), or an endotracheal tube with an in-line suction system and subglottic suctioning [23–26]. However, the impact of any given individual component remains unclear [26]. Recently, there has been a shift in focus from VAP to ventilator-associated events in order to improve the objectivity and reproducibility of surveillance and to encourage programs to consider a broader array of complications in mechanically ventilated patients. Prospective intervention studies have found that minimizing sedation, increasing the use of spontaneous awakening and breathing trials, and applying conservative fluid management can lower the rate of ventilator-associated events and decrease the duration of MV [27].

Intraoperative Ventilator Settings

A growing body of evidence is now available in the setting of abdominal surgery particularly for high-risk surgical patients showing the clinical benefits of protective lung ventilation, which combines intraoperative low-tidal volume MV with PEEP and intermittent recruitment maneuvers [28, 29]. In abdominal surgery with high-risk patients, the IMPROVE study, a multi-center, randomized, double-blind trial, compared an optimized strategy of ventilation called protective ventilation (tidal volume 6–8 mL/kg predicted body weight and PEEP 6–8 cm H_2O with systematic alveolar recruitment maneuvers every 30 min) with a traditional strategy called non-protective ventilation (tidal volume 10–12 mL/kg predicted body weight, without PEEP or recruitment maneuvers). Protective ventilation decreased the overall rate of a composite criterion including onset of pulmonary complications (pneumonia or need for either noninvasive or invasive ventilation) or extra-pulmonary complications (sepsis, septic shock, and death) from 27.5 to 10.5% and reduced the length of hospital stay by 2 days [30]. Liver transplant patients were not included in this study. However, LT is a high-risk abdominal procedure associated with a high risk of postoperative pulmonary complications [9, 31]. These complications are associated with a significant increase in morbidity and mortality. These risks are further increased for liver transplant candidates coming from the ICU with preoperative mechanical ventilation and frequent additional renal or neurological dysfunctions. Overall, it seems reasonable to consider protective lung ventilation a suitable strategy for intraoperative MV in liver transplant candidates [28, 29].

Conclusion

There has been significant improvement in the perioperative management of liver transplant candidates. However, candidates requiring critical care remain a challenge for intensivists and anesthesiologists. Liver transplantation may be a life-saving procedure for these very high-risk surgical patients. There is very little research focusing specifically on MV for these patients, yet evidence relating to the more general ICU or surgical population is probably strong enough to be appropriate. Continuing a protective ventilatory strategy from the preoperative ICU period to the intraoperative period may be an important pathway to further improvements in the outcomes of these patients.

Key Points

1. When a critically ill cirrhotic patient becomes a liver transplant candidate, pulmonary care should be considered as a continuum pathway from the preoperative to the intra- and post-operative periods.
2. Patients with end-stage liver disease (ESLD) requiring mechanical ventilation do not all suffer from ARDS. Acute lung injury is frequent in this population. The beneficial effect of a lung-protective ventilation strategy that includes combining low-tidal volume and positive end-expiratory pressure (PEEP) has been demonstrated in several evaluations. Even if ESLD patients are frequently excluded from clinical studies, there is no reason not to apply protective ventilation as a standard of care for all patients requiring mechanical ventilation (MV).
3. ESLD patients are highly susceptible to infections, which underlines the importance of ventilator-associated pneumonia (VAP) prevention in LT candidates requiring MV. The most efficient way to reduce VAP is to reduce the duration of MV or to avoid it altogether.
4. Noninvasive ventilation, which uses a facial mask as an interface between the patient and ventilator to deliver PEEP and inspiratory pressure support, could be an important therapeutic option in this patient population.
5. In prospective interventional studies, it has been found that minimizing sedation and increasing the use of spontaneous awakening, breathing trials, and conservative fluid management can decrease ventilator-associated event rates and shorten the duration of MV.
6. Continuing a protective ventilatory strategy from the preoperative ICU period to the intraoperative period may be an important pathway to further improvements in the outcomes of these patients.

References

1. Das V, et al. Cirrhotic patients in the medical intensive care unit: early prognosis and long-term survival. Crit Care Med. 2010;38(11):2108–16.
2. Galbois A, et al. Prognostic scores for cirrhotic patients admitted to an intensive care unit: which consequences for liver transplantation? Clin Res Hepatol Gastroenterol. 2013;37(5):455–66.
3. Weil D, et al. Prognosis of cirrhotic patients admitted to intensive care unit: a meta-analysis. Ann Intensive Care. 2017;7(1):33.
4. Majumdar A, et al. Declining mortality in critically ill patients with cirrhosis in Australia and New Zealand between 2000 and 2015. J Hepatol. 2017;67:1185.
5. Levesque E, et al. Outcome of patients with cirrhosis requiring mechanical ventilation in ICU. J Hepatol. 2014;60(3):570–8.
6. Annamalai A, et al. Predictors of mortality in the critically ill cirrhotic patient: is the model for end-stage liver disease enough? J Am Coll Surg. 2017;224(3):276–82.
7. Levesque E, et al. Liver transplantation in patients with end-stage liver disease requiring intensive care unit admission and intubation. Liver Transpl. 2015;21(10):1331–2.
8. Huang CT, et al. Pre-operative risk factors predict post-operative respiratory failure after liver transplantation. PLoS One. 2011;6(8):e22689.

9. Kleine M, et al. Respiratory risk score for the prediction of 3-month mortality and prolonged ventilation after liver transplantation. Liver Transpl. 2013;19(8):862–71.
10. Yuan H, et al. Prognostic impact of mechanical ventilation after liver transplantation: a national database study. Am J Surg. 2014;208(4):582–90.
11. Knaak J, et al. Liver transplantation in patients with end-stage liver disease requiring intensive care unit admission and intubation. Liver Transpl. 2015;21(6):761–7.
12. Chan KC, et al. Patterns of perioperative thoracic fluid indices changes in liver transplantation with or without postoperative acute lung injury. J Formos Med Assoc. 2017;116(6):432–40.
13. Frat JP, et al. High-flow oxygen through nasal cannula in acute hypoxemic respiratory failure. N Engl J Med. 2015;372(23):2185–96.
14. Lin SM, et al. Does high-flow nasal cannula oxygen improve outcome in acute hypoxemic respiratory failure? A systematic review and meta-analysis. Respir Med. 2017;131:58–64.
15. Zhao H, et al. High-flow nasal cannula oxygen therapy is superior to conventional oxygen therapy but not to noninvasive mechanical ventilation on intubation rate: a systematic review and meta-analysis. Crit Care. 2017;21(1):184.
16. Serpa Neto A, et al. Association between use of lung-protective ventilation with lower tidal volumes and clinical outcomes among patients without acute respiratory distress syndrome: a meta-analysis. JAMA. 2012;308(16):1651–9.
17. Jaber S, et al. The intensive care medicine research agenda for airways, invasive and noninvasive mechanical ventilation. Intensive Care Med. 2017;43:1352.
18. Fan E, et al. An Official American Thoracic Society/European Society of Intensive Care Medicine/Society of Critical Care Medicine clinical practice guideline: mechanical ventilation in adult patients with acute respiratory distress syndrome. Am J Respir Crit Care Med. 2017;195(9):1253–63.
19. Weiss E, et al. Type I interferon signaling in systemic immune cells from patients with alcoholic cirrhosis and its association with outcome. J Hepatol. 2017;66(5):930–41.
20. Strnad P, et al. Liver – guardian, modifier and target of sepsis. Nat Rev Gastroenterol Hepatol. 2017;14(1):55–66.
21. Blackwood B, et al. Protocolized versus non-protocolized weaning for reducing the duration of mechanical ventilation in critically ill adult patients. Cochrane Database Syst Rev. 2014;(11):CD006904.
22. Caroff DA, Szumita PM, Klompas M. The relationship between sedatives, sedative strategy, and healthcare-associated infection: a systematic review. Infect Control Hosp Epidemiol. 2016;37(10):1234–42.
23. Khan R, et al. The impact of implementing multifaceted interventions on the prevention of ventilator-associated pneumonia. Am J Infect Control. 2016;44(3):320–6.
24. Neuville M, et al. Bundle of care decreased ventilator-associated events-implications for ventilator-associated pneumonia prevention. J Thorac Dis. 2017;9(3):430–3.
25. Klompas M, et al. Associations between ventilator bundle components and outcomes. JAMA Intern Med. 2016;176(9):1277–83.
26. Wang L, et al. Semi-recumbent position versus supine position for the prevention of ventilator-associated pneumonia in adults requiring mechanical ventilation. Cochrane Database Syst Rev. 2016;(1):CD009946.
27. Cocoros NM, Klompas M. Ventilator-associated events and their prevention. Infect Dis Clin N Am. 2016;30(4):887–908.
28. Futier E, Marret E, Jaber S. Perioperative positive pressure ventilation: an integrated approach to improve pulmonary care. Anesthesiology. 2014;121(2):400–8.
29. Ball L, et al. Intraoperative mechanical ventilation: state of the art. Minerva Anestesiol. 2017;83(10):1075–88.
30. Futier E, et al. A trial of intraoperative low-tidal-volume ventilation in abdominal surgery. N Engl J Med. 2013;369(5):428–37.
31. Pedersen MR, et al. Pretransplant factors and associations with postoperative respiratory failure, ICU length of stay, and short-term survival after liver transplantation in a high MELD population. J Transp Secur. 2016;2016:6787854.

Chapter 4
Hemodynamic Changes and Modulation in Inpatients with Acute and Chronic Liver Failure

Ahmed M. Mukhtar

Hemodynamic Changes in Patients with Acute Liver Failure

Patients on the waiting list for a liver transplant are frequently admitted to an intensive care unit (ICU) due to decompensation of the liver function [1]. Hemodynamic management of this patient population can be very challenging. There are two distinct types of acute liver dysfunction that might require ICU admission: acute liver failure (ALF) and acute on chronic liver failure (ACLF). Although both types of liver dysfunction are presented with multi-system involvement, the underlying pathophysiological changes responsible for hemodynamic instability differ significantly between the conditions, which each requires specific management.

Acute Liver Failure (ALF)

ALF is a rapid decline in the liver function of a previously healthy liver caused by massive hepatic necrosis [2].

Hemodynamic Derangement in ALF

Most patients with acute liver failure develop hemodynamic instability [3]. There are several causes of hemodynamic instability in these patients, but most importantly, patients with ALF have relative or absolute hypovolemia due to inadequate fluid intake and/or capillary leak with transudation of fluid into extravascular space [4].

A. M. Mukhtar (✉)
Department of Anesthesia and Critical Care, Cairo University, Cairo, Egypt
e-mail: ahmed.mukhtar@kasralainy.edu.eg

D. Bezinover, F. Saner (eds.), *Critical Care for Potential Liver Transplant Candidates*,
https://doi.org/10.1007/978-3-319-92934-7_4

The second common cause of hemodynamic instability is systemic vasodilatation because of excess nitric oxide production [5]. Vasodilatation leads to hyperdynamic circulation and low mean arterial pressure, which may be severe and similar to those seen in patients with septic shock [6]. Patients with ALF are also at high risk of sepsis and septic shock [7] as well as relative adrenal insufficiency, which may reduce the response to α-adrenergic agents [8].

Hemodynamic Management of Patients with ALF

A. Hemodynamic target

- Mean arterial pressure (MAP)
  The appropriate MAP target in critically ill patients, especially those with ALF, has been a topic of debate for many years. However, in young patients without preexisting comorbidities and no evidence of increased intracranial pressure (ICP), a MAP of 60–65 mmHg is adequate [2]. Higher MAP $\geq$ 80 mmHg may be required in a subset of patients with elevated ICP to maintain adequate cerebral perfusion pressure (CPP) (CPP = MAP – ICP) [9]. Another group of patients who may benefit from high MAP are those with preexisting chronic hypertension, as high MAP minimizes the incidence of acute kidney injury (AKI). A SEPSISPAM study has demonstrated that a target MAP of 80–85 mmHg decreased the incidence of AKI among patients with septic shock with preexisting chronic hypertension [10].

B. Hemodynamic management

1. Fluid resuscitation
   Fluid resuscitation is the first step in the hemodynamic management of patients with ALF. The goal of fluid therapy is to maintain adequate MAP with subsequent optimization of cardiac output in order to improve tissue perfusion. Although fluid depletion should be avoided in these patients, fluid excess and positive balance are detrimental and associated with high morbidity and mortality [11]. That is why careful assessment of volume status for these patients is important during hemodynamic management. A stepwise approach to hemodynamic management is illustrated in Fig. 4.1.

   (a) Assessment of volume status

   - *Central venous pressure (CVP)*
     Several studies have demonstrated very limited utility of CVP to guide fluid resuscitation in critically ill patients [13]. However, high CVP, i.e., above 20 mmHg, should be avoided in patients with ALF because it may impede venous drainage from the brain [14].
   - *Central venous saturation (ScVO2)*
     ScVO2 is a surrogate marker for mixed venous oxygen saturation (SVO2) and indicates the balance between oxygen delivery and consumption. However, when CO is high, the changes in SVO2 are poorly

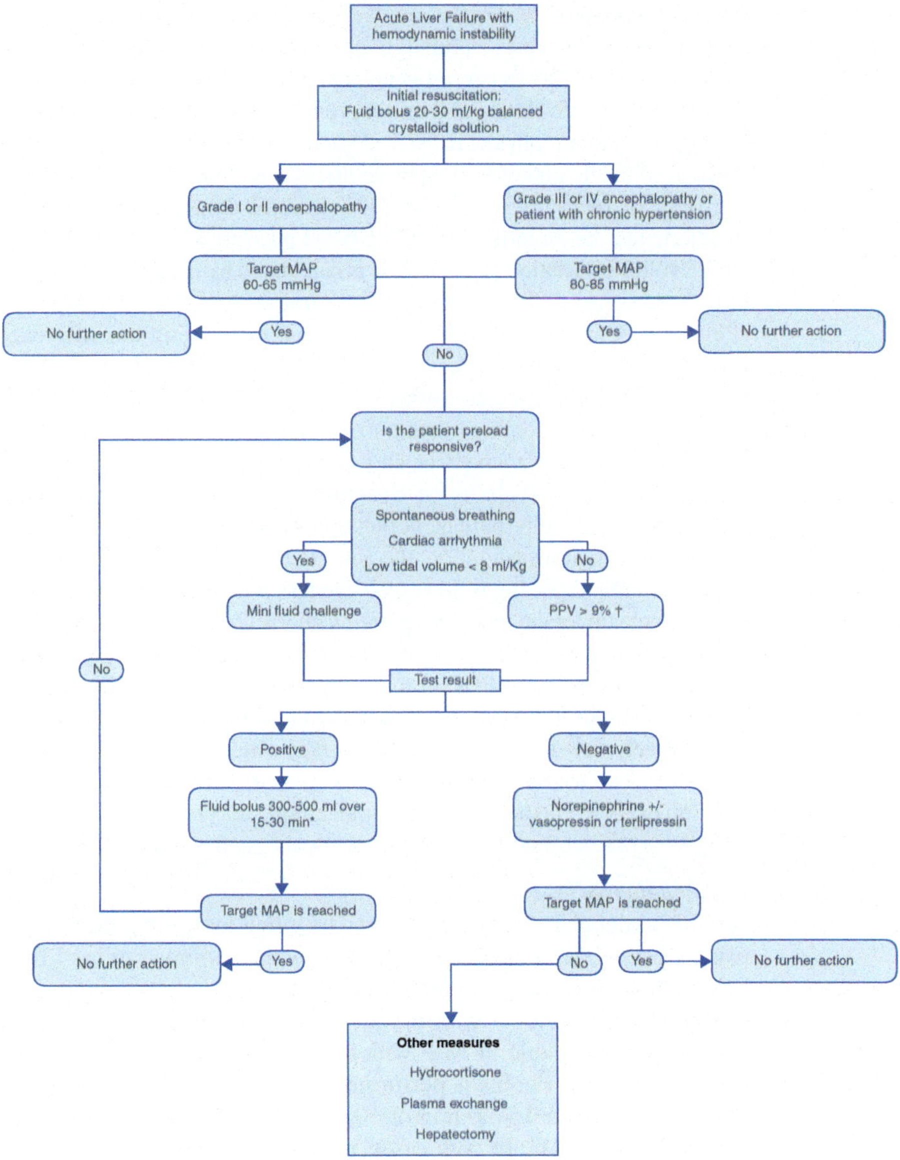

Fig. 4.1 Stepwise approach to hemodynamic management of a patient with ALF. *The decision to expand volume should be weighed against the risk of volume overload. †A PPV cutoff value of 9% was based on a single study [12]

correlated with changes in CO [15]. Because CO is high in patients with ALF, ScVO2 cannot guide fluid resuscitation in these patients. ScVO2 may be high even if the patient is hypovolemic and fluid-responsive [16].

- *Dynamic measure*
  Recent surviving-sepsis campaign guidelines recommend the use of dynamic measures over central venous pressure to guide fluid therapy in patients with septic shock, and this approach has gained wide acceptance among critical care physicians [17]. Dynamic measures are based on the concept of cyclic changes of right-ventricular preload and afterload during positive pressure ventilation [18]. Several dynamic measures are mentioned in the literature, including pulse pressure variation (PPV) and stroke volume variation (SVV). PPV is calculated by dividing the highest pulse pressure (PP) (PPmax − PPmin) by the average PP (PPmax + PPmin/2) [19]. SVV is calculated by dividing the difference between maximum stroke volume (SV) and minimum SV (SVmax − SVmin) by their average (SVmax + SVmin/2) in a time window of 30 s. SVV requires continuous cardiac output monitoring such as via pulse contour analysis or an esophageal Doppler monitor. In the setting of ALF, the validity of dynamic measures for assessing fluid responsiveness in this patient population has been tested in only one study [12]. In that investigation, the authors found that only PPV and not SVV was able to predict fluid responsiveness with a cutoff value of 9%, with the area under the receiver operating characteristic curve 0.752 [95% confidence interval, 0.565–0.889]; $P = 0.005$] [12]. The explanation for the modest accuracy of PPV in this study is multifactorial. The smaller volume of bolus fluid used during the fluid challenge (5 mL/kg) and the relatively low tidal volume (7.6 mL/kg) might explain this finding. Moreover, low arterial resistance in these patients and the complex computation of SVV via the pulse contour technique may explain the inability of SVV to predict fluid responsiveness in patients with ALF [12].

- *Fluid challenge*
  A fluid challenge is usually performed by either increasing the preload using a passive leg raising test (PLR) or by the administration of fluid bolus. PLR induces a transient increase in the preload through translocation of venous blood from the lower limbs to the chest. However, PLR is less applicable in ALF with a high grade of hepatic encephalopathy [20]. Fluid bolus is performed by either infusing 250–500 cc of crystalloids over 15–30 min or 100 cc of colloids over 1 min (mini fluid challenge) [21]. In both cases, real-time changes to cardiac output should be measured by continuous CO monitoring.

(b) Choice of fluid
In critically ill patients, the evidence supports the use of crystalloids over colloids during initial fluid resuscitations [17]. However, in patients with ALF, there is no evidence to support specific fluid therapy. Because of the increasing risk of worsening brain edema, a hypotonic solution such as ringer lactate should be avoided in patients with ALF. Furthermore, there is an increased risk of elevated blood lactate levels because of the decreased capacity of the liver to metabolize lactate in patients with

ALF. However, the general critical care literature supports the use of a balanced crystalloid solution over normal saline because of the increased risk of hyperchloremic acidosis and acute kidney injury [22].

2. Vasopressor therapy
   The use of vasopressor should be considered when hypotension persists despite adequate fluid resuscitation. Several vasopressor agents can be used to achieve the target MAP.

   - Norepinephrine
     Norepinephrine should be the agent of choice for patients with ALF, as it increases MAP without a concomitant increase in heart rate [2].

   - Vasopressin and terlipressin
     Vasopressin is arginine vasopressin (AVP), a non-peptide molecule that acts by stimulating V1 and V2 receptors [23]. Terlipressin (triglycyl-lysine-vasopressin) is a synthetic analogue of arginine vasopressin and has a half-life of ~6 h [24].
     Vasopressin or terlipressin should be considered when a high dose of norepinephrine is required to achieve the target MAP. One previous study demonstrated that both vasopressin and terlipressin may exacerbate cerebral edema in patients with ALF [25]. However, in a more recent study, no detrimental effect was found to arise from infusing terlipressin on ICP when compared to norepinephrine [26].

3. Other measures

   - Hydrocortisone
     The incidence of adrenal insufficiency exceeds 60% in patients with ALF [8]. Administration of 200–300 mg/day of hydrocortisone may decrease vasopressor requirements in ALF patients with vasopressor-resistant shock [27].

   - Plasma exchange (PE)
     Plasma exchange is an established treatment modality for various autoimmune conditions, and evidence supporting its use in the treatment of ALF is growing. Plasma is separated from cells in an extracorporeal device, which uses either a filter or centrifuge. The plasma is then replaced with either human albumin solution (HAS), fresh frozen plasma (FFP), or a combination of the two. In several studies, it has been demonstrated that PE in the first 3 days after ICU admission may improve the hemodynamics of patients with ALF [28, 29]. In a recent randomized controlled study, it was found that high-volume PE improved the free survival rate of patients with ALF. This improvement was achieved mainly because of the removal of inflammatory mediators, antibodies, and albumin-bound toxins with a subsequent improvement in arterial pressure and a decreased requirement for norepinephrine infusion [30].

   - Hepatectomy
     The reversal of circulatory failure related to vasopressor-resistant shock after the removal of a native liver is noted in several case reports [31].

Acute on Chronic Liver Failure (ACLF)

Acute hepatic decompensation in patients with end-stage liver disease is the major cause of cirrhotic patient admission to the ICU. The precipitating factors for liver decompensation include gastrointestinal hemorrhage, sepsis, trauma, and surgery. However, on many occasions, the precipitating factors remain unidentified. In all these cases, acute hepatic decompensation is often termed ACLF. Although there are multiple definitions of ACLF, it can be described as a rapid progression to multiple organ dysfunctions in patients with preexisting chronic liver disease.

Hemodynamic Derangement in ACLF

Understanding pathophysiological changes in patients with ESLD is essential for successful hemodynamic management of patients with ACLF.

- *Portal hypertension and hyperdynamic state*
  Portal hypertension, increased splanchnic blood flow, and development of portosystemic collaterals are the main pathognomonic features of patients with ESLD. There is increased splanchnic blood flow caused mainly by a vasodilation of arterial splanchnic vessels, both in splenic and mesenteric vascular beds. Excess nitric oxide production due to shear forces between portal and systemic circulation is the pivotal factor involved in profound splanchnic vasodilatation. Bacterial translocation from the gut is another mechanism responsible for increased NO production in these patients [32]. Excess NO, together with increased pro-inflammatory mediators, precipitates a specific hemodynamic state characterized by high cardiac output, low systemic vascular resistance, and low MAP, which typically resembles the hyperdynamic state of patients with sepsis. During acute decompensation, the hyperdynamic state worsens with an increase in portal pressure and exacerbation of systemic hypotension.
- *Abnormal distribution of blood volume*
  Patients with ESLD have abnormally distributed blood volume with more than 37% concentrated in the abdomen. This is significantly higher than the abdominal blood volume of healthy subjects, whose abdominal organs contain less than 30% of their total blood volume.
- *Blunted response to fluid bolus*
  Total vascular compliance is markedly different between healthy subjects and patients with ESLD. Whereas total vascular compliance in healthy individuals is 0.5–1 mL/mmHg/kg body weight, it is estimated to be 1.5–2.5 mL/mmHg/kg body weight in patients with liver cirrhosis. This difference in vascular compliance means the responses to volume loading differ radically between these patient populations. For instance, fluid loading in a healthy subject is associated

with an increase in central blood volume and a subsequent increase in systemic blood pressure [33] (Fig. 4.2). But in patients with ESLD, fluid loading is associated with pooling of blood to splanchnic circulation, with a minimal effect on central blood volume and cardiac output [35] (Fig. 4.3). Collection of blood in the splanchnic circulation is associated with portal hyperemia and increased portal pressure, which may aggravate bleeding and gastrointestinal hemorrhage. Because of this, the traditional approach of optimizing hemodynamics via aggressive volume resuscitation is unlikely to be the best strategy to employ during resuscitation of patients with ESLD.

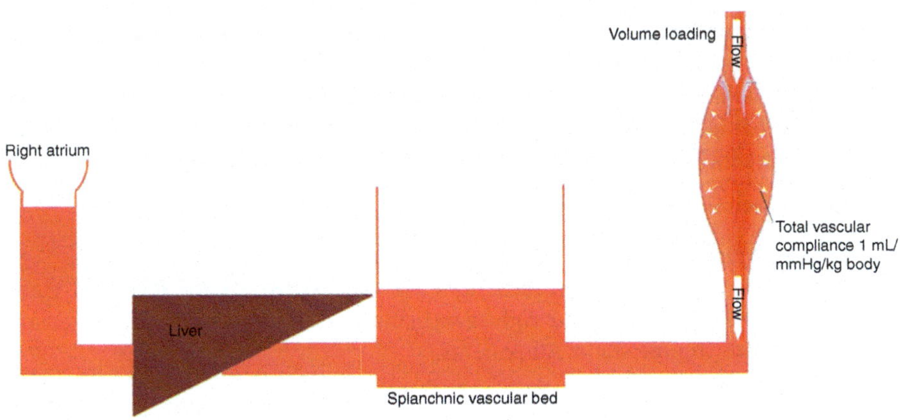

Fig. 4.2 Fluid loading in a healthy subject. Low vascular compliance combined with decreased pooling of blood in splanchnic circulation is associated with increased central venous pressure. (With permission [34])

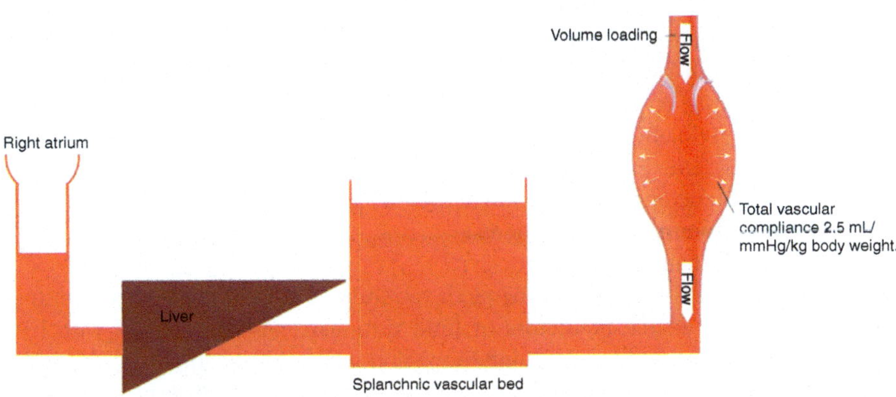

Fig. 4.3 Fluid loading in a cirrhotic patient. High vascular compliance combined with increased pooling of blood in splanchnic circulation is associated with a minimal increase in central venous pressure. (With permission [34])

Hemodynamic Management of Patients with ACLF

Sepsis is the most important cause of hemodynamic instability in patients with ACLF. This section will focus on the hemodynamic management of ACLF patients with septic shock, with special emphasis on the modulation of splanchnic circulation. The approach to hemodynamic management of patients with ACLF is illustrated in Fig. 4.4.

A. Hemodynamic target
   Recent surviving-sepsis campaign guidelines recommend early fluid administration with 30 ml/kg and maintaining MAP above 65 mmHg. Lactate clearance should be used as a guide for successful resuscitation [17]. In relation to cirrhotic patients with septic shock, the data are limited, and hemodynamic therapy may need specific protocol-guided management that takes into consideration the pathophysiological changes of these patients. For example, it has been demonstrated that lactate clearance is significantly impaired during early resuscitation of septic shock in patients with preexisting liver dysfunction [37].

B. Hemodynamic management
   1. Assessment of cardiac function
      Echocardiography is a robust tool for the assessment of left- and right-ventricular function and right-ventricular systolic pressure and to ensure adequate volume status for patients.
   2. Fluid resuscitation
      Because of the aforementioned pathophysiological changes, septic shock is fluid-responsive in only ~12% of cirrhotic patients [38]. That is the reason why the assessment of volume status is an essential step during the early hemodynamic management of these patients.

      (a) Volume assessment
         - Central venous pressure
           In addition to the general limitations of CVP in guiding fluid therapy, high intra-abdominal pressure in cirrhotic patients, due to ascites, may erroneously increase the reading of CVP despite ventricular preload [39]. In a recent study, CVP failed to predict fluid responsiveness in patients with liver cirrhosis [40]. The dynamic rather than static approach to cardiac preload assessment can help to guide fluid therapy in these patients.
         - Dynamic measures
           - PPV, SVV, and the pleth variability index (PVI) were found to be reliable predictors of fluid responsiveness in patients with liver cirrhosis undergoing living donor liver transplantation [40]. In this study, the cutoff values for PPV, SVV, and PVI were 10% (sensitivity 78.3%, specificity 79.5%) and 12% (sensitivity 69.6%, specificity 71.8%) for predicting fluid responsiveness [40]. However, in patients with tense ascites and high intra-abdominal

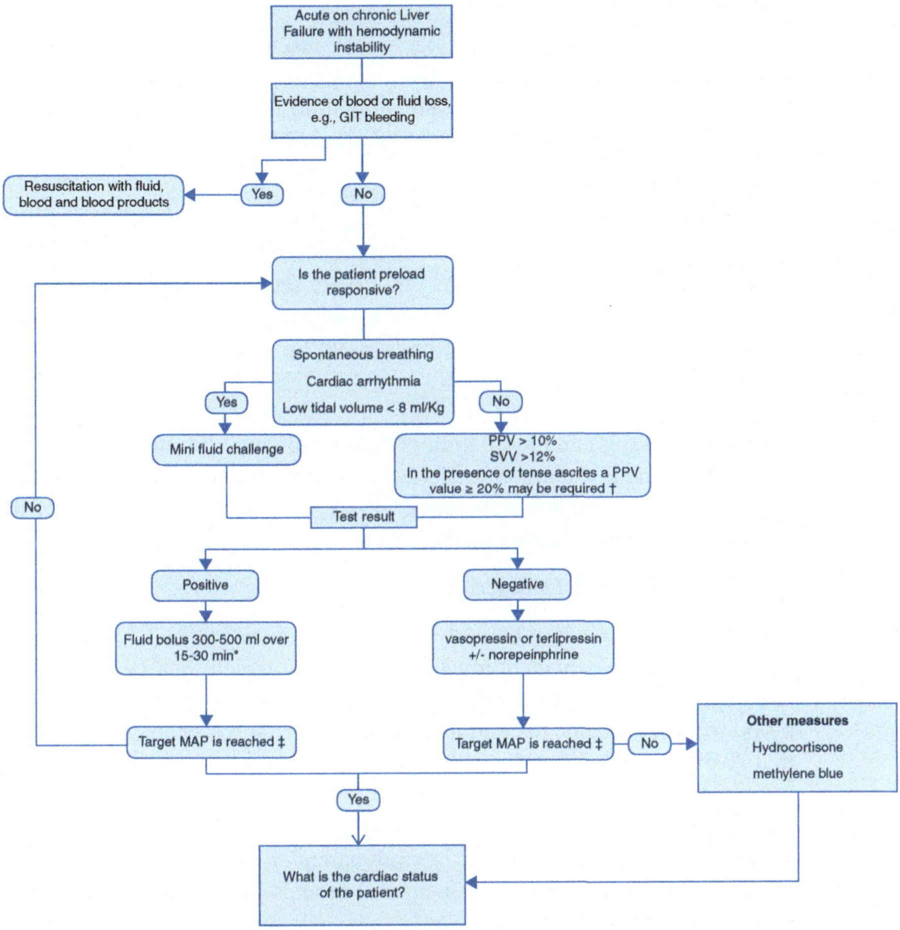

Fig. 4.4 Stepwise approach to hemodynamic management of a patient with ACLF. *The decision to expand volume should be weighed against the risk of volume overload. †A PPV cutoff value of 20% is based on an animal study [36]. ‡Although a target MAP of 65 mmHg is considered sufficient in general in critically ill patients, it still remains poorly defined in cirrhotic patients

pressure, the threshold values of PPV and SVV to discriminate responders and non-responders might be as high as 20% [36].

– Inferior vena cava (IVC) diameter
  The variation of the IVC diameter measured by transthoracic echocardiography has been reported to detect preload responsiveness with reasonable accuracy [41]. However, in patients with liver cirrhosis, interpretations of caval physiology may be hindered by conditions that restrict the physiologic variability of the IVC, such as liver fibrosis and elevated intra-abdominal pressure [42].

- Preload challenge
  - The PLR test is not reliable in the presence of tense ascites and/or abdominal hypertension [34].
  - Both the conventional and mini fluid challenge can be used, as previously described, with real-time CO measurements.

(b) Type of fluid
The role of human albumin in cirrhotic patients with septic shock has not been investigated. However, in patients with ESLD, improved arterial pressure and improved outcomes were seen in patients with spontaneous bacterial peritonitis who received albumin [43]. This indicates that albumin-containing solutions should be included in the fluid therapy used with this population.

3. Vasopressor therapy and modulation of splanchnic circulation
   - Norepinephrine is the first line of vasopressor therapy to correct refractory hypotension in patients with septic shock [17]. However, patients with ESLD are known to be less responsive to vasopressors [44].
     - Vasopressin (AVP) and terlipressin
   - An effective approach to hemodynamic management in ACLF is splanchnic modulation by splanchnic vasoconstrictors, which may be an alternative approach to volume loading. Splanchnic vasoconstrictors redistribute blood from splanchnic to central circulation [45]. It has been demonstrated that AVP significantly reduces both portal pressure and portal flow while maintaining intestinal perfusion, which may be beneficial in minimizing the incidence of gastrointestinal hemorrhage [46]. Terlipressin has demonstrated splanchnic and systemic hemodynamic effects similar to those produced by AVP when examined in animal models [47], and also in patients with liver cirrhosis [48].
   - Kiszka-Kanowitz et al. [49] reported that when administered to cirrhotic patients, terlipressin increased the volume of blood in the liver and the thoracic regions by 12% and 6%, respectively, resulting in an increase in mean arterial pressure as well as a reduction in hyperdynamic circulation. The effect of intraoperative terlipressin infusion on splanchnic and systemic hemodynamics has been evaluated in patients undergoing living donor liver transplantation [50]. The authors found that when compared to controls, patients receiving terlipressin had higher MAP and SVR. More recently, the efficacy of terlipressin compared to norepinephrine was evaluated in cirrhotic patients with septic shock [38]. The authors found that a larger proportion of patients (92%) in the terlipressin group achieved the target MAP > 65 mmHg at 48 h compared to those in the norepinephrine group (69%) $P = 0.005$). Terlipressin additionally reduces the incidence of variceal bleeding to a greater extent than does norepinephrine (0% vs 9.5%, $P = 0.01$) [38].

4. Other measures
   (a) Adrenal function
   Surviving-sepsis campaign guidelines recommend corticosteroid therapy (intravenous hydrocortisone 200 mg/day in four divided doses for a week before slowly tapering) for non-cirrhotic patients with vasopressor-dependent septic shock [17]. The effect of steroid therapy in cirrhotic patients with septic shock has been investigated in many studies [51–53]. Most of these evaluations demonstrated that hydrocortisone therapy is associated with a significant reduction in vasopressor doses and higher rates of shock reversal. However, the effect on survival remains controversial.
   (b) Methylene blue
   As previously mentioned, the main cause of vasopressor-resistant shock is the overproduction of nitric oxide (NO) mediated by the release of cytokines and endotoxins [54]. Administration of methylene blue, which is a NO inhibitor, has been demonstrated to be effective in reversing the course of hemodynamic deterioration and in preventing the development of severe septic shock [55]. The efficacy of methylene blue in reverting vasoplegia during and after liver transplantation has been investigated in several case reports [56–58]. The reported dosages of methylene blue are variable, but in general it ranges from 1 to 2 mg/kg bolus with or without a subsequent infusion for 6 h.

Key Points

1. There are two distinct types of acute liver dysfunction that might require ICU admission: acute liver failure (ALF) and acute on chronic liver failure (ACLF).
2. Hemodynamic instability in patients with ALF is mainly associated with hypovolemia and/or systemic vasodilatation, which can be severe, as seen in patients with septic shock.
3. In patients with ALF and no evidence of increased intracranial pressure (ICP), a mean arterial pressure (MAP) of 60–65 mmHg will adequately maintain normal cerebral perfusion. However, MAP ≥ 80 mmHg may be required in a subset of patients with elevated ICP. Fluid resuscitation is the mainstay of therapy in patients with ALF. If hypotension persists after adequate fluid resuscitation, vasopressor therapy should be initiated.
4. In patients with ACLF, sepsis is the most important cause of hemodynamic instability. A poor response to a fluid challenge is associated with several causes, including abnormal distribution of blood volume, splanchnic vasodilatation, and increased vascular compliance.
5. The use of vasopressors is the mainstay therapy in patients with ACLF. Another effective approach to hemodynamic management in ACLF is the administration of splanchnic vasoconstrictors to redistribute blood from portal to central circulation.

References

1. Findlay JY, Fix OK, Paugam-burtz C, et al. Critical care of the end-stage liver disease patient awaiting liver transplantation. Liver Transpl. 2011;17:496–510.
2. Wendon J, Cordoba J, Dhawan A, et al. Clinical practice guidelines EASL clinical practical guidelines on the management of acute (fulminant) liver failure q clinical practice guidelines [Internet]. J Hepatol. 2017;66:1047–81. Available from: https://doi.org/10.1016/j.jhep.2016.12.003.
3. Ford RM, Sakaria SS, Subramanian RM. Critical care management of patients before liver transplantation [Internet]. Transplant Rev. 2010;24:190–206. Available from: https://doi.org/10.1016/j.trre.2010.05.003.
4. Wang D-W. Advances in the management of acute liver failure [Internet]. World J Gastroenterol. 2013;19:7069. Available from: http://www.wjgnet.com/1007-9327/full/v19/i41/7069.htm.
5. Siniscalchi A, Dante A, Spedicato S, et al. Hyperdynamic circulation in acute liver failure: reperfusion syndrome and outcome following liver transplantation. Transplant Proc. 2010;42:1197–9.
6. Ellis A, Wendon J. Circulatory, respiratory, cerebral, and renal derangements in acute liver failure: pathophysiology and management. Semin Liver Dis. 1996;16:379–88.
7. Vaquero J, Polson J, Chung C, et al. Infection and the progression of hepatic encephalopathy in acute liver failure. Gastroenterology. 2003;125:755–64.
8. Harry R, Auzinger G, Wendon J. The clinical importance of adrenal insufficiency in acute hepatic dysfunction. Hepatology. 2002;36:395–402.
9. Kandiah PA, Olson JC, Subramanian RM. Emerging strategies for the treatment of patients with acute hepatic failure [Internet]. Curr Opin Crit Care. 2016;22:1. Available from: http://content.wkhealth.com/linkback/openurl?sid=WKPTLP:landingpage&an=00075198-900000000-99374.
10. Asfar P, Meziani F, Hamel J-F, et al. High versus low blood-pressure target in patients with septic shock. N Engl J Med. 2014;370:1583–93.
11. Acheampong A, Vincent J. A positive fluid balance is an independent prognostic factor in patients with sepsis [Internet]. Crit Care. 2015;19:1–7. Available from: https://doi.org/10.1186/s13054-015-0970-1.
12. Audimoolam VK, Mcphail MJW, Willars C, et al. Predicting fluid responsiveness in acute liver. Anesth Analg. 2017;124:480–6.
13. Marik PE, Cavallazzi R. Does the central venous pressure predict fluid responsiveness? An updated meta-analysis and a plea for some common sense*. Crit Care Med. 2013;41:1774–81.
14. Scheuermann K, Thiel C, Thiel K, et al. Correlation of the intracranial pressure to the central venous pressure in the late phase of acute liver failure in a porcine model. Acta Neurochir Suppl. 2012;114:387–91.
15. el-Masry A, Mukhtar AM, el-Sherbeny AM, et al. Comparison of central venous oxygen saturation and mixed venous oxygen saturation during liver transplantation. Anaesthesia. 2009;64:378–82.
16. Lee YK, Hwang SY, Shin TG, et al. Prognostic value of lactate and central venous oxygen saturation after early resuscitation in sepsis patients. PLoS One. 2016;11:e0153305.
17. Rhodes A, Evans LE, Alhazzani W, et al. Surviving sepsis campaign: international guidelines for management of sepsis and septic shock: 2016. Intensive Care Med. 2017;43:304–77.
18. Hasanin A. Fluid responsiveness in acute circulatory failure. J Intensive Care. 2015;19(3):50.
19. Yang X, Du B. Does pulse pressure variation predict fluid responsiveness in critically ill patients? A systematic review and meta-analysis. Crit Care. 2014;18:650.
20. Monnet X, Rienzo M, Osman D, et al. Passive leg raising predicts fluid responsiveness in the critically ill. Crit Care Med. 2006;34:1402–7.
21. Muller L, Toumi M, Bousquet P-J, et al. An increase in aortic blood flow after an infusion of 100 ml colloid over 1 minute can predict fluid responsiveness. Anesthesiology. 2011;115:541–7.

22. Krajewski ML, Raghunathan K, Paluszkiewicz SM, et al. Meta-analysis of high- versus low-chloride content in perioperative and critical care fluid resuscitation. Br J Surg. 2015;102:24–36.
23. Barrett LK, Singer M, Clapp LH. Vasopressin: mechanisms of action on the vasculature in health and in septic shock. Crit Care Med. 2007;35:33–40.
24. Nilsson G, Lindblom P, Ohlin M, et al. Pharmacokinetics of terlipressin after single i.v. doses to healthy volunteers. Drugs Exp Clin Res. 1990;16:307–14.
25. Shawcross DL, Davies NA, Mookerjee RP, et al. Worsening of cerebral hyperemia by the administration of terlipressin in acute liver failure with severe encephalopathy. Hepatology. 2004;39:471–5.
26. Eefsen M, Dethloff T, Frederiksen H-J, et al. Comparison of terlipressin and noradrenalin on cerebral perfusion, intracranial pressure and cerebral extracellular concentrations of lactate and pyruvate in patients with acute liver failure in need of inotropic support [Internet]. J Hepatol. 2007;47:381–6. Available from: https://www.ncbi.nlm.nih.gov/pubmed/17599633.
27. Harry R, Auzinger G, Wendon J. The effects of supraphysiological doses of corticosteroids in hypotensive liver failure. Liver Int. 2003;23:71–7.
28. Clemmesen JO, Kondrup J, Nielsen LB, et al. Effects of high-volume plasmapheresis on ammonia, urea, and amino acids in patients with acute liver failure. Am J Gastroenterol. 2001;96:1217–23.
29. Clemmesen JO, Gerbes AL, Gülberg V, et al. Hepatic blood flow and splanchnic oxygen consumption in patients with liver failure. Effect of high-volume plasmapheresis. Hepatology. 1999;29:347–55.
30. Larsen FS, Schmidt LE, Bernsmeier C, et al. High-volume plasma exchange in patients with acute liver failure: an open randomised controlled trial. J Hepatol. 2016;64:69–78.
31. Guirl MJ, Weinstein JS, Goldstein RM, et al. Two-stage total hepatectomy and liver transplantation for acute deterioration of chronic liver disease: a new bridge to transplantation. [Internet]. Liver Transplant. 2004;10:564–70. Available from: http://doi.wiley.com/10.1002/lt.20134.
32. Bellot P, García-Pagán JC, Francés R, et al. Bacterial DNA translocation is associated with systemic circulatory abnormalities and intrahepatic endothelial dysfunction in patients with cirrhosis. [Internet]. Hepatology. 2010;52:2044–52. [cited 2014 Nov 10] Available from: http://www.ncbi.nlm.nih.gov/pubmed/20979050.
33. Henriksen JH. Volume adaptation in chronic liver disease: on the static and dynamic location of water, salt, protein and red cells in cirrhosis. [Internet]. Scand J Clin Lab Invest. 2004;64:523–33. [cited 2014 Nov 10] Available from: http://www.ncbi.nlm.nih.gov/pubmed/15370457.
34. The passive leg-raising maneuver cannot accurately predict fluid responsiveness in patients with intra-abdominal hypertension [Internet]. Available from: https://www.ncbi.nlm.nih.gov/pubmed/20639753.
35. Hadengue A, Moreau R, Gaudin C, et al. Total effective vascular compliance in patients with cirrhosis: a study of the response to acute blood volume expansion. Hepatology. 1992;15:809–15.
36. Jacques D, Bendjelid K, Duperret S, et al. Pulse pressure variation and stroke volume variation during increased intra-abdominal pressure: an experimental study. Crit Care. 2011;15:R33.
37. Sterling SA, Puskarich MA, Jones AE. The effect of liver disease on lactate normalization in severe sepsis and septic shock: a cohort study. Clin Exp Emerg Med. 2015;2:197–202.
38. Choudhury A, Kedarisetty CK, Vashishtha C, et al. A randomized trial comparing terlipressin and noradrenaline in patients with cirrhosis and septic shock. Liver Int. 2017;37:552–61.
39. Hollenberg SM. The circulatory system in liver disease [Internet]. Crit Care Clin. 2017;32:331–42. Available from: https://doi.org/10.1016/j.ccc.2016.02.004.
40. Wu C, Cheng Y, Liu Y, et al. Predicting stroke volume and arterial pressure fluid responsiveness in liver cirrhosis patients using dynamic preload variables. A prospective study of diagnostic accuracy. Eur J Anaesthesiol. 2016;33:645–52.
41. Monnet X, Marik PE, Teboul J-L. Prediction of fluid responsiveness: an update [Internet]. Ann Intensive Care. 2016;6:111. Available from: http://annalsofintensivecare.springeropen.com/articles/10.1186/s13613-016-0216-7.

42. Kitamura H, Kobayashi C. Impairment of change in diameter of the hepatic portion of the inferior vena cava – a sonographic sign of liver fibrosis or cirrhosis. J Ultrasound Med. 2005;24:355–9.
43. Fernández J, Monteagudo J, Bargallo X, Jiménez W, Bosch J, Arroyo V, Navasa M. A randomized unblinded pilot study comparing albumin versus hydroxyethyl starch in spontaneous bacterial peritonitis. Hepatology. 2005;42:627–34.
44. Albillos A, Rossi I, Cacho G, et al. Enhanced endothelium-dependent vasodilation in patients with cirrhosis. Am J Phys. 1995;268:G459–64.
45. Mukhtar A, Dabbous H. Modulation of splanchnic circulation: role in perioperative management of liver transplant patients. World J Gastroenterol. 2016;22:1582–92.
46. Wagener G, Gubitosa G, Renz J, et al. Vasopressin decreases portal vein pressure and flow in the native liver during liver transplantation. [Internet]. Liver Transpl. 2008;14:1664–70. [cited 2014 Nov 10] Available from: http://www.ncbi.nlm.nih.gov/pubmed/18975276.
47. Moreau R, Cailmail S, Lebrec D. Effects of vasopressin on haemodynamics in portal hypertensive rats receiving clonidine. Liver. 1994;14:45–9.
48. Freeman JG, Cobden I, Lishman AH, et al. Controlled trial of terlipressin ('Glypressin') versus vasopressin in the early treatment of oesophageal varices. Lancet. 1982;2:66–8.
49. Kiszka-Kanowitz M, Henriksen JH, Hansen EF, et al. Effect of terlipressin on blood volume distribution in patients with cirrhosis [Internet]. Scand J Gastroenterol. 2004;39:486–92. [cited 2014 Nov 10] Available from: http://informahealthcare.com/doi/abs/10.1080/00365520310008728.
50. Mukhtar A, Salah M, Aboulfetouh F, et al. The use of terlipressin during living donor liver transplantation: effects on systemic and splanchnic hemodynamics and renal function. [Internet]. Crit Care Med. 2011;39:1329–34. [cited 2014 Aug 22] Available from: http://www.ncbi.nlm.nih.gov/pubmed/21336108.
51. Marik PE, Gayowski T, Starzl TE, et al. The hepatoadrenal syndrome: a common yet unrecognized clinical condition. Crit Care Med. 2005;33:1254–9.
52. Fernández J, Escorsell A, Zabalza M, et al. Adrenal insufficiency in patients with cirrhosis and septic shock: effect of treatment with hydrocortisone on survival. Hepatology. 2006;44:1288–95.
53. Arabi YM, Aljumah A, Dabbagh O, et al. Low-dose hydrocortisone in patients with cirrhosis and septic shock: a randomized controlled trial. CMAJ. 2010;182:1971–7.
54. Evans T, Carpenter A, Kinderman H, et al. Evidence of increased nitric oxide production in patients with the sepsis syndrome. Circ Shock. 1993;41:77–81.
55. Hosseinian L, Weiner M, Levin MA, et al. Methylene blue: magic bullet for vasoplegia? Anesth Analg. 2016;122:194–201.
56. Cheng SS, Berman GW, Merritt GR, et al. The response to methylene blue in patients with severe hypotension during liver transplantation. J Clin Anesth. 2012;24:324–8.
57. Fischer GW, Bengtsson Y, Scarola S, et al. Methylene blue for vasopressor-resistant vasoplegia syndrome during liver transplantation [Internet]. J Cardiothorac Vasc Anesth. 2010;24:463–6. Available from: http://linkinghub.elsevier.com/retrieve/pii/S1053077008002292.
58. Ramamoorthy S, Patel S, Bradburn E, et al. Use of methylene blue for treatment of severe sepsis in an immunosuppressed patient after liver transplantation [Internet]. Case Rep Transplant. 2013;2013:1–4. Available from: http://www.hindawi.com/journals/crit/2013/203791/.

Chapter 5
Management of Hyponatremia in End-Stage Liver Disease

Vanessa G. Henke, Michael P. Bokoch, and Linda L. Liu

Introduction

In end-stage liver disease (ESLD), hemodynamic changes associated with neurohormonal adaptations reduce the ability of the kidneys to excrete free water. The net gain of free water relative to sodium, which causes hyponatremia, is a common feature of ESLD and a strong independent predictor of mortality among patients on the wait list for liver transplantation (LT). Unfortunately, the peri-transplantation period is often associated with large fluctuations in serum sodium concentration, which increases the risk of neurologic complications. Consequently, the therapeutic goals and management strategies for hyponatremia vary greatly between the pre-transplantation, intraoperative, and post-transplantation periods. In this chapter, the definition, prognosis, pathophysiology, and treatment of hyponatremia in patients with cirrhosis are reviewed.

Definition and Prevalence

Hyponatremia is usually defined as a serum sodium concentration ($[Na^+]_{serum}$) < 135 mEq/L. With this definition, the prevalence of hyponatremia is reported as between 2 and 5% in general hospitalized patients [1] and at 7.8% in surgical patients [2]. When compared to the general population, the prevalence of hyponatremia is much higher among patients with cirrhosis. Serum sodium concentration measured ≤ 135 mEq/L in 49% of patients with cirrhosis [3]. Because the incidence is so high, investigators often use a lower number as

V. G. Henke · M. P. Bokoch · L. L. Liu (✉)
Department of Anesthesia and Perioperative Care, University of California, San Francisco, School of Medicine, San Francisco, CA, USA
e-mail: linda.liu@ucsf.edu

D. Bezinover, F. Saner (eds.), *Critical Care for Potential Liver Transplant Candidates*,
https://doi.org/10.1007/978-3-319-92934-7_5

clinically significant hyponatremia, which is defined by $[Na^+]_{serum} \leq 130$ mEq/L [1]. Even with this definition change, $[Na^+]_{serum} \leq 130$ mEq/L is reported in 22% of patients. In the subset of cirrhotic patients who were hospitalized, the incidence of $[Na^+]_{serum} \leq 135$ or ≤ 130 mEq/L was even higher at 57% and 28%, respectively [3].

Prognostic Significance

Morbidity

The severity of hyponatremia correlates with the severity of cirrhosis, and worsening hyponatremia in decompensated cirrhosis is often a marker of disease progression. An acute drop in serum sodium may reflect fluid shifts, worsening systemic vasodilation, as well as gastrointestinal or renal losses due to thiazide diuretic use or worsening renal function. One study identified significant associations between hyponatremia and refractory ascites, increased creatinine and the need for paracentesis [3]. Compared to ESLD patients with normal sodium levels, ESLD patients with hyponatremia were at significantly greater risk of major complications related to portal hypertension including increased risk for hepatic encephalopathy [odds ratio (OR) 3.4, 95% confidence interval (CI) 2.35–4.92], as well as hepatorenal syndrome (OR 3.5, 95% CI 2.04–5.82) and spontaneous bacterial peritonitis (OR 2.4, 95% CI 1.41–3.93) [3].

Hepatic encephalopathy (HE) is a serious complication related to ESLD. It has been demonstrated that a serum sodium concentration < 130 mEq/L is a strong predictor of clinically relevant episodes of HE [4]. One hypothesis is that in chronic cirrhosis, low-grade cerebral edema due to astrocyte swelling reflects both hyperammonemia and hyponatremia [5]. This hypothesis is supported by data showing more profound slowing of the electroencephalogram with worsening hyponatremia in patients with cirrhosis [6]. This mild-to-moderate hyponatremia can significantly impair neurological function but rarely causes overt cerebral edema with elevated intracranial pressure.

For patients with ESLD and ascites, especially those who are not transplant candidates, the severity of hyponatremia is also a strong predictor of impaired health-related quality of life that declines even before $[Na^+]_{serum}$ reaches the threshold value of <130 mEq/L [7]. A similar association has not been found with other measures of liver dysfunction, such as the Child-Pugh score, serum bilirubin, albumin, prothrombin time, or the Model for End-Stage Liver Disease (MELD) score [8]. The exact mechanism for this phenomenon is not known, although animal studies have demonstrated that mild cerebral edema has multiple effects on the central nervous system and may play a role here by affecting a patient's sense of well-being [9, 10].

Mortality

Multiple investigations have demonstrated that in ESLD, hyponatremia is associated with increased mortality independent of other predictive factors [11–13]. According to an evaluation of 6,769 patients awaiting LT, the hazard ratio (HR) for death increased by 1.05 with each 1 mEq/L drop in $[Na^+]_{serum}$ between 140 and 125 mEq/L [14], with the greatest prognostic significance noted among patients with the lowest MELD scores. Another study included results showing a striking 12% increase in the risk of death within 3 months of listing for LT for each 1 mEq/L decrease in serum sodium between 120 and 135 mEq/L [15]. Among patients with acute-on-chronic liver failure and hyponatremia, the relative risk of dying at 90 days was significantly higher (HR 6.85, 95% CI 3.85–12.19) than for patients who had neither of these factors [16].

Given these data, in 2016, hyponatremia was incorporated into the allocation algorithm by the Organ Procurement and Transplantation Network and the United Network for Organ Sharing. For patients with an initial MELD score greater than 11, a modified MELD-Na formula is now applied, resulting in higher scores if $[Na^+]_{serum}$ is less than 137 mEq/L and with no incremental score increases when $[Na^+]_{serum}$ drops below 125 mEq/L [17]. This modification is a key driver of organ allocation policy both in the United States and internationally [17]. Preliminary data suggest that this transition to include sodium in the MELD calculation results in more equitable allocation of organs without a negative impact on post-LT survival [18, 19].

While the effects of hyponatremia on wait-list mortality have been well studied, it remains undetermined whether hyponatremia affects post-transplant outcomes. The most recent data from a large American registry demonstrated no difference in post-transplant survival for patients with $[Na^+]_{serum} \leq 130$ [20]. In fact, when the authors divided the groups into mild hyponatremia (125–130 mEq/L), moderate hyponatremia (120–124 mEq/L), and severe hyponatremia (<120 mEq/L), none of the patients had a statistically significant difference in survival compared with their counterparts with normal $[Na^+]_{serum}$. Similar results were reported in a Chinese Liver Transplant Registry where no significant differences were found between the normal group ($[Na^+]_{serum}$ between 135 and 150 mEq/L) and two hyponatremia groups: $[Na^+]_{serum}$ between 125 and 130 mEq/L ($p = 0.113$) and $[Na^+]_{serum}$ between 130 and 135 mEq/L ($p = 0.461$) [21]. A statistically significant lower survival rate for the patients with severe hyponatremia ($[Na^+]_{serum} \leq 125$ mEq/L) compared with the patients in the normal sodium group ($p = 0.023$) was reported. In contrast, two earlier European evaluations demonstrated a higher risk-adjusted mortality at 3 months post-transplant for patients with pre-transplant $[Na^+]_{serum} < 130$ mEq/L [22, 23]. In those studies, patients with hyponatremia were also found to be at increased risk of post-transplant neurologic dysfunction, infection, and renal failure. More data are needed before a plausible explanation for the conflicting results and a definitive statement can be made.

Pathophysiology

ESLD is associated with the development of portosystemic shunts and increased synthesis of prostaglandins and nitric oxide. These factors reduce systemic vascular resistance, resulting in a drop in arterial pressure and an increase in cardiac output [24] (Fig. 5.1). The systemic and splanchnic vasodilation induces a decrease in effective circulating blood volume with subsequent activation of the sympathetic nervous and renin-angiotensin-aldosterone systems. These changes result in systemic vasoconstriction and sodium reabsorption, respectively [25]. Reabsorption of sodium in the proximal tubules reduces sodium delivery to the ascending loop of Henle, which can blunt the urinary diluting capabilities of the kidneys and impair water excretion [26].

At the level of the carotid sinus baroreceptors, the reduction of effective circulating blood volume triggers non-osmotic secretion of the antidiuretic hormone (ADH) from the posterior pituitary. Circulating ADH binds to vasopressin V2 receptors in the renal collecting duct with subsequent stimulation of water-permeable channels in the apical plasma membrane, which increases water reabsorption and leads to a dilutional hypotonic hyponatremia [27].

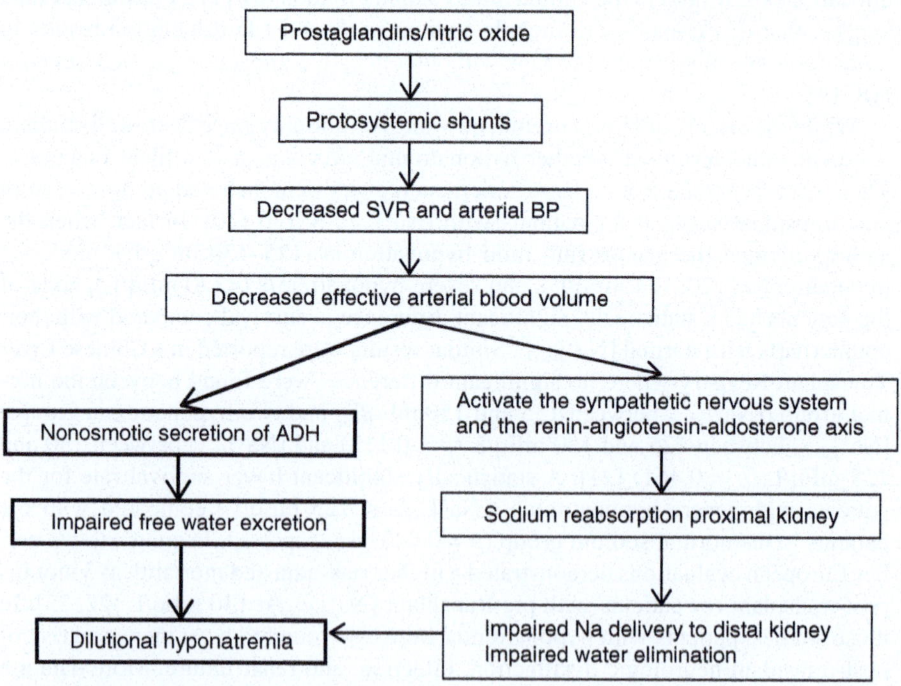

Fig. 5.1 The pathophysiology of hyponatremia in patients with end-stage liver disease

Diagnosis

The diagnostic analysis and basis for treatment of hyponatremia in ESLD are predicated based on an understanding of tonicity and the normal mechanisms governing sodium and water homeostasis. Net retention or excretion of free water is the main determinant of serum sodium concentration, because water freely traverses cell membranes. To defend against large changes in cell volume triggered by the net movement of water, serum tonicity is tightly regulated by osmoreceptors in the hypothalamus. Increased tonicity leads to decreased cell stretch, which increases the firing rate of these hypothalamic neurons, leading to increased thirst and increased release of ADH from the posterior pituitary. Normally, the circulating ADH level rapidly declines to zero when the serum tonicity drops. Under conditions of decreased effective circulating blood volume associated with cirrhosis, baroreceptor-mediated ADH secretion can continue. This inability to suppress ADH release despite low serum tonicity causes hypotonic hyponatremia.

The diagnostic workup begins by assessing the patient for non-hypotonic causes of hyponatremia (Fig. 5.2). The differentiation between hypotonic and non-hypotonic hyponatremia is important, because non-hypotonic hyponatremia does not cause cerebral edema, which has major implications for prognosis and treatment. While serum tonicity is the physiologically relevant entity, it cannot be measured directly. Serum osmolality is the measurable entity.

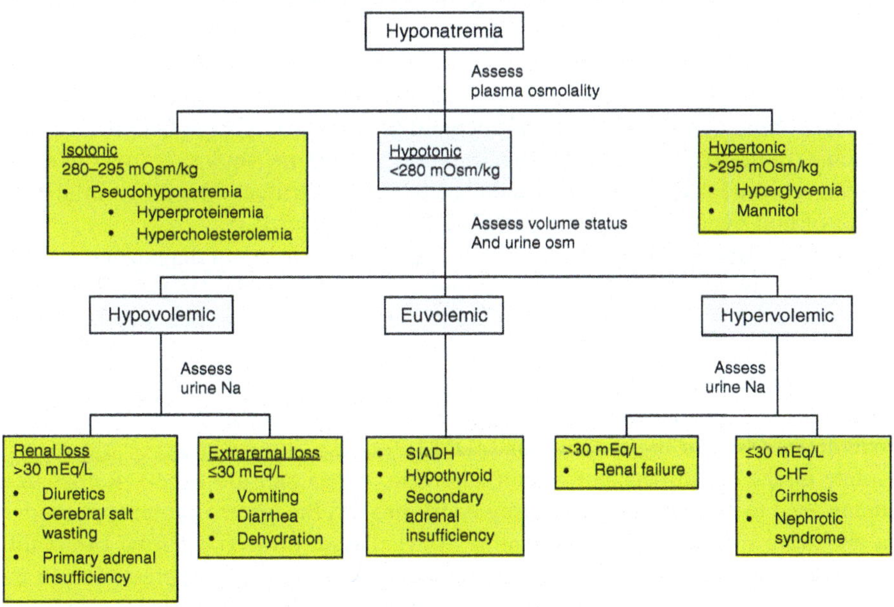

Fig. 5.2 Algorithm to diagnose hyponatremia

Table 5.1 Types of non-hypotonic hyponatremia

Tonicity	Pathophysiology	Examples
Isotonic or hypertonic	Effective osmoles	Glucose Maltose Mannitol Sorbitol Glycine Hyperosmolar radiocontrast media Histidine-tryptophan-ketoglutarate
Isotonic	Pseudohyponatremia	Monoclonal gammopathies, IVIG Severe hypertriglyceridemia Hypercholesterolemia Mixed dyslipidemia

IVIG intravenous immunoglobulin

Tonicity and osmolality often trend in similar directions, but there are situations when the two are divergent. Serum tonicity describes the osmotic gradient generated by effective solutes or osmoles that are impermeable to cell membranes and, therefore, drive water movement in and out of cells. Ineffective osmoles (such as urea and ingested alcohols and glycols) cross cell membranes, contributing to serum osmolality without affecting serum tonicity and, therefore, do not cause hyponatremia. Serum osmolality can reflect the concentrations of both effective and ineffective osmoles. To rule out non-hypotonic causes of hyponatremia, a patient history and physical examination are helpful, and serum osmolality may also be measured. Serum osmolality is not always part of the standard evaluation of hyponatremia, but it should be measured when non-hypotonic hyponatremia is suspected.

Hypertonic hyponatremia (>295 mOsm/kg) is due to hyperglycemia, mannitol, glycine, or sorbitol. Isotonic hyponatremia (280–295 mOsm/kg) is most likely to be due to pseudohyponatremia, which is a laboratory artifact. The differential diagnosis of non-hypotonic hyponatremia is listed in Table 5.1.

For the patient with hypotonic hyponatremia, the important diagnostic question is whether the serum ADH level is inappropriately elevated or whether hypotonic hyponatremia is due to excess free water intake and appropriate suppression of ADH secretion. In this rare situation, despite appropriate suppression of ADH, the capacity of the kidneys to excrete free water is insufficient to keep up with the rapid ingestion of large amounts of solute-free water. This is caused by either primary polydipsia (as seen in psychosis or MDMA "ecstasy" intoxication) or low dietary solute intake (as in beer potomania, anorexia, or tea and toast diet). Rather than being used to measure the circulating ADH directly, the urine osmolality is used as a surrogate marker for the circulating ADH. Dilute urine (i.e., urine osmolality < 100 mOsm/kg) implies that circulating ADH is completely suppressed as in the case of excess free water intake, and concentrated urine (i.e., urine osmolality > 100 mOsm/kg) implies that ADH secretion is present, as in the case of cirrhosis.

Further diagnosis of hypotonic hyponatremia separates patients by volume status based on the history and a physical examination to determine the patient's extracellular fluid (ECF) volume. Recent or ongoing use of diuretics and significant renal dysfunction both limit the predictive value of urine chemistries, highlighting the importance of the exam and clinical assessment in refining the differential diagnosis.

The differential for hypotonic hyponatremia and elevated ECF volume on exam includes cirrhosis, congestive heart failure, or nephrotic syndrome. In cases with normal ECF volume, the syndrome of inappropriate ADH secretion (SIADH), secondary adrenal insufficiency, or myxedema coma should be considered. In the case of contracted ECF volume or hypovolemia, possible causes include vomiting, diarrhea, or third-spacing as the etiology of the hyponatremia when $[Na^+]_{urine} < 30$ mEq/L. If $[Na^+]_{urine} > 30$ mEq/L and ECF is low, the use of diuretic, cerebral salt-wasting, or primary adrenal insufficiency should be taken into consideration as possible etiologies.

It is important to remember that patients can present with multiple causes of hyponatremia. Some of the diagnoses may require conflicting therapies, which may have important implications. For instance, a cirrhotic patient may develop worsening hyponatremia because of hypovolemia from vomiting or diarrhea, which requires intravenous fluid replacement. A careful history and physical exam should be useful in distinguishing between hypovolemic and hypervolemic hyponatremia, and a fluid restriction treatment plan should not be instituted as a standard response.

Treatment of Hyponatremia: General Principles

The clinical significance of hyponatremia depends on the severity and the length of time during which the condition has developed. Acute hyponatremia results in cerebral edema that can progress from nausea, confusion, and headache to severe symptoms such as somnolence, seizures, and signs of brainstem herniation with subsequent coma and cardiorespiratory arrest. Adaptive processes within the neurons (reduced generation of intracellular osmoles like myoinositol, taurine, and sodium) help reduce the osmotic gradient with plasma [28]. Because this adaptive process generally takes about 48 h, hyponatremia is considered to be chronic after that time point. Chronic hyponatremia, therefore, generally leads to milder symptoms and is not as urgent a situation [29]. Extreme hyponatremia ($[Na^+]_{serum} < 110$ mEq/L), even if chronic, is usually symptomatic. However, unless such levels are reached, chronic hyponatremia rarely causes seizures or the other life-threatening complications listed above [30]. Once adaptation is completed, brain cells can again sustain damage if the serum sodium concentration now increases too rapidly. Breakdown of the myelin sheath insulating individual neurons with rapid sodium correction can result in osmotic demyelination syndrome (ODS).

Acute symptomatic hyponatremia is considered a medical emergency (Table 5.2). Sodium correction with a bolus or infusion of hypertonic saline (usually 3% NaCl) should be based on the severity of symptoms [31] and strive to correct severe symptoms of cerebral herniation, seizures, or coma. Rapid sodium correction leading to osmotic demyelination syndrome is not as concerning because the osmotic adaptive processes are not completely developed with acute hyponatremia. Patients should be closely monitored in a critical care setting with frequent sodium checks to avoid overcorrection.

Table 5.2 General treatment recommendations for hyponatremia

Classification of hyponatremia	Treatment recommendations	Comments
Acute or symptomatic	Severe symptoms: bolus 3% NaCl Moderate symptoms: infuse 3% NaCl (0.5–2 ml/kg/h)	48 h is usually the cutoff to differentiate between acute and chronic hyponatremia Severe symptoms: vomiting, seizures, respiratory arrest, coma Moderate symptoms: headache, nausea, confusion
Chronic		
Hypovolemic: dehydration	Isotonic saline	
Euvolemic – SIADH	Fluid restriction (first line) Demeclocycline, urea, Vaptans (second line)	
Hypervolemic: cirrhosis, CHF, nephrotic syndrome	Fluid restriction Vaptans	In cirrhosis, restrict vaptans to patients where benefit outweighs risk of worsening liver function

SIADH syndrome of inappropriate antidiuretic hormone, *CHF* congestive heart failure

General recommendations for the treatment of chronic hyponatremia are to limit the rate of correction. The management of chronic hyponatremia depends on the suspected etiology. Hypovolemic hyponatremia should be treated by resuscitation with isotonic saline [32]. Euvolemic and hypervolemic hyponatremia are best treated with fluid restriction or correction of the underlying endocrine disorder.

Total sodium correction should not exceed 6–8 mEq/L/day in either acute or chronic hyponatremia patients because of the concern for ODS. Although the risk for developing ODS is low, especially in patients with acute hyponatremia, there is no additional benefit to correcting sodium faster than the recommended limits as long as the symptoms of cerebral edema resolve.

Osmotic Demyelination Syndrome

Osmotic demyelination syndrome (ODS) was initially referred to as central pontine myelinolysis. The name change occurred due to the discovery that the demyelination does not involve just the central pons but can involve extrapontine structures as well [33]. Because it may take up to a week to regenerate normal intracellular levels of osmotically active organic solutes, rapid sodium correction can lead to the programmed death of myelin-producing oligodendrocytes [34]. ODS, while rare, may present with devastating neurologic consequences such as quadriparesis, locked-in syndrome, and death 2–6 days after overcorrection of hyponatremia.

ODS is typically associated with overcorrection of severe hyponatremia ($[Na^+]_{serum}$ < 120 mEq/L) that has been present for 2–3 days, but no absolutely safe cutoffs for sodium correction are known. Other risk factors include alcoholism, liver disease, malnutrition, and hypokalemia [35]. ODS has been reported in less severe hyponatremia ($[Na^+]_{serum} > 120$ mEq/L), especially in patients whose sodium levels increased drastically after liver transplantation (LT), but this is even more rare [36]. The overall incidence of ODS after LT is reported as 0.5–1% at some centers, with preoperative hyponatremia and perioperative sodium fluctuations identified as risk factors [36, 37]. It is impossible to follow neurologic symptoms intraoperatively during LT to determine when sodium correction is excessive, but the guideline is to limit sodium changes to < 8 mEq/L in 24 h.

While this complication can be neurologically devastating, some patients do recover from ODS despite prolonged periods with neurologic deficits. ODS is potentially reversible even in quadriplegic, ventilator-dependent patients. In a retrospective analysis of 36 patients with severe ODS, there was a lower than expected 1-year mortality of 31%, and 56% of the survivors demonstrated a marked recovery (Rankin score ≤ 1) [38].

Treatment of Hyponatremia: Liver Transplant Patients

The goals for sodium management are based on the phase of perioperative care. While there are no data showing that increasing the serum sodium concentration in patients with cirrhosis improves outpatient morbidity or mortality, every effort should be made during the intraoperative period to maintain serum sodium levels close to the patient's baseline level. LT is a critical time for fluid and electrolyte shifts, and transplant anesthesiologists must often undertake efforts to limit a dangerous and rapid rise in serum sodium that may lead to ODS. Thus, intraoperative efforts often focus on limiting the rise or even driving down the sodium concentration, in apparent contradiction to preoperative goals.

Pre-transplant Period

While it is clear that the severity of chronic hyponatremia correlates with complications and impaired survival in patients with decompensated cirrhosis, treatment of asymptomatic, stable chronic hyponatremia in this population is not recommended, because there is no proven benefit. The usual rate at which hyponatremia develops in cirrhosis is slow, allowing ample time for brain tissue to equilibrate to the hypotonic state. It is rare for patients to experience moderate-to-severe neurologic symptoms (i.e., hepatic encephalopathy Grade 3 or higher [39], new-onset encephalopathy, seizures, focal deficit, stupor, or coma) [40] due to just hyponatremia unless the serum sodium concentration falls acutely or below an absolute value of 120 mEq/L. As such, treatment of hyponatremia is not indicated if these conditions are absent – unless transplant is likely to be imminent (within hours to days) (Fig. 5.3). If this is the case, treatment of moderate hyponatremia ($[Na^+]_{serum} < 130$ mEq/L) may be indicated to prepare the patient for the sodium swings expected in the perioperative period.

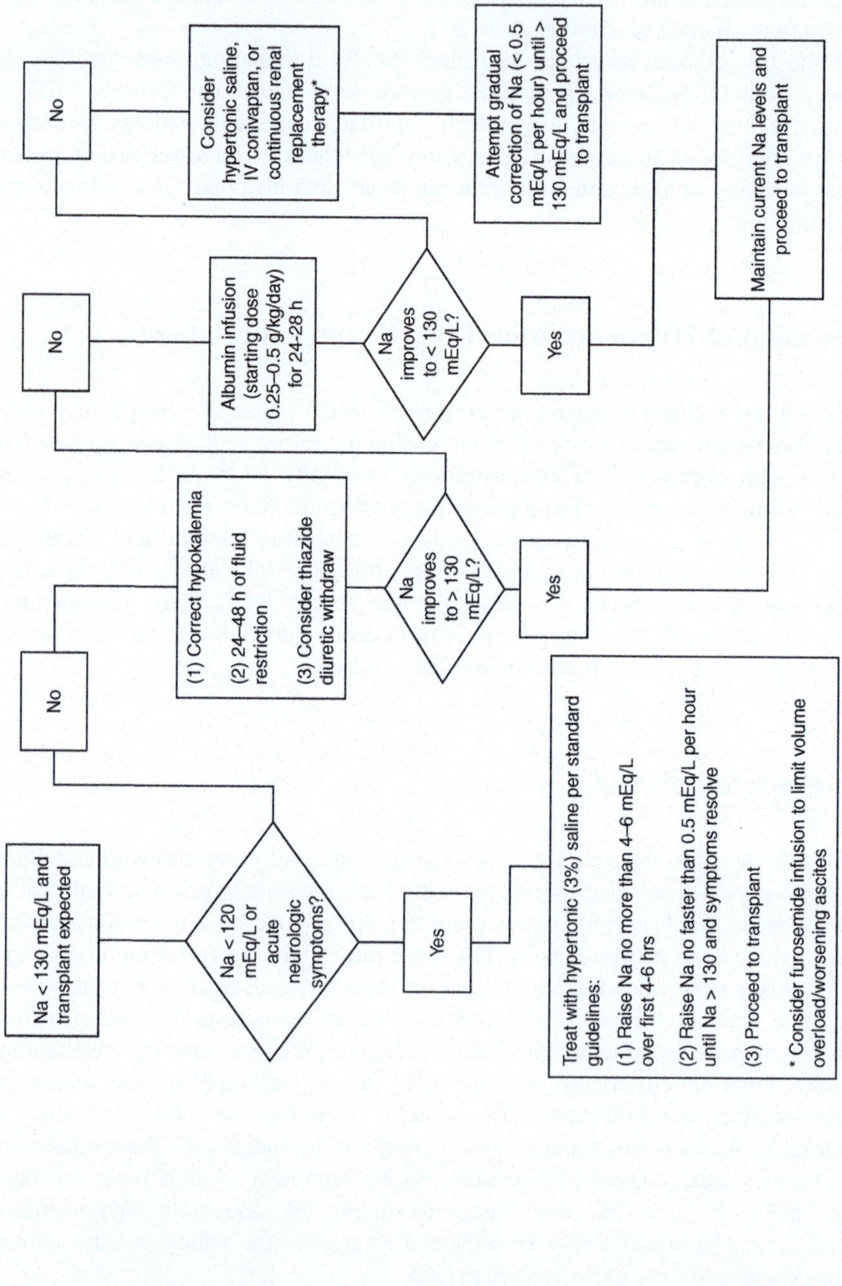

Fig. 5.3 Pre-transplant management of sodium in hospitalized hyponatremic patients around the time of liver transplantation

Diuresis and Fluid Restriction

For patients with compensated cirrhosis, the treatments for mild-to-moderate hyponatremia in the chronic setting are few and of little utility. In most instances, the etiology, as discussed earlier, is dilutional. Diuretic withdrawal can be considered if hyponatremia is severe, but caution is recommended for patients on chronic stable therapy. Thiazides are the most likely class of diuretics to cause hyponatremia [41], because they cause sodium secretion in excess of free water. Loop diuretics, on the other hand, increase free water clearance, which makes them an important component of ascites therapy in cirrhosis, and are potentially useful for the management of hyponatremia in some settings [42]. Fluid restriction is another option, as limiting the intake of free water to less than 1–1.5 L/day will ameliorate the effects of elevated circulating ADH. Fluid restriction is uncomfortable for patients, and patient compliance is poor in the outpatient setting [43].

Salt Tablets and Potassium Replacement

Hyponatremia in cirrhosis reflects an inappropriate excess of total body water, not a lack of sodium. Adding a sodium load may worsen the edematous state. Sodium chloride tablets are generally contraindicated, as the sodium load will worsen ascites and edema. It is generally recommended that patients with cirrhosis follow a diet of moderate sodium restriction (2–3 g per day) [44, 45]. A simple measure that mitigates hyponatremia is to ensure that potassium is adequately repleted. Hypokalemia is common in cirrhosis, especially among patients on diuretics. Serum potassium and sodium levels are closely linked, and potassium administration leads to a series of transcellular shifts of fluid and electrolytes that result in an increase in serum sodium [42, 43, 46].

Vaptans

The most promising drug introduced in recent years is "vaptans" or V2 vasopressin receptor antagonists. These agents block V2 receptors in the renal collecting ducts and increase free water clearance by producing a selective water diuresis. They have been shown to raise serum sodium in patients with hypervolemic hyponatremia [47] but not to reduce ascites or major complications of cirrhosis [48]. Predictable side effects include increased thirst and polyuria, which may increase discomfort for outpatients [49]. In a recent meta-analysis, the use of vaptans led to improved sodium levels without mortality benefit (RR = 1.06, 95% CI: 0.9–1.26) [50]. A large trial of V2 antagonists in patients with polycystic kidney disease demonstrated a higher rate of elevated transaminases in patients receiving tolvaptan [49]. In response to this result, the US Food and Drug Administration issued a 2013 statement warning against the use of tolvaptan in patients with liver disease. Based on the lack of clear benefit, drug costs, and lingering questions about risk, the routine use of vaptans in patients with cirrhosis is not recommended [51]. One proposed exception may be in the scenario where a hyponatremic patient with ESLD is awaiting imminent liver transplantation. The use of vaptans, particularly intravenous conivaptan [52], may pose little risk of additional hepatic injury yet provide the benefit of correcting the hyponatremia prior to surgery to decrease the risk of ODS [53]. As such, there are currently no good pharmacologic options to treat mild or moderate asymptomatic hyponatremia in cirrhosis, and more studies are necessary before a recommendation can be made based on clinical evidence.

Other Medications

A variety of other drug classes have been used to treat hyponatremia in cirrhosis, with limited efficacy. Demeclocycline, a tetracycline analog, blocks the effect of ADH on the renal collecting ducts and raises the serum sodium. However, it is not recommended due to an unacceptably high incidence of nephrotoxicity [54]. Niravoline, a kappa-opioid agonist, increases free water clearance but may cause neurologic side effects such as confusion and personality disorders [55].

Peri-transplant Period

The time around the LT operation is a highly dynamic period for sodium homeostasis in patients with ESLD. Patients often present with decompensated cirrhosis, acute elevations in MELD-Na, and worsening hyponatremia in the days or weeks just prior to transplant. Successful transplantation results in rapid resolution of portal hypertension and hemodynamic and renal function [56]. Typically, these changes are accompanied by rapid postoperative normalization of the serum sodium.

Intraoperatively during LT, the magnitude of blood loss and volume replacement puts the patient at risk for overly rapid correction of sodium [43]. Consistent risk factors for developing ODS after LT include (1) large sodium increases during surgery (> 12–14 mEq/L) [37, 57, 58] or in the perioperative period (> 20 mEq/L per 48 h) [59] and (2) a large volume of isotonic crystalloid or blood product infusions during transplant [57, 58]. Some series suggest that moderate to severe preoperative hyponatremia ($([Na^+]_{serum} < 125$ mEq/L) is itself a risk factor for ODS and post-transplant neurologic complications [40, 57, 58]. Hyperosmolarity, independent of sodium derangements, is also likely to pose a risk of ODS, which argues for adequate control of postoperative hyperglycemia [37, 59].

Perioperative physicians should strive to identify all patients at risk for overly rapid correction of sodium during LT. Almost all patients experience some rise in sodium during transplant, but those starting with moderate or severe hyponatremia have larger increases (a mean rise of 11 ± 3.6 mEq/L for patients starting with $[Na^+]_{serum} < 130$ mEq/L, versus 5.3 ± 4.5 mEq/L for those with $[Na^+]_{serum} > 130$ mEq/L) [60]. Larger intraoperative sodium increases are also associated with increased transfusion of packed red blood cells and fresh frozen plasma and administration of sodium bicarbonate. Given the low incidence of ODS, recent case series have not demonstrated increased mortality among patients who have experienced a rise in sodium >10 mEq/L during LT, but these patients do tend to have prolonged intubation, prolonged intubation, prolonged intensive care unit and hospital stays, and post-transplant altered mental status [56, 60].

Possible Treatment Options

Given the risks of entering the operating room for LT with severe hyponatremia ($[Na^+]_{serum} < 120$ mEq/L), consideration should be given to gradually correcting hyponatremia (no greater than 0.5 mEq/L per hour) to $[Na^+]_{serum} > 130$ mEq/L if possible in the days prior to transplant (Fig. 5.3). If conservative measures fail (no improvement in sodium after 24–48 h of fluid restriction), albumin infusion over several days may raise the sodium level. It is likely that albumin raises sodium by expanding intravascular volume, increasing free water clearance, and decreasing circulating ADH [61].

Hypertonic saline (usually 3% NaCl) infusion is effective in raising serum sodium but should be used with caution [24]. The associated sodium load tends to worsen ascites and edema and is associated with the risk of overly rapid correction or circulatory overload [62]. Consequently, hypertonic saline should be considered only if liver transplantation is thought to be imminent within days to hours. The goal rate of hypertonic saline infusion can be calculated, but these equations only provide an estimate [62]. Weight-based estimates of total body water may not be accurate in patients with cirrhosis, and frequent sodium checks are mandatory while therapy is in progress. Concurrent diuresis with furosemide may be useful to prevent volume overload and enhance free water clearance [62].

Continuous renal replacement therapy with isotonic saline infusion can be considered for gradual correction of severe hyponatremia in oliguric or severely volume-overloaded patients [63, 64].

Despite all the listed options, the data are unclear as to whether the perioperative correction of serum sodium improves overall outcomes. Hackworth et al., in a small retrospective study, were unable to find a survival benefit at 6 months in patients with a history of $[Na^+]_{serum} < 130$ mEq/L who had resolved hyponatremia versus those who had remained hyponatremic at the time of transplant [65]. It is possible that there may be a benefit to improving severe hyponatremia ($[Na^+]_{serum} < 120$ mEq/L) so that intraoperative sodium shifts would be less dramatic, but the treatment endpoint (i.e., the target sodium goal) is unknown.

Intraoperative Period

Intraoperative sodium management requires an understanding of the sodium content of the crystalloids, colloids, and blood products that are typically given during surgery [66]. All isotonic crystalloids and albumin have sodium content >130 mEq/L, whereas lactated Ringers have the lowest and normal (0.9%) saline the highest sodium content (Table 5.3). Fresh frozen plasma, which is often transfused in high volumes during LT, has markedly higher sodium content (170 ± 1.4 mEq/L) than do packed red blood cells (119 ± 4 mEq/L). It has been demonstrated that the administration rate of crystalloid and blood products strongly correlated with the rate of intraoperative sodium rise over the course of LT [57]. Sodium bicarbonate, routinely used at some centers for the management of metabolic acidosis, constitutes a significant sodium load (50 mEq per 50 mL ampule of 8.4% sodium bicarbonate).

For patients at risk of rapid sodium overcorrection, consideration should be given to limit the perioperative sodium load. It has been reported in a small patient series that the use of hypotonic crystalloid infusion (0.45% saline), limited use of bicarbonate (< 1 mEq/kg), and administration of furosemide to promote natriuresis during LT can limit the intraoperative sodium rise [67]. Dextrose 5% can be used as an entirely sodium-free infusion during the dissection and anhepatic phase but should be switched to half-normal (0.45%) saline during the neohepatic phase due to the marked hyperglycemia that can accompany good allograft function [68]. It is not uncommon for some centers to administer 1–3 L of hypotonic crystalloid to balance the sodium load in at-risk patients. The use of sodium bicarbonate during LT should be limited, and compensation for metabolic acidosis can be at least partially achieved by establishing a respiratory alkalosis using ventilator changes. Diuretics can be useful in promoting natriuresis in patients with preserved renal function [42]. To limit the intraoperative sodium load for coagulopathic patients at high risk of sodium overcorrection, consideration should be given to the use of prothrombin complex concentrates or fibrinogen concentrates as substitutes for FFP and cryoprecipitate. Although there is no clinical evidence evaluating this practice, the substitution does make physiologic sense given the decrease in sodium load.

Table 5.3 Sodium concentration in common intravenous fluids used intraoperatively

Solution	Na^+ (mEq/L)	K^+ (mEq/L)	Cl^- (mEq/L)	Other components
D5W	0	0	0	Dextrose (50 g/L)
LR	130	4	109	Lactate, calcium
Plasmalyte	140	5	98	Magnesium, acetate, gluconate
0.9% NS	154	0	154	
Albumin 5% [79]	130–160	<1	109–136	Albumin (50 g/L)
PRBC [66]	119 ± 4	45 ± 6	100 ± 3	
FFP [66]	170 ± 1.4	3.3 ± 0.2	73 ± 2	
Platelets [66]	172 ± 1.8	1.7 ± 0.1	91 ± 1	
8.4% bicarbonate	1000			

No matter which strategy is implemented, frequent sodium checks should be performed intraoperatively to guide adjustments in fluid therapy, particularly if sodium is rising faster than 1 mEq/L per hour. If overcorrection occurs, measures should be taken to reduce the sodium concentration toward preoperative values. Desmopressin, also known as DDAVP, is a V2 receptor agonist that acts on the renal collecting ducts and drives free water absorption. Desmopressin (usual dose 0.03 mcg/kg IV) with hypotonic fluids has been proposed as a treatment option to re-lower the serum sodium in an attempt to prevent ODS [69]. However, a systematic review of this strategy found only observational studies with a total of 80 patients, none of whom had liver failure. Although desmopressin has not been studied in liver transplantation, it could be considered a rescue option when sodium overcorrection occurs [70].

Postoperative Period

If the patient is found to have worrisome neurologic symptoms in the immediate post-transplant period (such as seizures, focal deficits, stupor, or coma), it may be associated with the beginning of cerebral herniation. Therefore, the intensivist should consider reducing the serum sodium concentration. Unfortunately, the clinical diagnosis of ODS is challenging in the post-transplant period. These patients often manifest postoperative encephalopathy not necessarily related to ODS and are also prone to vascular and infectious complications of the central nervous system that may confound the diagnosis [71]. A high index of suspicion and early magnetic resonance imaging to detect subclinical ODS are advised in post-LT patients who have experienced large sodium fluctuations.

Studies have reported success with lowering sodium using desmopressin and dextrose 5% following overly rapid correction of hyponatremia [72, 73], but evidence of improved neurologic outcomes with this technique has been reported only in rat models and case reports [74, 75]. Finally, plasmapheresis and intravenous immunoglobulins have been described as a rescue therapy for ODS in a patient 2 weeks after LT [76]. Currently, the optimal treatment for patients who have developed neurologic symptoms after rapid sodium correction is unclear, and in the absence of other effective therapies, lowering sodium back closer to baseline seems to have physiologic plausibility.

Acute Liver Failure Patients

In contrast to chronic liver failure, acute liver failure (ALF) induces rapid-onset hyperammonemia, leading to astrocyte swelling, cytotoxic brain edema, and intracranial hypertension because of insufficient time for adaptations to occur at the cellular level [77]. Hyponatremia in the setting of ALF and hyperammonemia is particular dangerous, as it exacerbates the osmotic gradient driving water into the brain and worsens cerebral edema with the development of intracranial hypertension. Current guidelines recommend aggressive correction of hyponatremia in ALF patients using hypertonic saline with or without renal replacement therapy, with a goal of maintaining relative hypernatremia in the range of 140–145 mEq/L [78]. ALF patients managed with this strategy were shown in a small randomized trial (30 patients) to have improved intracranial pressure and lower vasopressor requirements [64]. Note that the sodium goal for ALF is significantly higher than the pre-transplant goal for patients with chronic liver disease ($[Na^+]_{serum}$ > 130 mEq/L) because of the difference in pathophysiology.

Conclusion

Hyponatremia is common among patients with end-stage liver disease and is associated with increased mortality. Unfortunately, the treatments for mild-to-moderate hyponatremia in the chronic setting (diuretics, fluid restriction, and vaptans) are not ideal given that the underlying pathophysiology continues to persist (non-osmotic secretion of ADH). Intraoperatively, the goals shift to maintaining sodium levels near baseline levels and refraining from correcting sodium rapidly due to the serious risks. These competing targets make hyponatremia a challenging problem for the perioperative physician. Appropriate treatment plans depend on understanding the pathophysiology, the phase of care, and the risks and benefits of sodium correction.

Key Points

1. Hyponatremia is common among patients with end-stage liver disease and is associated with increased mortality.
2. The outpatient treatments for mild-to-moderate hyponatremia (diuretics, fluid restriction, and vaptans) are not ideal given that the underlying pathophysiology of non-osmotic ADH secretion is not fixed.
3. Intraoperative goals are to maintain sodium levels near baseline levels and to refrain from correcting sodium rapidly due to concern about osmotic demyelinating syndrome.
4. Postoperatively, the optimal treatment for patients who have developed neurologic symptoms after rapid sodium correction is unclear, and in the absence of other effective therapies, lowering sodium back closer to baseline may be the best option.

References

1. Upadhyay A, Jaber BL, Madias NE. Incidence and prevalence of hyponatremia. Am J Med. 2006;119:S30–5. https://doi.org/10.1016/j.amjmed.2006.05.005.
2. Leung AA, McAlister FA, Rogers SO Jr, Pazo V, Wright A, Bates DW. Preoperative hyponatremia and perioperative complications. Arch Intern Med. 2012;172:1474–81. https://doi.org/10.1001/archinternmed.2012.3992.
3. Angeli P, Wong F, Watson H, Gines P, Investigators C. Hyponatremia in cirrhosis: results of a patient population survey. Hepatology. 2006;44:1535–42. https://doi.org/10.1002/hep.21412.
4. Guevara M, Baccaro ME, Torre A, Gomez-Anson B, Rios J, Torres F, et al. Hyponatremia is a risk factor of hepatic encephalopathy in patients with cirrhosis: a prospective study with time-dependent analysis. Am J Gastroenterol. 2009;104:1382–9. https://doi.org/10.1038/ajg.2009.293.
5. Gines P, Guevara M. Hyponatremia in cirrhosis: pathogenesis, clinical significance, and management. Hepatology. 2008;48:1002–10. https://doi.org/10.1002/hep.22418.
6. Amodio P, Del Piccolo F, Petteno E, Mapelli D, Angeli P, Iemmolo R, et al. Prevalence and prognostic value of quantified electroencephalogram (EEG) alterations in cirrhotic patients. J Hepatol. 2001;35:37–45.
7. Sola E, Watson H, Graupera I, Turon F, Barreto R, Rodriguez E, et al. Factors related to quality of life in patients with cirrhosis and ascites: relevance of serum sodium concentration and leg edema. J Hepatol. 2012;57:1199–206. https://doi.org/10.1016/j.jhep.2012.07.020.
8. Saab S, Ibrahim AB, Shpaner A, Younossi ZM, Lee C, Durazo F, et al. MELD fails to measure quality of life in liver transplant candidates. Liver Transpl. 2005;11:218–23. https://doi.org/10.1002/lt.20345.
9. Sterns RH, Silver SM. Brain volume regulation in response to hypo-osmolality and its correction. Am J Med. 2006;119:S12–6. https://doi.org/10.1016/j.amjmed.2006.05.003.
10. Cordoba J, Gottstein J, Blei AT. Chronic hyponatremia exacerbates ammonia-induced brain edema in rats after portacaval anastomosis. J Hepatol. 1998;29:589–94.
11. Heuman DM, Abou-Assi SG, Habib A, Williams LM, Stravitz RT, Sanyal AJ, et al. Persistent ascites and low serum sodium identify patients with cirrhosis and low MELD scores who are at high risk for early death. Hepatology. 2004;40:802–10. https://doi.org/10.1002/hep.20405.
12. Biggins SW, Rodriguez HJ, Bacchetti P, Bass NM, Roberts JP, Terrault NA. Serum sodium predicts mortality in patients listed for liver transplantation. Hepatology. 2005;41:32–9. https://doi.org/10.1002/hep.20517.
13. Ruf AE, Kremers WK, Chavez LL, Descalzi VI, Podesta LG, Villamil FG. Addition of serum sodium into the MELD score predicts waiting list mortality better than MELD alone. Liver Transpl. 2005;11:336–43. https://doi.org/10.1002/lt.20329.
14. Kim WR, Biggins SW, Kremers WK, Wiesner RH, Kamath PS, Benson JT, et al. Hyponatremia and mortality among patients on the liver-transplant waiting list. N Engl J Med. 2008;359:1018–26. https://doi.org/10.1056/NEJMoa0801209.
15. Londono MC, Cardenas A, Guevara M, Quinto L, de Las Heras D, Navasa M, et al. MELD score and serum sodium in the prediction of survival of patients with cirrhosis awaiting liver transplantation. Gut. 2007;56:1283–90. https://doi.org/10.1136/gut.2006.102764.
16. Cardenas A, Sola E, Rodriguez E, Barreto R, Graupera I, Pavesi M, et al. Hyponatremia influences the outcome of patients with acute-on-chronic liver failure: an analysis of the CANONIC study. Crit Care. 2014;18:700. https://doi.org/10.1186/s13054-014-0700-0.
17. Machicao VI. Model for end-stage liver disease-sodium score: the evolution in the prioritization of liver transplantation. Clin Liver Dis. 2017;21:275–87. https://doi.org/10.1016/j.cld.2016.12.014.
18. Fisher RA, Heuman DM, Harper AM, Behnke MK, Smith AD, Russo MW, et al. Region 11 MELD Na exception prospective study. Ann Hepatol. 2012;11:62–7.

19. Sharma P, Schaubel DE, Goodrich NP, Merion RM. Serum sodium and survival benefit of liver transplantation. Liver Transpl. 2015;21:308–13. https://doi.org/10.1002/lt.24063.
20. Leise MD, Yun BC, Larson JJ, Benson JT, Yang JD, Therneau TM, et al. Effect of the pretransplant serum sodium concentration on outcomes following liver transplantation. Liver Transpl. 2014;20:687–97. https://doi.org/10.1002/lt.23860.
21. Wang P, Huang G, Tam N, Wu C, Fu S, Hughes BP, et al. Influence of preoperative sodium concentration on outcome of patients with hepatitis B virus cirrhosis after liver transplantation. Eur J Gastroenterol Hepatol. 2016;28:1210–5. https://doi.org/10.1097/MEG.0000000000000690.
22. Londono MC, Guevara M, Rimola A, Navasa M, Taura P, Mas A, et al. Hyponatremia impairs early posttransplantation outcome in patients with cirrhosis undergoing liver transplantation. Gastroenterology. 2006;130:1135–43. https://doi.org/10.1053/j.gastro.2006.02.017.
23. Dawwas MF, Lewsey JD, Neuberger JM, Gimson AE. The impact of serum sodium concentration on mortality after liver transplantation: a cohort multicenter study. Liver Transpl. 2007;13:1115–24. https://doi.org/10.1002/lt.21154.
24. Urso C, Brucculeri S, Caimi G. Employment of vasopressin receptor antagonists in management of hyponatraemia and volume overload in some clinical conditions. J Clin Pharm Ther. 2015;40:376–85. https://doi.org/10.1111/jcpt.12279.
25. Asbert M, Gines A, Gines P, Jimenez W, Claria J, Salo J, et al. Circulating levels of endothelin in cirrhosis. Gastroenterology. 1993;104:1485–91.
26. Bernardi M, Ricci CS, Santi L. Hyponatremia in patients with cirrhosis of the liver. J Clin Med. 2014;4:85–101. https://doi.org/10.3390/jcm4010085.
27. Spasovski G, Vanholder R, Allolio B, Annane D, Ball S, Bichet D, et al. Clinical practice guideline on diagnosis and treatment of hyponatraemia. Eur J Endocrinol. 2014;170:G1–47. https://doi.org/10.1530/EJE-13-1020.
28. Sterns RH, Hix JK, Silver SM. Management of hyponatremia in the ICU. Chest. 2013;144:672–9. https://doi.org/10.1378/chest.12-2600.
29. Sterns RH, Nigwekar SU, Hix JK. The treatment of hyponatremia. Semin Nephrol. 2009;29:282–99. https://doi.org/10.1016/j.semnephrol.2009.03.002.
30. Sterns RH, Hix JK, Silver S. Treating profound hyponatremia: a strategy for controlled correction. Am J Kidney Dis. 2010;56:774–9. https://doi.org/10.1053/j.ajkd.2010.04.020.
31. Verbalis JG, Goldsmith SR, Greenberg A, Schrier RW, Sterns RH. Hyponatremia treatment guidelines 2007: expert panel recommendations. Am J Med. 2007;120:S1–21. https://doi.org/10.1016/j.amjmed.2007.09.001.
32. Hoorn EJ, Zietse R. Diagnosis and treatment of hyponatremia: compilation of the guidelines. J Am Soc Nephrol. 2017;28:1340–9. https://doi.org/10.1681/ASN.2016101139.
33. Norenberg MD. Central pontine myelinolysis: historical and mechanistic considerations. Metab Brain Dis. 2010;25:97–106. https://doi.org/10.1007/s11011-010-9175-0.
34. Gankam Kengne F, Nicaise C, Soupart A, Boom A, Schiettecatte J, Pochet R, et al. Astrocytes are an early target in osmotic demyelination syndrome. J Am Soc Nephrol. 2011;22:1834–45. https://doi.org/10.1681/ASN.2010111127.
35. Verbalis JG, Goldsmith SR, Greenberg A, Korzelius C, Schrier RW, Sterns RH, et al. Diagnosis, evaluation, and treatment of hyponatremia: expert panel recommendations. Am J Med. 2013;126:S1–42. https://doi.org/10.1016/j.amjmed.2013.07.006.
36. Yun BC, Kim WR, Benson JT, Biggins SW, Therneau TM, Kremers WK, et al. Impact of pretransplant hyponatremia on outcome following liver transplantation. Hepatology. 2009;49:1610–5. https://doi.org/10.1002/hep.22846.
37. Crivellin C, Cagnin A, Manara R, Boccagni P, Cillo U, Feltracco P, et al. Risk factors for central pontine and extrapontine myelinolysis after liver transplantation: a single-center study. Transplantation. 2015;99:1257–64. https://doi.org/10.1097/TP.0000000000000496.
38. Louis G, Megarbane B, Lavoue S, Lassalle V, Argaud L, Poussel JF, et al. Long-term outcome of patients hospitalized in intensive care units with central or extrapontine myelinolysis. Crit Care Med. 2012;40:970–2. https://doi.org/10.1097/CCM.0b013e318236f152.
39. Ferenci P, Lockwood A, Mullen K, Tarter R, Weissenborn K, Blei AT. Hepatic encephalopathy--definition, nomenclature, diagnosis, and quantification: final report of the working party

at the 11th World Congresses of Gastroenterology, Vienna, 1998. Hepatology. 2002;35:716–21. https://doi.org/10.1053/jhep.2002.31250.

40. Lee J, Kim DK, Lee JW, Oh KH, Oh YK, Na KY, et al. Rapid correction rate of hyponatremia as an independent risk factor for neurological complication following liver transplantation. Tohoku J Exp Med. 2013;229:97–105.
41. Hix JK, Silver S, Sterns RH. Diuretic-associated hyponatremia. Semin Nephrol. 2011;31:553–66. https://doi.org/10.1016/j.semnephrol.2011.09.010.
42. Rose BD, Post TW. Clinical physiology of acid-base and electrolyte disorders. 5th ed. Medical Publishing Division: McGraw-Hill; 2001.
43. John S, Thuluvath PJ. Hyponatremia in cirrhosis: pathophysiology and management. World J Gastroenterol. 2015;21:3197–205. https://doi.org/10.3748/wjg.v21.i11.3197.
44. European Association for the Study of the L. EASL clinical practice guidelines on the management of ascites, spontaneous bacterial peritonitis, and hepatorenal syndrome in cirrhosis. J Hepatol. 2010;53:397–417. https://doi.org/10.1016/j.jhep.2010.05.004.
45. Runyon BA. Introduction to the revised American Association for the Study of Liver Diseases Practice Guideline management of adult patients with ascites due to cirrhosis 2012. Hepatology. 2013;57:1651–3. https://doi.org/10.1002/hep.26359.
46. Rose BD. New approach to disturbances in the plasma sodium concentration. Am J Med. 1986;81:1033–40.
47. Schrier RW, Gross P, Gheorghiade M, Berl T, Verbalis JG, Czerwiec FS, et al. Tolvaptan, a selective oral vasopressin V2-receptor antagonist, for hyponatremia. N Engl J Med. 2006;355:2099–112. https://doi.org/10.1056/NEJMoa065181.
48. Wong F, Watson H, Gerbes A, Vilstrup H, Badalamenti S, Bernardi M, et al. Satavaptan for the management of ascites in cirrhosis: efficacy and safety across the spectrum of ascites severity. Gut. 2012;61:108–16. https://doi.org/10.1136/gutjnl-2011-300157.
49. Torres VE, Chapman AB, Devuyst O, Gansevoort RT, Grantham JJ, Higashihara E, et al. Tolvaptan in patients with autosomal dominant polycystic kidney disease. N Engl J Med. 2012;367:2407–18. https://doi.org/10.1056/NEJMoa1205511.
50. Dahl E, Gluud LL, Kimer N, Krag A. Meta-analysis: the safety and efficacy of vaptans (tolvaptan, satavaptan and lixivaptan) in cirrhosis with ascites or hyponatraemia. Aliment Pharmacol Ther. 2012;36:619–26. https://doi.org/10.1111/apt.12025.
51. Rozen-Zvi B, Yahav D, Gheorghiade M, Korzets A, Leibovici L, Gafter U. Vasopressin receptor antagonists for the treatment of hyponatremia: systematic review and meta-analysis. Am J Kidney Dis. 2010;56:325–37. https://doi.org/10.1053/j.ajkd.2010.01.013.
52. O'Leary JG, Davis GL. Conivaptan increases serum sodium in hyponatremic patients with end-stage liver disease. Liver Transpl. 2009;15:1325–9. https://doi.org/10.1002/lt.21836.
53. Abbasoglu O, Goldstein RM, Vodapally MS, Jennings LW, Levy MF, Husberg BS, et al. Liver transplantation in hyponatremic patients with emphasis on central pontine myelinolysis. Clin Transpl. 1998;12:263–9.
54. Miller PD, Linas SL, Schrier RW. Plasma demeclocycline levels and nephrotoxicity. Correlation in hyponatremic cirrhotic patients. JAMA. 1980;243:2513–5.
55. Gadano A, Moreau R, Pessione F, Trombino C, Giuily N, Sinnassamy P, et al. Aquaretic effects of niravoline, a kappa-opioid agonist, in patients with cirrhosis. J Hepatol. 2000;32:38–42.
56. Brandman D, Biggins SW, Hameed B, Roberts JP, Terrault NA. Pretransplant severe hepatic encephalopathy, peritransplant sodium and post-liver transplantation morbidity and mortality. Liver Int. 2012;32:158–64. https://doi.org/10.1111/j.1478-3231.2011.02618.x.
57. Lee EM, Kang JK, Yun SC, Kim KH, Kim SJ, Hwang KS, et al. Risk factors for central pontine and extrapontine myelinolysis following orthotopic liver transplantation. Eur Neurol. 2009;62:362–8. https://doi.org/10.1159/000242426.
58. Morard I, Gasche Y, Kneteman M, Toso C, Mentha A, Meeberg G, et al. Identifying risk factors for central pontine and extrapontine myelinolysis after liver transplantation: a case-control study. Neurocrit Care. 2014;20:287–95. https://doi.org/10.1007/s12028-013-9928-9.
59. Wszolek ZK, McComb RD, Pfeiffer RF, Steg RE, Wood RP, Shaw BW Jr, et al. Pontine and extrapontine myelinolysis following liver transplantation. Relationship to serum sodium. Transplantation. 1989;48:1006–12.

60. Hudcova J, Ruthazer R, Bonney I, Schumann R. Sodium homeostasis during liver transplantation and correlation with outcomes. Anesth Analg. 2014;119:1420–8. https://doi.org/10.1213/ANE.0000000000000415.
61. McCormick PA, Mistry P, Kaye G, Burroughs AK, McIntyre N. Intravenous albumin infusion is an effective therapy for hyponatraemia in cirrhotic patients with ascites. Gut. 1990;31:204–7.
62. Adrogue HJ, Madias NE. Hyponatremia. N Engl J Med. 2000;342:1581–9. https://doi.org/10.1056/NEJM200005253422107.
63. Larner AJ, Vickers CR, Adu D, Buckels JA, Elias E, Neuberger J. Correction of severe hyponatraemia by continuous arteriovenous haemofiltration before liver transplantation. BMJ. 1988;297:1514–5.
64. Murphy N, Auzinger G, Bernel W, Wendon J. The effect of hypertonic sodium chloride on intracranial pressure in patients with acute liver failure. Hepatology. 2004;39:464–70. https://doi.org/10.1002/hep.20056.
65. Hackworth WA, Heuman DM, Sanyal AJ, Fisher RA, Sterling RK, Luketic VA, et al. Effect of hyponatraemia on outcomes following orthotopic liver transplantation. Liver Int. 2009;29:1071–7. https://doi.org/10.1111/j.1478-3231.2009.01982.x.
66. Langer T, Ferrari M, Zazzeron L, Gattinoni L, Caironi P. Effects of intravenous solutions on acid-base equilibrium: from crystalloids to colloids and blood components. Anaesthesiol Intensive Ther. 2014;46:350–60. https://doi.org/10.5603/AIT.2014.0059.
67. Ghaffaripour S, Jannatmakan F, Firoozifar M. Practical protocol for management of severe hyponatremia in patients undergoing liver transplant surgery. Prog Transplant. 2015;25:106. https://doi.org/10.7182/pit2015186.
68. Atchison SR, Rettke SR, Fromme GA, Janossy TA, Kunkel SE, Williamson KR, et al. Plasma glucose concentrations during liver transplantation. Mayo Clin Proc. 1989;64:241–5.
69. MacMillan TE, Tang T, Cavalcanti RB. Desmopressin to prevent rapid sodium correction in severe hyponatremia: a systematic review. Am J Med. 2015;128:1362 e15–24. https://doi.org/10.1016/j.amjmed.2015.04.040.
70. Brinson EL, Yu JS, Liu LL, Bokoch MP. Desmopressin reverses overly rapid serum sodium correction in a hyponatremic patient undergoing living donor liver transplantation: a case report. A A Pract. 2018;11(3):82–4.
71. Bonham CA, Dominguez EA, Fukui MB, Paterson DL, Pankey GA, Wagener MM, et al. Central nervous system lesions in liver transplant recipients: prospective assessment of indications for biopsy and implications for management. Transplantation. 1998;66:1596–604.
72. Rafat C, Schortgen F, Gaudry S, Bertrand F, Miguel-Montanes R, Labbe V, et al. Use of desmopressin acetate in severe hyponatremia in the intensive care unit. Clin J Am Soc Nephrol. 2014;9:229–37. https://doi.org/10.2215/CJN.00950113.
73. Perianayagam A, Sterns RH, Silver SM, Grieff M, Mayo R, Hix J, et al. DDAVP is effective in preventing and reversing inadvertent overcorrection of hyponatremia. Clin J Am Soc Nephrol. 2008;3:331–6. https://doi.org/10.2215/CJN.03190807.
74. Soupart A, Ngassa M, Decaux G. Therapeutic relowering of the serum sodium in a patient after excessive correction of hyponatremia. Clin Nephrol. 1999;51:383–6.
75. Oya S, Tsutsumi K, Ueki K, Kirino T. Reinduction of hyponatremia to treat central pontine myelinolysis. Neurology. 2001;57:1931–2.
76. Saner FH, Koeppen S, Meyer M, Kohnle M, Herget-Rosenthal S, Sotiropoulos GC, et al. Treatment of central pontine myelinolysis with plasmapheresis and immunoglobulins in liver transplant patient. Transpl Int. 2008;21:390–1. https://doi.org/10.1111/j.1432-2277.2007.00608.x.
77. Butterworth RF. Pathogenesis of hepatic encephalopathy and brain edema in acute liver failure. J Clin Exp Hepatol. 2015;5:S96–S103. https://doi.org/10.1016/j.jceh.2014.02.004.
78. Wendon J, Cordoba J, Dhawan A, Larsen FS, Manns M, Nevens F, et al. EASL 2017 clinical practice guidelines on the management of acute (fulminant) liver failure. J Hepatol. 2017;66:1047–81. https://doi.org/10.1016/j.jhep.2016.12.003.
79. Lai A, Zeller M, Millen T, Kavsak P, Lamontagne F, Cook D, et al. Chloride concentration of commonly available 5% human albumin solutions. In: Paper presented at the Society of Critical Care Medicine 46th Critical Care Congress, Honolulu, 2016.

Chapter 6
Sepsis and Septic Shock in Cirrhotic Patients

Antonios Katsounas

Introduction

Patients with liver cirrhosis are considered to be more susceptible to both spontaneous and healthcare-associated (HCA) infections. It is likely that the cause of this phenomenon is excessive pro-inflammatory cytokine responses, which play a fundamental role in the development of severe liver dysfunction with subsequent multi-organ failure. Effective prevention and early detection strategies, as well as proper clinical management, are of crucial importance for the reduction of morbidity and mortality in this very vulnerable population. This chapter expands on and summarizes the current published literature, which pays particular attention to sepsis-related organ dysfunction in patients with chronic liver diseases.

Immune Dysfunction, Gut Barrier Disruption, and Vasoplegia in Patients with Liver Cirrhosis

Overall, prior to admission to clinical facilities, 25–35% of cirrhotic patients acquire infections that persist during hospitalization, and this trend has increased over the last 5 years. Infections occur 4–5× more frequently in hospitalized patients with cirrhosis in comparison to those without this disease [1]. The risk of infection is more serious in patients with decompensated cirrhosis than in those with stable liver disease [1]. Around 40–60% of cirrhotic patients experiencing gastrointestinal bleeding during hospitalization develop infections [2]. Further, bacterial infections are considered a cause of death in up to 50% of all fatal outcomes in patients with

A. Katsounas (✉)
Division of Infectious Diseases, Department of Gastroenterology, Hepatology and Infectious Diseases, University Hospital Magdeburg, Magdeburg, Germany
e-mail: antonios.katsounas@med.ovgu.de

D. Bezinover, F. Saner (eds.), *Critical Care for Potential Liver Transplant Candidates*,
https://doi.org/10.1007/978-3-319-92934-7_6

cirrhosis [3]. This is not surprising because chronic liver disease is responsible for increased susceptibility to infections.

The molecular mechanisms of this phenomenon may involve compromised macrophage Fc_{γ}-receptor-mediated neutralization of antibody-coated bacteria, functional deficiencies of the complement factors C3 and C4, and impaired antigen presentation ability resulting from the downregulation of monocyte human leukocyte antigen–DR expression [4]. Furthermore, neutrophil cells with downregulated phagocytic killing behavior against germs like *Escherichia coli* or *Staphylococcus aureus* have been identified in patients with alcohol-related cirrhosis [5]. In the presence of portal hypertension, this state of immune dysfunction alters the composition of gut microbiota with a subsequent increase in bacterial translocation from the gastrointestinal tract to the extraintestinal sites. Portal hypertension also leads to hypersplenism, which, in turn, results in a more advanced attenuation of an antimicrobial defense capacity through over-elimination of circulating immune cells. In addition, cirrhotic patients show a diminished synthesis of bile fluid and a prolonged intestinal transit time. These two factors in combination with abnormal production of antibacterial peptides, along with an attenuated secretion of gastric acid, favor intestinal microbial overgrowth. Translocation of bacteria through a "leaky gut" along with decreasing hepatic clearance of bacterial antigens (lipopolysaccharides (LPS) or endotoxins) may lead to a systemic overload of toll-like receptor TLR-ligands and (through activation of TLR pathways) to a massive production of cytokines, which further enhances inflammatory activity [6]. This, in turn, favors a systemic cytokine "blast" and a further secretion of reactive oxygen species (ROS) in large amounts, which accelerates the development of increased intestinal permeability and leads to the formation of a "circulus vitiosus" [7, 8]. There is substantial evidence for the regulatory potential of the C-X3-C Motif Chemokine Receptor 1 (CX3CR1) in intestinal macrophages with regard to maintaining the integrity of the gut barrier [9]. Damage to this barrier (favoring bacterial translocation and, thus, hepatic inflammation/dysfunction) can lead to enhanced splanchnic vasodilation with subsequent further intestinal injury. Indeed, uncontrolled release of vasodilatory inflammatory mediators in combination with endothelial damage and an arginine-vasopressin system dysfunction may cause a vasoplegic syndrome. Nitric oxide (NO) induced by $Ca2^{+}$-independent isoforms of nitric oxide synthase (iNOS) activates soluble guanylyl cyclase (sGC). In turn, sGC is responsible for increasing intracellular cyclic guanosine monophosphate (cGMP) production, which leads to the relaxation of vascular smooth muscles and vascular unresponsiveness along with hypotension. In this setting, it is much more challenging to improve microcirculation and tissue perfusion than it is to solely increase blood pressure using vasopressors. To this end, sufficient support with fluids along with albumin is fundamental. Recent studies have shown that reversing the endothelial nitric oxide synthase (eNOS) uncoupling reaction can diminish ROS levels, increase NO bioavailability, and, thus, attenuate the endothelial "functio laesa" [10]. However, it is very likely that vascular failure during sepsis has a multifactorial background, especially in patients with end-stage liver disease. A concerted research effort focused on the underlying molecular mechanisms for vasoplegia could make a significant contribution to a more meaningful selection of therapeutic targets in this highly vulnerable patient group.

From a pathophysiological point of view, the degree of inflammation markedly affects the outcomes of cirrhotic patients with bacterial infections and sepsis. This is strongly supported by recent findings clearly identifying C-reactive protein (CRP) and white blood cell (WBC) count as independent predictive factors of in-hospital survival [11, 12].

Sepsis in Patients with Liver Cirrhosis

Epidemiological Data on Infections in Patients with Liver Cirrhosis

Infections and immune dysfunction are common etiologies for prolonged liver injury and terminal organ failure [13]. Many patients experience repeated episodes of systemic infections that gradually impair intrinsic liver function before leading to end-stage disease. During the last decade, liver cirrhosis itself has been identified as a risk factor for hospitalization due to severe infection and sepsis-related mortality [14]. Early and accurate detection of infections and identification of their primary source are considered to be essential for targeted therapy, which, in turn, has a significant impact on patient survival (Table 6.1) [15].

According to current studies, spontaneous bacterial peritonitis, urinary tract infections, and pneumonia are the most common bacterial diseases in cirrhotic patients [11]. The origin of infections, i.e., hospital-acquired (HA) vs. community-acquired (CA), and the bacterial types, i.e., Gram-positive and Gram-negative strains, demonstrate a balanced distribution [11]. *Escherichia coli*, *Enterococcus faecium*, and *Klebsiella pneumoniae* count as the most frequently isolated microbial pathogens that cause spontaneous bacterial peritonitis (SBP). Among all patients with SBP, 30–35% of cases are caused by multidrug-resistant (MDR) bacteria [11].

Table 6.1 Site and type of infections in patients with liver cirrhosis

Sites of Infection	Type of isolated bacteria
1. Spontaneous Bacterial Peritonitis	1. Escherichia coli
2. Urinary Tract Infection	2. Enterococcus faecium
3. Pneumonia	3. Klebsiella pneumoniae
4. Primary bacteremia	4. Enterococcus faecalis
5. Skin	5. Fungi
6. Soft tissue	6. Staphylococcus aureus

Definition: Sepsis, Septic Shock, and Applicable Prognostic Scores in Patients with Liver Cirrhosis

Based on the Sepsis-3 criteria, sepsis is defined as a life-threatening organ dysfunction triggered by a dysregulated host response to infection [16–18]. Organ dysfunction can be determined by an increase in the total Sequential Organ Failure Assessment (SOFA) score of ≥ 2 points (i.e., Delta SOFA ≥ 2 points) due to an infection [16–18] (Table 6.2). The baseline SOFA score can be set to zero unless the patient is known to have a preexisting (acute or chronic) organ dysfunction before the onset of infection [16–18].

There are significant differences between the SOFA score and the Chronic Liver Failure-Sequential Organ Failure Assessment (CLIF-SOFA) score. CLIF-SOFA (Table 6.3) was developed to assess 30-day mortality rates in patients with acute decompensation of cirrhosis – defined by the development of complications (e.g., bacterial infection, hepatic encephalopathy, gastrointestinal bleeding, and ascites). However, CLIF-SOFA differs from the SOFA score in the consideration of two parameters: coagulation and the Glasgow Coma Scale (GCS) score [20].

Septic shock is defined as hypotension requiring the use of vasopressors to maintain MAP ≥ 65 mm Hg and a serum lactate level > 2 mmol/l despite adequate fluid resuscitation. For patients meeting these criteria, the hospital mortality rate exceeds 40% [16–18]. Timely and accurate identification of patients at risk for sepsis and septic shock must, therefore, be prioritized. In order to identify adult patients with a possible infection and an expected poor outcome, a new scoring tool quick SOFA (qSOFA) has been introduced. The qSOFA provides simple bedside measures and is considered to be positive when patients meet ≥ 2 of the following three criteria: alteration of consciousness, respiratory rate ≥ 22/min, and systolic blood pressure ≤ 100 mm Hg. According to recent findings [7], cirrhotic patients with a positive qSOFA score meet significantly more Sepsis-3 criteria [16–18] than do those with a negative qSOFA score [16–18].

Based on these observations, a novel algorithm focused on the implementation of Sepsis-3 criteria and the qSOFA has been proposed to assist clinicians with the management of hospitalized patients facing the challenge of concomitant liver cirrhosis and bacterial infection (Fig. 6.1).

According to this algorithm, both Sepsis-3 criteria and the qSOFA should be applied if a baseline SOFA score is unavailable. A patient who meets both screening criteria should be admitted to the ICU, due to a predicted worse outcome. On the other hand, a patient who does not meet the criteria for either scale has the best prognosis. If the situation is uncertain, the SOFA score should be closely monitored for further clinical decisions and management [7].

It has been demonstrated that the CLIF Consortium Acute Decompensation score (CLIF-CADs), used to establish a prognosis for hospitalized cirrhotic patients without acute-on-chronic liver failure, is capable of predicting mortality more

Table 6.2 SOFA score modified from Vincent et al. [19]

	Score				
System	0	1	2	3	4
Respiration					
Pap2/FIO_2, mm Hg (kPa)	≤ 400 m (53.3)	< 400 m (53.3)	< 300 m (40)	< 200 m (26.7) with respiratory support	< 100 m (13.3) with respiratory support
Coagulation					
Platelets, $\times 10^3/\mu L$	≥ 150	< 150	< 100 m	< 50	< 20 m
Liver					
Bilirubin mg/dl (μmol/L)	<1.2	1.2–1.9 (20–32)	2.0–5.9 (33–101)	6.0–11.9 (102–204)	> 12.0 (204)
Cardiovascular					
	MAP ≥ 70 mm Hg	MAP < 70 mm Hg	Dopamine < 5 or dobutamine (any dose)	Dopamine 5.1–15 or epinephrine ≤ 0.1 or norepinephrine ≤ 0.1	Dopamine > 15 or epinephrine > 0.1 or norepinephrine > 0.1
Central nervous system					
Glasgow Coma Scale Score	15	13–14	10–12	6–9	< 6
Renal					
Creatinine, mg/dL (μmol/L)	< 1.2 (110)	1.2–1.9 (110–170)	2.0–3.4 (171–299)	3.5–4.9 (300–440)	> 5.0 (≥ 441)
Urine output (mL/day)				< 500	< 200

Catecholamine doses are given as μg/kg/min for at least 1 h. Glasgow Coma Scale scores range from 3 to 15; higher score values indicate better neurological function

FIO_2 fraction of inspired oxygen, *MAP* mean arterial pressure, *PaO_2* partial pressure of oxygen

Table 6.3 CLIF-SOFA modified from Jalan et al. [21]

	CLIF-SOFA score				
Organ/system	0	1	2	3	4
Liver					
Bilirubin (mg/dl)	< 1.2	1.20–1.99	2.0–5.99	6.0–11.9	≥ 12.0 (204)
Kidney					
Creatinine (mg/dL)	< 1.2	1.20–1.99	2.0–3.49	3.5–4.99	≥ 5.0
Cerebral					
Hepatic encephalopathy (HE) grade	No HE	HE grade1	HE grade 2	HE grade 3	HE grade 4
Coagulation					
INR	< 1.1	1.1–1.25	1.26–1.5	1.51–2.5	> 2.5 or Platelets ≤ 20 × 10^3/µl
Circulation					
MAP (mmHg)	≥ 70	< 70	Dopamine < 5 or dobutamine or terlipressin	Dopamine 5.1–15 or epinephrine ≤ 0.1 or norepinephrine ≤ 0.1	Dopamine > 15 or epinephrine > 0.1 or norepinephrine > 0.1
Lungs					
PaO_2/FiO_2	> 400	≤ 400	≤ 300	≤ 200	≤ 100
or SpO_2/FiO_2	> 512	358–512	215–357	90–214	≤ 89

Overall, scores range from 0 to 24. The use of dobutamine or terlipressin, at any dose, is sufficient for a score of 2 for circulation. Doses of catecholamines are given as µg/kg/min

HE hepatic encephalopathy, *INR* international normalized ratio, *MAP* mean arterial pressure, PaO_2 partial pressure of arterial oxygen, FIO_2 fraction of inspired oxygen, SpO_2 pulse oximetric saturation

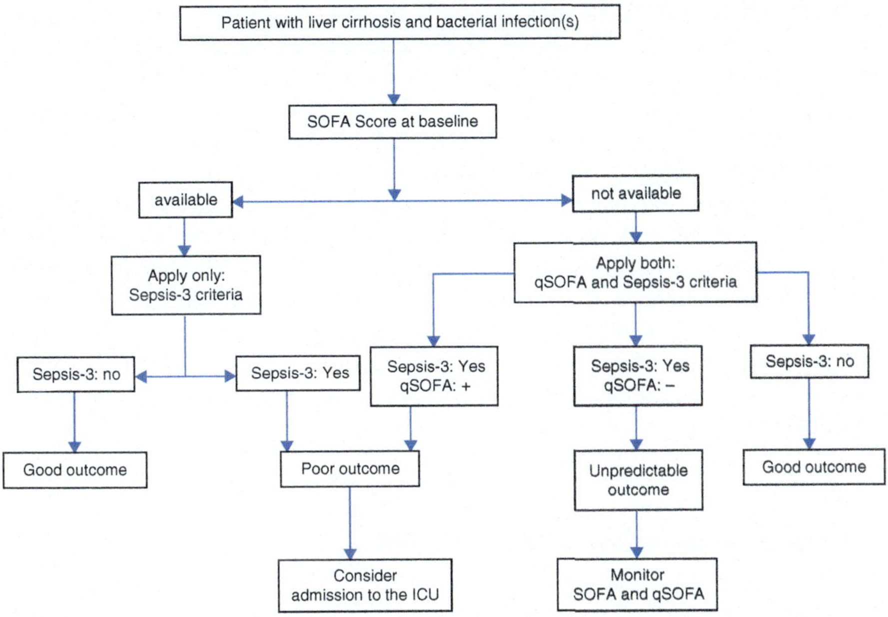

Fig. 6.1 Flowchart for the implementation of Sepsis-3 criteria in the clinical management of patients with cirrhosis and systemic infections. *ICU* intensive care unit. (Figure modified from Piano et al. [11])

accurately. This is likely because in CLIF-CADs both the organ dysfunction-specific variables (e.g., international normalized ratio, creatinine, and serum sodium concentration) and the degree of inflammation (e.g., WBC count) during systemic bacterial infections are taken into account [12].

Treatment/Hemodynamics and Sepsis-Related Complications of Cirrhosis

In patients with cirrhosis, therapy is aimed at preventing and correcting organ hypoperfusion along with fast identification and elimination of the infectious sources. Fluid substitution should be the primary therapeutic option to improve perfusion and enable the maintenance of stable function of vital organs [17]. Hypotensive patients with an adequate intravascular volume status should receive additional treatment with vasopressors to stabilize mean arterial pressure (MAP) (measured by direct arterial pressure monitoring) above 65 mmHg and urine output above 0.5 ml/kg/h [22]. Some recommendations for the management of hemodynamics are based on a measurement of central venous pressure (CVP) [22] and the goal of achieving central venous oxygen saturation (ScvO2) > 70%. Several studies have shown that albumin supplementation using a dose of 1.0–1.5 g/kg may delay the onset of renal failure, especially in cirrhotic patients with an infection not related to SBP [23, 24]. However, these results are controversial [25–28]. In the ongoing debate on the potential beneficial effect of albumin administration in these patients, clinicians should be aware of the anti-oxidant/anti-inflammatory, immunomodulatory properties and functional role of albumin as a carrier molecule for many endogenous/exogenous substances, in addition to its physiological effect as a plasma expander [29]. Beyond that, caution should be exercised; that is, treatment with highly protein-bound antibiotics should not be initiated without considering what is likely to be the unfavorable influence of hypoalbuminemia on the pharmacokinetics of these drugs [30]. All these complications of cirrhosis, including hepatic encephalopathy [31, 32], hepatorenal syndrome [33], hepato- and porto-pulmonary hypertension [34], malnutrition and impaired gluconeogenesis [35], must be optimally managed in order to support a cirrhotic patient through sepsis [36].

Treatment/Anti-infective Management

Bacterial infections may cause fatal complications such as septic and/or hepatic encephalopathy, decompensation of ascites along with hypervolemic hyponatremia, gastrointestinal bleeding, renal failure, and acute-on-chronic or acute-on-cirrhosis liver failure. In patients with SBP, ascites removal equals source control! Most importantly, after the ascetic fluid has been drained from the abdominal cavity, a blood culture evaluation should be performed immediately in order to improve diagnostic accuracy [37]. It is important to consider that antibiotics may not reach a sufficient level to treat an infection localized in the peritoneal compartment if dose administration follows standard recommendations. Therapeutic drug monitoring should be performed along with systemic substitution of albumin, as stated above. It is essential to consider the patient's previous and current antibiotic regimen. For example, if levofloxacin was used for SBP prophylaxis, it is crucial to consider that fluoroquinolones might no longer be effective as a viable therapeutic alternative. In more than 50% of cases, empirical treatment includes ≥ 2 antibiotics [11]. Quinolones, third-generation cephalosporins, carbapenems, piperacillin/tazobactam, and glycopeptides are the most frequently used substances, and empirical antibiotic treatment can be considered effective in approximately 80–85% of cases [11] (Table 6.4). While almost all of these patients achieve final resolution of infection, 15–20% develop a reinfection during hospitalization [11]. Indeed, empirical treatment should be based on valid clinical and microbiological (prognosis-related) scores and, therefore, requires good knowledge of local epidemiology including common bacterial resistance profiles and rates as well as the history of infection(s) in individual patients with chronic liver disease. With regard to the increasing prevalence of resistance to quinolones and colonization/infection with MDR bacteria, in 2014 the European Association for the Study of the Liver (EASL) published recommendations for the management of bacterial infections in cirrhotic patients [21].

Table 6.4 Common empirical antibiotic approaches for patients with severe liver disease and bacterial infection(s) modified from Gustot et al. [38]

Site/type of infection	No severe sepsis or shock		
	CA infections	HCA and HA infections	
		Prevalence of MDR bacteria	
		Low	High
SBP	Third-generation Cephalosporins (i.v.)	Piperacillin/ Tazobactam (i.v.)	Meropenem (i.v.) ± Glycopeptide (i.v.)[a] or Linezolid/ Daptomycin (i.v.)[b]
SMB			
UI			
PNE	Third-generation Cephalosporins (i.v.) + Macrolide (oral/i.v.) Or Levofloxacin (oral/i.v.)		Meropenem (i.v.) or Ceftazidime (i.v.) + Ciprofloxacin (i.v.) ± Glycopeptide (i.v.)[a] or Linezolid (i.v.)[a]
STI	Amoxicillin/Clavulanic Acid (i.v.)		Meropenem or Ceftazidime + Glycopeptide (i.v.)[a] or Linezolid/ Daptomycin (i.v.)[b]
Site/type of infection	**Severe sepsis or shock**		
	Empirical antibiotic treatment of severe sepsis or shock should be administered with the local rate of MDR pathogens taken into account		

MDR multidrug resistant, *CA* community-acquired, *HCA* healthcare-associated, *HA* hospital-acquired, *SBP* spontaneous bacterial peritonitis, *SBM* spontaneous bacteremia, *UI* urinary infections, *PNE* pneumonia, *STI* soft tissue infections

[a]Use of antibiotics with proven activity against methicillin-resistant *Staphylococcus aureus* (MRSA) should be considered in patients with risk factors such as previous and/or current nasal MRSA carriage, ventilator-associated pneumonia, and previous antibiotic therapy. In areas with a high prevalence of MDR *Pseudomonas aeruginosa*, the addition of nebulized colistin or amikacin should be carefully evaluated

[b]In areas with a high prevalence of vancomycin-resistant enterococci (VRE), the use of linezolid/ daptomycin should be carefully evaluated

Future Challenge

Antimicrobial Resistance [39]

In patients with liver cirrhosis, the course of bacterial infections can be severe with a fourfold increase in mortality in comparison to other groups. Early and thorough administration of carefully selected anti-infective treatments is essential for the effective clinical management of these patients, especially considering that their risk of developing an MRD-associated infection is increased due to frequent hospitalization and repeated exposure to antibiotics. In order to limit the spread of MDR organisms, rational management should be implemented to help establish an equilibrium between granting all necessary access to antimicrobial drugs and preventing both the overuse and the misuse of these:

1. For example, development of cost-efficient, bedside diagnostic tools is needed to support faster and more evidence-based decisions related to antibiotic therapies. This should help clinicians to avoid less precise empirical clinical practices.
2. It is equally important to de-escalate antibiotic regimes to single antibiotic drugs as promptly as possible. More hospital antibiotic stewardship (ABS) programs should be promoted and implemented across in-hospital settings.
3. Alternatives to antibiotics should be more intensively investigated and clinically evaluated. The paradigm of microbiota transfer via fecal transplantation as an effective technique to manage vancomycin-resistant *Clostridium difficile* infections has proven to be a true drug-free strategy for managing bacterial infections resistant to antibiotics.
4. During the last three decades, no new classes of antibiotics have been discovered and only a few novel agents are in development. Greater investment in this field is an absolute priority in order to boost basic and clinical research focused on developing new antimicrobials [40].

There is an obvious need to strengthen the understanding of antimicrobial resistance and to gain additional knowledge through focused research on diagnostic innovations, novel antimicrobials, and/or new alternative drug-free therapies.

Key Points

1. Bacterial infections are considered to be the cause of death in up to 50% of all fatalities in patients with liver cirrhosis.
2. Spontaneous bacterial peritonitis (SBP), urinary tract infections, and pneumonia are the most common bacterial infections in cirrhotic patients. *Escherichia coli*, *Enterococcus faecium*, and *Klebsiella pneumoniae* are the most frequently isolated microbial pathogens associated with SBP, which is caused by multidrug-resistant (MDR) bacteria in 30–35% of patients. In SBP, ascites removal is equivalent to source control!
3. Immune dysfunction, gut barrier disruption, and vasoplegia share common pathophysiologic mechanisms in patients with liver cirrhosis.
4. In cirrhotic patients with sepsis-related hypotension, it is very challenging to improve microcirculation and tissue perfusion based solely on administering vasopressors. Adequate fluid resuscitation including albumin is essential.
5. The SOFA score and the CLIF-SOFA score differ, as the latter includes two additional parameters: coagulation and the Glasgow Coma Scale (GCS).
6. Hospital antibiotic stewardship (ABS) programs should be promoted and implemented across in-hospital settings in order to better position clinicians to face the challenge of antimicrobial resistance.

References

1. Borzio M, et al. Bacterial infection in patients with advanced cirrhosis: a multicentre prospective study. Dig Liver Dis. 2001;33(1):41–8.
2. Bernard B, et al. Antibiotic prophylaxis for the prevention of bacterial infections in cirrhotic patients with gastrointestinal bleeding: a meta-analysis. Hepatology. 1999;29(6):1655–61.
3. Tandon P, Garcia-Tsao G. Bacterial infections, sepsis, and multiorgan failure in cirrhosis. Semin Liver Dis. 2008;28(1):26–42.
4. Wasmuth HE, et al. Patients with acute on chronic liver failure display "sepsis-like" immune paralysis. J Hepatol. 2005;42(2):195–201.
5. Rajkovic IA, Williams R. Abnormalities of neutrophil phagocytosis, intracellular killing and metabolic activity in alcoholic cirrhosis and hepatitis. Hepatology. 1986;6(2):252–62.
6. Katsounas A, et al. Altered expression of SHIP, a toll-like receptor pathway inhibitor, is associated with the severity of liver fibrosis in chronic hepatitis C virus infection. J Infect Dis. 2011;204(8):1181–5.
7. Strnad P, et al. Liver - guardian, modifier and target of sepsis. Nat Rev Gastroenterol Hepatol. 2017;14(1):55–66.
8. Prin M, Bakker J, Wagener G. Hepatosplanchnic circulation in cirrhosis and sepsis. World J Gastroenterol. 2015;21(9):2582–92.
9. Schneider KM, et al. CX3CR1 is a gatekeeper for intestinal barrier integrity in mice: limiting steatohepatitis by maintaining intestinal homeostasis. Hepatology. 2015;62(5):1405–16.
10. Sharawy N. Vasoplegia in septic shock: do we really fight the right enemy? J Crit Care. 2014;29(1):83–7.
11. Piano S, Bartoletti M, Tonon M, et al. Assessment of Sepsis-3 criteria and quick SOFA in patients with cirrhosis and bacterial infections. Gut. Published Online First: 31 Aug 2017. https://doi.org/10.1136/gutjnl-2017-314324
12. Jalan R, et al. The CLIF consortium acute decompensation score (CLIF-C ADs) for prognosis of hospitalised cirrhotic patients without acute-on-chronic liver failure. J Hepatol. 2015;62(4):831–40.
13. Scaglione S, et al. The epidemiology of cirrhosis in the United States: a population-based study. J Clin Gastroenterol. 2015;49(8):690–6.
14. Foreman MG, Mannino DM, Moss M. Cirrhosis as a risk factor for sepsis and death: analysis of the National Hospital Discharge Survey. Chest. 2003;124(3):1016–20.
15. Gustot T, et al. Severe sepsis in cirrhosis. Hepatology. 2009;50(6):2022–33.
16. Singer M, et al. The third international consensus definitions for sepsis and septic shock (Sepsis-3). JAMA. 2016;315(8):801–10.
17. Shankar-Hari M, et al. Developing a new definition and assessing new clinical criteria for septic shock: for the third international consensus definitions for sepsis and septic shock (Sepsis-3). JAMA. 2016;315(8):775–87.
18. Seymour CW, et al. Assessment of clinical criteria for Sepsis: for the third international consensus definitions for sepsis and septic shock (Sepsis-3). JAMA. 2016;315(8):762–74.
19. Vincent JL, et al. The SOFA (sepsis-related organ failure assessment) score to describe organ dysfunction/failure. On behalf of the working group on sepsis-related problems of the European Society of Intensive Care Medicine. Intensive Care Med. 1996;22(7):707–10.
20. Moreau R, et al. Acute-on-chronic liver failure is a distinct syndrome that develops in patients with acute decompensation of cirrhosis. Gastroenterology. 2013;144(7):1426–37, 1437.e1–9.
21. Jalan R, et al. Bacterial infections in cirrhosis: a position statement based on the EASL Special Conference 2013. J Hepatol. 2014;60(6):1310–24.
22. Rhodes A, et al. Surviving sepsis campaign: international guidelines for management of sepsis and septic shock: 2016. Intensive Care Med. 2017;43(3):304–77.
23. Merli M, et al. Albumin infusion in cirrhotic patients with infections other than spontaneous bacterial peritonitis: end of the story? J Hepatol. 2015;63(3):767–8.
24. Thevenot T, et al. Effect of albumin in cirrhotic patients with infection other than spontaneous bacterial peritonitis. A randomized trial. J Hepatol. 2015;62(4):822–30.

25. Guevara M, et al. Albumin for bacterial infections other than spontaneous bacterial peritonitis in cirrhosis. A randomized, controlled study. J Hepatol. 2012;57(4):759–65.
26. Sort P, et al. Effect of intravenous albumin on renal impairment and mortality in patients with cirrhosis and spontaneous bacterial peritonitis. N Engl J Med. 1999;341(6):403–9.
27. Thevenot T, Monnet E, Di Martino V. Effect of albumin on survival in septic cirrhotic patients other than spontaneous bacterial peritonitis. The question remains open. J Hepatol. 2013;58(3):638–9.
28. Guevara M, Arroyo V, Gines P. Reply to: "effect of albumin on survival in septic cirrhotic patients other than spontaneous bacterial peritonitis. The question remains open". J Hepatol. 2013;58(3):640.
29. Caraceni P, et al. Clinical indications for the albumin use: still a controversial issue. Eur J Intern Med. 2013;24(8):721–8.
30. Roberts JA, et al. Individualised antibiotic dosing for patients who are critically ill: challenges and potential solutions. Lancet Infect Dis. 2014;14(6):498–509.
31. Iacobone E, et al. Sepsis-associated encephalopathy and its differential diagnosis. Crit Care Med. 2009;37(10 Suppl):S331–6.
32. Ferenci P, et al. Hepatic encephalopathy--definition, nomenclature, diagnosis, and quantification: final report of the working party at the 11th World Congresses of Gastroenterology, Vienna, 1998. Hepatology. 2002;35(3):716–21.
33. Tandon P, et al. Relevance of new definitions to incidence and prognosis of acute kidney injury in hospitalized patients with cirrhosis: a retrospective population-based cohort study. PLoS One. 2016;11(8):e0160394.
34. Schiffer E, et al. Hepatopulmonary syndrome increases the postoperative mortality rate following liver transplantation: a prospective study in 90 patients. Am J Transplant. 2006;6(6):1430–7.
35. Kauffmann RM, et al. Provision of balanced nutrition protects against hypoglycemia in the critically ill surgical patient. JPEN J Parenter Enteral Nutr. 2011;35(6):686–94.
36. Findlay JY, et al. Critical care of the end-stage liver disease patient awaiting liver transplantation. Liver Transpl. 2011;17(5):496–510.
37. Koulaouzidis A, et al. Spontaneous bacterial peritonitis. Postgrad Med J. 2007;83(980):379–83.
38. Gustot T, et al. Sepsis in alcohol-related liver disease. J Hepatol. 2017;67(5):1031–50.
39. Fernández J, Bert F, Nicolas-Chanoine M-H. The challenges of multi-drug-resistance in hepatology. J Hepatol. 2016;65(5):1043–54.
40. The challenge of antimicrobial resistance. The Lancet Gastroenterology & Hepatology. 1(3):173. https://www.thelancet.com/pdfs/journals/langas/PIIS2468-1253(16)30121-2.pdf

Chapter 7
The Hemostatic System in Patients with Cirrhosis, Monitoring of Coagulation and Management of Bleeding

Daniel Dirkmann

The hemostatic system consists of several components including endothelial cells, platelets and other blood cells, plasmatic pro- and anti-coagulant factors, and hepatocytes and hepatic stellate cells, as well as fibrinolytic and antifibrinolytic enzymes [1]. Complex feedback and feedforward mechanisms and cross-interactions between primary, secondary, and tertiary hemostasis regulate the delicate balance between coagulation and fibrinolysis. Disturbances in either part of the hemostatic system may lead to both bleeding and clotting.

Chronic and acute liver failure (LF) can directly and indirectly impact the entire hemostatic system. Historically, liver failure is associated with coagulopathy and bleeding diathesis [2, 3]. However, a significant proportion of these patients suffering liver failure also suffer thrombotic complications, demonstrating a rather thrombotic diathesis [4–8].

The current understanding of the alterations to the hemostatic system evoked by cirrhosis and/or liver failure suggests that changes to pro- and anti-coagulant as well as to pro- and anti-fibrinolytic mechanisms result in a rebalanced but highly vulnerable and unstable state of hemostasis [9–12].

Plasmatic Pro- and Anti-coagulant Factors

One of the most apparent effects of liver disease on coagulation is on plasmatic coagulation factors, resulting in prolonged coagulation times of various assays (e.g., prothrombin time and activated partial thromboplastin time). Almost all plasmatic coagulation factors (F) (i.e., factors II, V, VII, IX, X, XI, and XIII) are synthetized in

D. Dirkmann (✉)
Department of Anesthesiology and Intensive Care Medicine,
University Hospital Essen, Essen, Germany
e-mail: Daniel.Dirkmann@uk-essen.de

D. Bezinover, F. Saner (eds.), *Critical Care for Potential Liver Transplant Candidates*,
https://doi.org/10.1007/978-3-319-92934-7_7

the liver. Accordingly, decreased hepatic production of these factors, due to chronic or acute LF, leads to decreased plasma concentrations of these procoagulant factors. Vitamin K deficiency is also common in patients with liver disease and may further exacerbate already low concentrations of what are referred to as the vitamin K-dependent coagulation factors, such as F II, F VII, F IX, and F X [3, 13]. This decrease in plasmatic coagulation factors is counterbalanced by a concurrent decrease in the natural anticoagulant plasma proteins such as antithrombin III (AT III) and α_2-antiplasmin, as well as vitamin K-dependent factors, protein C (PC) and protein S (PS) [3, 14]. Simultaneously, patients with end-stage liver disease (ESLD) show a considerable increase in the plasma concentration of the endothelium-produced F VIII and its carrier protein, von Willebrand factor (vWF). While the reason for the reduced concentrations of AT III and the vitamin K-dependent proteins C and S is decreased liver synthetic capacity and vitamin K deficiency, it is likely that the increased concentration of the F VIII-vWF complex is induced by profound endothelial dysfunction due to the release of cytokines and endotoxins. Another cause of diminished hepatic clearance of F VIII is reduced expression of low-density lipoprotein receptor-related protein [3, 15]. Inflammatory cytokines have been demonstrated to inhibit the synthesis of the vWF cleaving protease ADAMTS13 (a disintegrin and metalloprotease with thrombospondin type 1 motif 13), which is synthetized in hepatic stellate cells and the endothelium [16], resulting in its markedly reduced activity in patients with acute and chronic LF [17]. This leads to an increased concentration of unusually large vWF multimers and, thus, to a further increase in the F VIII plasma concentration, which affects thrombin generation capacity [15].

While chronic LD is usually associated with a gradual reduction over time in all pro- and anti-coagulant factors synthetized in the liver, their decrease in acute LF is characterized by a more rapid onset, and concentration depends on the half-life of each of the respective factors. Therefore, acute LF is accompanied by a more rapid drop in the concentration of both factors V and VII, followed by factors II and X. It should be noted that the concentrations of factors IX and XI seem to be preserved in acute LF but not in chronic LF [18].

Thrombocytopenia and Platelet Function

Numerous mechanisms may affect platelet concentration and function in patients with ESLD. A decreased platelet count is the most frequent alteration due to diminished production and increased consumption. Low platelet concentration results from reduced hepatic production of thrombopoietin, with subsequent diminished production of platelets by the megakaryocytes of the bone marrow [19]. Furthermore, myelodepression, seen in hepatitis C virus (HCV) infection [20], and folate deficiency, commonly encountered in alcohol abuse [21], may contribute to decreased platelet formation. In addition, it has been reported that immune-mediated thrombocytopenia is associated with chronic LD due to hepatitis B virus (HBV), HCV infection [22], and primary biliary cirrhosis [23]. Pharmacotherapy for HBV and

HCV infections may also induce or aggravate thrombocytopenia [24]. Consumption of platelets is associated with hypersplenism related to portal hypertension with subsequent sequestration in the spleen. Furthermore, ADAMTS13 deficiency [25] also results in increased plasma concentrations of vWF and unusually large vWF multimers, which may contribute to platelet consumption due to the formation of platelet microthrombi. This thrombosis in microcirculation may induce sinusoidal microcirculatory disturbances with further worsening of liver injury and potentially induce multiple-organ failure [25–27]. The mechanism of thrombocytopenia is partly comparable to the mechanism observed in thrombotic thrombocytopenic purpura (TTP). In general, thrombocytopenia seems to be more severe in patients with concurrent cirrhosis and splenomegaly than in those with extrahepatic portal hypertension [28].

Impaired platelet aggregation in response to adenosine diphosphate, adrenaline, thrombin, and ristocetin has been described in both acute LF and chronic LD [29, 30]. Normal platelet adhesion could be demonstrated following correction of hematocrit and platelet count [30, 31]. Cholestatic liver diseases are usually associated with mild to moderate thrombocytopenia; however, platelet function seems to be preserved or possibly even enhanced as compared to that of patients without this condition [32].

As thrombocytopenia, at least in part, occurs in response to ADAMTS13 deficiency, which in turn leads to increased levels of larger and unusually large vWF multimers, low platelet counts seem to be the mechanism that can balance out increased platelet aggregation.

Hypo- and Dys-fibrinogenemia

Fibrinogen represents the vast majority of the procoagulant coagulation factors, and the thrombin-mediated generation of a dense, three-dimensional fibrin network is the final step in clot formation. The stability of the clot and its resistance to fibrinolysis are highly dependent on fibrinogen concentration and structure, the concentrations of pro- and anti-coagulants, and antifibrinolytics and local cellular properties [33, 34]. Plasma fibrinogen concentration is usually normal in patients with stable chronic LF and may even be increased. In contrast, fibrinogen levels are frequently decreased in patients with acute LF and decompensated chronic LF [10, 32, 35, 36]. Dysfibrinogenemia resulting from the accumulation of sialic acid residues, which are thought to impair fibrinogen polymerization, can be encountered in both acute LF and chronic LF [37].

Fibrinolysis

Most pro- and anti-fibrinolytic proteins are synthetized in the liver. As a consequence of impaired syntheses, concentrations of the antifibrinolytic proteins F XIII, α_2-antiplasmin, plasminogen activator inhibitor-1 (PAI-1), and TAFI are decreased in chronic LD. The plasma concentration of plasminogen is also decreased. In contrast, tissue plasminogen activator (tPA) (the most important activator of plasminogen) is synthetized in the endothelium, and its decreased hepatic clearance [38] results in increased plasma concentrations in patients with chronic LD. Furthermore, ascetic fluid has been demonstrated to have some fibrinolytic activity, and it is thought likely that the reabsorption of ascites via the thoracic duct contributes to increased fibrinolysis [39].

Both acute LF [40, 41] and cholestatic liver disease [35] result in a hypofibrinolytic state induced by increased plasma concentration of PAI-1.

The perceived imbalance of pro- and anti-fibrinolytic proteins led to the assumption that fibrinolysis is increased in chronic LD. Observations of increased plasma concentrations of thrombin-antithrombin complexes, d-dimer, and fibrinogen degradation products along with shortened euglobulin lysis time support this theory. However, it has also been hypothesized that these markers of fibrinolysis are elevated due to decreased hepatic clearance and not as a result of increased fibrinolysis [10], and no evidence for increased fibrinolytic potential using clot lysis time assays could be found in cirrhotic patients [42]. Similar to procoagulant and anticoagulant systems, the fibrinolytic system is also considered to be rebalanced. However, acute situations like sepsis, bleeding, and shock might easily disturb this fragile balance, with subsequent manifest hyperfibrinolysis [36].

Coagulation Tests in Patients with Cirrhosis and Liver Failure

The entire hemostatic system in patients with cirrhosis is considered rebalanced. In general, patients seem to be at a higher risk for thromboembolic events than for coagulopathic bleeding. However, standard coagulation assays fail to reflect this tendency or even to indicate thromboembolic risk. In fact, these assays frequently even suggest a hypocoagulable state and trigger prohemostatic therapies. Viscoelastic hemostasis assays (VHA) and assessment of thrombin generation may overcome several of the limitations associated with the standard tests for these patients. Proficiency in the interpretation of VHA and knowledge of its limitations may help to avoid unnecessary transfusions of blood products and coagulation factors and improve thromboprophylaxis in patients with ESLD.

Standard Laboratory Coagulation Assays

The prothrombin time (PT), the activated partial thromboplastin time (aPTT), assays that reflect plasma fibrinogen concentration, and platelet count are the most frequently used coagulation tests. However, the usefulness of these assays for estimating potential bleeding risk and managing coagulopathic and surgical bleeding is very limited due to their long turn-around times [43–45] and relatively narrow information value. In a recent meta-analysis, such standard laboratory tests (SLTs) were evaluated for their usefulness in the diagnosis and management of coagulopathic bleeding in the perioperative setting; only three prospective, nonrandomized studies, with a total of 108 patients, demonstrating that SLTs are useful in guiding coagulation management were identified [46]. Nevertheless, the use of SLT to guide bleeding management is still recommended [47, 48].

The prothrombin time (PT) was developed and is implemented to monitor anticoagulation with vitamin K antagonists (VKAs) [49]. Measurements are performed in plasma that is recalcified and activated by the addition of a thromboplastin (i.e., tissue factor and phospholipids), and the time until the onset of coagulation, registered by an optical or mechanical detector, is assessed. Due to the use of different types of thromboplastin, PT results in seconds are not comparable between different assays, such that standardization using the international sensitivity index (ISI) is required. The testing principle of the PT is based on the thrombin-mediated conversion of fibrinogen to fibrin, and both tests (PT and aPTT) end when about 5% of the overall thrombin has been generated. Due to its activation with the tissue factor, the PT mainly reflects thrombin generation via what is referred to as the extrinsic pathway of the coagulation cascade and, thus, mainly the activity of the vitamin K-dependent procoagulant factors (i.e., factors II, VII, and IX) and factor V, which are most severely affected in ESLD. However, test results are not affected by the activities of the vitamin K-dependent anticoagulant proteins C and S and so do not reflect the rebalancing of thrombin generation in patients with cirrhosis. Furthermore, the complex interactions of cells and coagulation factors are also not reflected by this test, as red and white blood cells are removed during preanalytic centrifugation.

The international normalized ratio (INR) is the standardized PT test and is independent of other testing methods. The clinical usefulness of the INR for predicting bleeding complications and the value of using the INR to guide prophylactic treatment prior to invasive procedures is poor [46]. In cirrhotic patients undergoing laparoscopic liver biopsy, no correlation between bleeding and the PT could be demonstrated [50]. Similar results have been demonstrated for patients undergoing liver transplantation [51]. However, PT is an excellent prognostic marker of liver failure and an independent predictor of survival in liver disease [52].

Similar to the PT, the aPTT was not invented to assess a patient's bleeding risk but to identify patients with deficient coagulation factors from what is considered an intrinsic pathway of the coagulation cascade (i.e., factors XII, XI, IX, and VIII) [53]. Furthermore, the aPTT is established as the standard way to monitor for anticoagulation with unfractionated heparin. Different aPTT assays demonstrate varying sensitivity to deficiencies in the coagulation factors [54] and heparin concentrations [55]. In chronic LD, many patients may present with normal aPTT values, despite deficiencies of several coagulation factors resulting from increased concentrations of liver-independent coagulation factors [56].

A decreased concentration of plasma fibrinogen is frequently found in patients with ESLD. This results from decreased fibrinogen synthesis as well as from the formation of dysfibrinogens [57]. It should be noted that measurements of fibrinogen concentration are strongly dependent on the assay used. In particular, the derived fibrinogen concentration, which is used to calculate the fibrinogen concentration based on PT measurements, can be expected to be markedly influenced by impaired synthesis of plasmatic coagulation factors. In contrast, the Clauss method has been shown to provide a reliable assessment of fibrinogen concentrations, irrespective of the severity of ESLD, and is suggested as the method of choice [58]. In stable liver disease, low fibrinogen concentrations are common and not well correlated with bleeding complications. However, during liver transplantation, low fibrinogen concentration is associated with an increased risk of excessive bleeding [59–61].

Thrombin Generation Assays

Ex vivo thrombin generation assays (TGAs) can be performed in various specimens such as platelet-poor plasma (PPP), platelet-rich plasma (PRP), or whole blood and are usually activated by small amounts of tissue factor [62]. The time course of thrombin generation is analyzed and described as the thrombogram. The main variables of TGAs are the lag time (i.e., the time until the initial thrombin formation is detected), the peak thrombin generation (indicating the maximum thrombin concentration during measurement), and the endogenous thrombin potential (ETP) as assessed by calculating the area under the thrombogram curve. Whereas standard plasmatic coagulation assays provide a single clotting time when about 5% of the overall thrombin is generated, TGAs reflect the total amount of thrombin formed and are thought to quantify the enzymatic work that thrombin can do during its lifetime [63].

Patients with cirrhosis demonstrate decreased TG in PPP corresponding to the decreased synthesis of plasmatic coagulation enzymes. However, this observation is attributable to the ex vivo character of the assay, which does not reflect the concurrent decrease in proteins C and S found in cirrhotic patients. In vivo, thrombin generation is regulated by the protein C system, which is activated by the thrombin-thrombomodulin complex located on endothelial cells [64]. Activation of the protein C system results in the cessation of thrombin generation by inactivating coagulation factors V and VIII and PAI-1. This results in increased fibrinolysis. In the presence of soluble thrombomodulin or a direct activator of protein C (Protac® (Pentapharm, Basel, Switzerland)), patients with acute or chronic liver failure demonstrated thrombin generation similar to that of healthy volunteers [41, 65–67]. Furthermore, the platelet count also markedly affects thrombin generation in both healthy controls and patients with cirrhosis [68–70]. In this context, it seems that platelet factor 4 is suggested in order to exert a modulatory effect on the thrombin-thrombomodulin complex, thereby enhancing protein C activation while inhibiting TAFI activation [71].

In summary, preserved thrombin generation in the presence of an activator of the protein C system underlines the limitations of conventional coagulation tests in patients with liver failure and means that the concept of rebalanced hemostasis should be emphasized. The role of platelets in thrombin generation might suggest that platelet transfusion should be considered in bleeding episodes with preserved thrombin generation. However, as TGAs are not available in either a routine or timely way, their application in clinical practice is limited at the present time.

Viscoelastic Hemostatic Assays

In 1948, several years before the invention of aPTT, the German professor Hartert published his description of a coagulation test capable of assessing the viscoelastic properties of coagulation in plasma or whole blood plotted against time [72]. In contrast to the standard laboratory assays, viscoelastic testing does not end when initial clotting occurs. This assay also reflects the dynamics of clot propagation, clot firmness, and potential clot lysis. Over time, Hartert's original method underwent modifications, and viscoelastic hemostatic assays (VHAs) became available as point-of-care tests, which have increasingly been used to guide coagulation management in liver transplantation and several other clinical settings such as cardiac and trauma surgery. The most commonly used contemporary VHAs, i.e., thrombelastometry (ROTEM®, Tem International GmbH, Munich, Germany) and thrombelastography (TEG®, Haemonetics, Niles, IL, USA), are usually conducted using whole blood and do not require centrifugation of the sampled blood. However, the semi-automated devices (ROTEM® delta and TEG® 5000) require several pipetting steps for each assay. Nevertheless, both devices are likewise considered suitable for deployment at the point of care, for example, in intensive care units and operating areas. Fully automated devices (ROTEM® sigma and TEG® 6S) have also been developed, providing similar results and full point-of-care capability.

The VHAs ROTEM and TEG differ significantly from each other with respect to measurement technique, assays used, and resulting variables. In general, the measurement technique of VHAs is based on the registration of the viscoelastic coagulation properties of whole blood. In the ROTEM system, a fixed pin oscillates in a cup, whereas in the TEG system, the cup oscillates around a pin connected to the detection unit by a torsion wire. Increasing viscosity of the blood sample hinders the oscillating movement, and the viscoelastic resistance of the blood clot is plotted against time, resulting in the typical tracing. The clotting time (CT) in ROTEM analyses and the corresponding reaction time (*r*) in TEG measurements principally reflect the initial thrombin generation, and the respective corresponding assays have been demonstrated to correlate to the plasmatic clotting times of SLTs (aPTT and PT) [73, 74]. Thromboelastometric clot formation time, corresponding to the TEG kinetic time (*k*) and the angle alpha, reflects the dynamics of clot formation. The thromboelastometric clot firmness values 5, 10, 15, and 20 min, CT, and the maximum clot firmness (MCF), corresponding to the maximum amplitude (MA) in TEG measurements, mainly reflect the clot firmness or viscosity as induced mainly by platelets and fibrin and to a much lesser degree by factor XIII and hematocrit. Finally, both devices provide variables reflecting clot lysis. The ROTEM system provides results for clot lysis as the percentage of the MCF present at 30, 45, and 60 min following CT (clot lysis index: CLI30, CLI45, and CLI60). However, the

TEG system provides lysis as the percentage of MA present at 30, 45, and 60 min following MA (LY30, LY45, and LY60, respectively).

In order to obtain a comprehensive picture of a patient's current hemostatic status, a panel of specific assays with extrinsic and intrinsic activation of coagulation, as well as assays with platelet inhibition and heparinase, are available for both devices, ROTEM and TEG. Furthermore, an extrinsically activated assay containing tranexamic acid is available for the ROTEM system, enabling in vitro assessment of the expected effects of an antifibrinolytic therapy in vivo. Although corresponding assays are available for TEG, there are several differences between the two systems, resulting in non-interchangeability of the respective tests. Whereas the semi-automated ROTEM system provides four channels for parallel measurements, the TEG 5000 system provides only two measurement channels. The superiority of performing parallel assays in comparison with a single kaolin-activated viscoelastic assay for the differential diagnosis of the underlying reason for a potential coagulopathy has clearly been demonstrated [75]. Furthermore, algorithms based on the use of kaolin-activated assays alone frequently result in platelet transfusion when reduced clot firmness is detected [76]. In contrast, coagulation management based on fast and parallel assays may help to avoid platelet transfusion when a reduction in clot firmness results from hypofibrinogenemia and/or impaired fibrin polymerization [77–82]. This seems to offer potential benefits for patients undergoing liver transplantation where platelet transfusion has been found to be associated with a significant increase in 1-year mortality [83]. However, the new TEG 6s system now available can be used to perform several assays simultaneously.

In contrast to SLTs with turn-around times above 45 min, thromboelastometric results for CT, CFT, angle alpha, and A5 are available within 10–20 min [43–45]. The early variables of clot firmness, available only for the ROTEM, have been shown to provide excellent correlation with the overall clot firmness achieved during measurements [77, 84] and to allow early detection of hyperfibrinolysis [85]. As short turn-around times appear to be of the utmost importance in enabling a targeted therapy and avoiding blind and potentially unnecessary and harmful transfusions, VHAs seem to be superior to SLTs. Furthermore, compared to SLTs, VHAs are significantly more accurate in predicting bleeding and thrombosis and have been shown to be superior in guiding hemostatic therapy during and after liver transplantation and major liver resections. Accordingly, VHAs are increasingly being used in high-volume centers and are recommended as the standard of care [86–89]. A recent Cochrane report demonstrated that coagulation management as guided by VHAs is associated with reduced transfusion requirements.

Platelet Function Tests

Platelet function tests can be used to assess the potential effects of antiplatelet drugs and other alterations in platelet function [96, 97]. In cardiac surgery, incorporating platelet function tests into transfusion algorithms based on VHAs has been found to be associated with less blood loss and lower transfusion requirements in comparison with VHAs alone [90]. However, data on the usefulness of platelet function tests in the bleeding management of patients with liver failure and in the liver transplantation setting are sparse. Although rapid changes of ADP-activated platelet aggregation have been demonstrated to be associated with liver graft damage and worse outcomes [91, 92], there are no data available demonstrating improvements in transfusions and/or coagulation management in this setting. The application of various platelet function tests in patients with liver failure and those undergoing liver transplantation is further hampered by low platelet counts [93] and anemia [94, 95], which may impact the results of platelet function tests. However, platelet function testing could theoretically help to guide platelet transfusion and avoid unnecessary and potentially harmful transfusions of platelets in this setting.

Management of Bleeding Episodes

Coagulation management in patients with cirrhosis can be associated with several problems. The key issue and also the main confounding factor for bleeding in patients with ESLD is portal hypertension [98]. A volume load of 1.5 L (which is equivalent to 6 FFPs) would raise the portal venous pressure up to 15 mmHg [99] with subsequent increased risk for bleeding. Administration of cryoprecipitate can also be associated with volume overload. Another problem associated with transfusion is a possibility of nosocomial infections [100]. In this situation, administration of prothrombin complex concentrate (PCC) might be the better option for selected patients. PCC can be used instead of FFP to manage coagulation using a small amount of fluid. A recent in vitro study indicates the improved thrombin generation potential of PCC compared to plasma transfusion [101, 102]. Considering that patients with ESLD are prone to both bleeding and clotting, monitoring coagulation is an absolute priority.

Bleeding risk assessment in patients with ESLD is difficult, and viscoelastic tests (VET) (ROTEM™/TEG™) seem to be significantly more reliable than SLTs. Wang et al. [87] conducted a randomized controlled trial (RCT) in 28 LT patients assigned either to VET or to SLT. The group managed using VETs received significantly less transfusion of FFPs (12.7 vs. 21.5 units) as compared to the group managed using SLTs. However, the 3-year survival rate was not affected.

In another RCT, TEG™ was compared with SLT. Of 60 patients, 30 were assigned to VET and 30 to SLT to evaluate bleeding risk and guide coagulation management before invasive procedures [103]. The trigger for an FFP transfusion was a prolonged *r*-time, and the trigger for platelets was an MA $\leq$ 40 mm, whereas in the SLT group, the triggers were an INR $\geq$ 1.8 and a platelet count $\leq$ 50/nl for FFP or platelet transfusion. In the VET-guided group, the transfusion rate for any blood product was 16% vs 100% in the SLT group. The hemoglobin level in the VET group was significantly higher than in the SLT group, although the bleeding episodes did not differ between the two groups.

Another study was conducted before VET and after VET implementation in liver transplantation to assess the transfusion rate [104]. The study results indicated a significant reduction in transfused blood products, and the number of transfusion-free transplants increased from 5 to 24% when VET was used. Other complications such as bleeding, reoperation, and kidney failure were significantly lower in the VET group.

Therapy of Thrombin Generation Impairment

The new cell-based coagulation system [105] is not conceived of as an extrinsic system and an intrinsic system. Instead, it introduced three subsequent steps: initiation, propagation, and amplification. The initiation starts with activation of F VII and the tissue factor, which triggers propagation and amplification. The aim of this process is a thrombin burst that increases the thrombin concentration 1,000-fold compared to the baseline. At the end, fibrinopeptides A and B are cleaved from fibrinogen, and a fibrin net is formed, which is strengthened by F XIII-induced cross-links. Activation depends on F II, V, IX, and X (prothrombin complex). If these factors are deficient, the CT in EXTEM will be delayed. However, fibrinogen deficiency will also delay the CT in EXTEM. For stratification, if fibrinogen or prothrombin complex is responsible for this delay, an evaluation of the FIBTEM channel is mandatory. If MCF in FIBTEM is $\geq$ 10 mm, then in actively bleeding patients, PCC should be administered.

A prothrombin complex deficiency should be treated with a four-factor PCC concentrate (Factors II, VII, IX, X) (25 I.U./kg - 40 I.U./kg depending on the CT EXTEM and the severity of the bleeding). Initially, the administration of AT III with a target serum level of 70%, prior to PCC infusion, was recommended in order to prevent thrombosis [106]. However, recently, another study indicated that a ROTEM-guided PCC application in bleeding patients is safe and not associated with an increased rate of thrombosis [79].

Treatment of Clot Firmness Impairment

The interaction between fibrinogen and platelets determines clot firmness. Fibrinogen comprises more than 90% of all plasmatic coagulation factors. All other factors are enzymes, which though necessary to accelerate the coagulation process, do not contribute to clot formation. Fibrinogen is the only coagulation factor that requires normal serum levels for sufficient clot formation, whereas for other factors just 30% activity will be enough for a regular coagulation process [107]. Fibrinogen deficiency can be traced by the FIBTEM channel. A recent study demonstrated that if MCF in EXTEM $\geq$ 40 mm and MCF in FIBTEM $\geq$ 9 mm, coagulopathy associated with nonsurgical bleeding is unlikely [79]. In a bleeding patient with hypofibrinogenemia, replacement should be performed according to the target increase of the MCF amplitude in FIBTEM. Solomon [108] reported that after replacement of 7.6 mg/kg of fibrinogen, the amplitude in MCF of FIBTEM increased by 1 mm. An alternative method for dose calculation is as follows:

Dose fibrinogen in g = (target FIBTEM MCF (mm) – current FIBTEM MCF (mm)) × body weight (kg)/140 [109].

For example, a bleeding patient FIBTEM-MCF = 4 mm; target MCF = 9 mm; body weight 80 kg: Dose of fibrinogen concentrate in g = (9–4) × 80/140 = 2.85 g.

Fibrinolysis

The incidence of fibrinolysis in liver transplantation is up to 84% [110]. The best way to assess fibrinolysis is via VET. In particular, ROTEM with four channels provides fibrinolysis tracing in EXTEM/INTEM and FIBTEM channels. If maximum lysis (ML) is higher than 15%, a fibrinolysis is assumed. However, in some cases, platelet retraction mimics ML in the EXTEM/INTEM channel. This is the reason why fibrinolysis should also be confirmed in the FIBTEM channel. Given that the FIBTEM channel contains cytochalasin, which destroys platelets, only real fibrinolysis will be demonstrated.

Lysis can be confirmed in the APTEM channel. This channel is similar to EXTEM with the addition of aprotinin, which inhibits lysis. Lack of lysis in this channel will confirm fibrinolysis. A recent study indicated that the clot firmness in extrinsically activated and thromboelastometric assays is associated with fibrinolysis and can help to improve its early detection. However, the addition of aprotinin to the assay fails to improve the early diagnosis of fibrinolysis [85].

Most fibrinolysis is self-limiting [79]. Antifibrinolytic treatment is required only in patients with significant clinical bleeding. In this case, tranexamic acid (TXA) of 30 mg/kg should be applied, and 30 min later the ROTEM analysis should be repeated. Based on the actual data, VET-guided factor concentrate coagulation management seems superior to a blind FFP transfusion.

Thromboprophylaxis in Patients with Cirrhosis/Liver Dysfunction

Patients with ESLD are at risk for venous thromboembolism (VTE). An adequate VTE prophylaxis seems necessary despite prolonged clotting times suggesting auto-anticoagulation. According to the most recent American College of Chest Physicians (ACCP) guidelines, VTE prophylaxis can be performed by pharmacological and/or mechanical approaches (compression stockings, intermittent pneumatic compression). These guidelines do not provide a clear recommendation on

VTE prophylaxis in patients with liver disease, which is due to a lack of data and the complexity of the problem. In most studies on VTE prophylaxis, patients with liver dysfunction are specifically excluded on the assumption of an increased bleeding risk in this cohort. Nevertheless, according to the ACCP guideline, low-molecular-weight heparins are the preferred anticoagulant in patients with liver disease and coagulopathy requiring VTE prophylaxis.

A randomized controlled trial demonstrated that enoxaparin (4,000 U subcutaneously once daily) significantly reduced the incidence of portal vein thrombosis and liver decompensation [111]. Another cohort study demonstrated the safety of both prophylactic and therapeutic enoxaparin use in 84 consecutive patients with cirrhosis [112]. However, the latter study also found that standard doses were too low to achieve the targeted anti-Xa activity, which likely resulted from an increased dissolution volume and impaired AT III synthesis [112]. In patients with cirrhotic portal vein thrombosis [113] or non-cirrhotic [114] portal vein thrombosis, anticoagulation resulted in an improved rate of recanalization and appeared to be safe, even in patients with acute variceal bleeding [113].

The direct thrombin inhibitor Argatroban should be used with caution in patients with liver dysfunction and/or hyperbilirubinemia, as it is mainly metabolized in the liver and eliminated in the feces through biliary excretion [115, 116].

Although mechanical VTE prophylaxis can be used in most patients, the utilization of mechanical prophylaxis seems to be rare in intensive care units.

Key Points

1. Patients with end-stage liver disease have a rebalanced coagulation profile due to a decrease in both coagulation and anticoagulation factors.
2. Patients with end-stage liver disease are prone to thromboses, mostly because of profound endothelial dysfunction.
3. Standard laboratory tests do not reflect the actual coagulation profile, and viscoelastic testing should be used instead.
4. Thromboprophylaxis should be considered in this patient population.

References

1. Stassen JM, Arnout J, Deckmyn H. The hemostatic system. Curr Med Chem. 2004;11(17):2245–60.
2. Pereira SP, Langley PG, Williams R. The management of abnormalities of hemostasis in acute liver failure. Semin Liver Dis. © 1996 by Thieme Medical Publishers, Inc; 1996;16(4):403–14.
3. Amitrano L, Guardascione MA, Brancaccio V, Balzano A. Coagulation disorders in liver disease. Semin Liver Dis. 2002;22(1):83–96.
4. Ishitani M, Angle J, Bickston S, Caldwell S, Isaacs R, Pruett T. Liver transplantation: incidence and management of deep venous thrombosis and pulmonary emboli. Transplant Proc. 1997;29(7):2861–3.

5. Northup PG, McMahon MM, Ruhl AP, Altschuler SE, Volk-Bednarz A, Caldwell SH, et al. Coagulopathy does not fully protect hospitalized cirrhosis patients from peripheral venous thromboembolism. Am J Gastroenterol. 2006;101(7):1524–8; quiz 1680.
6. Valla DC. Thrombosis and anticoagulation in liver disease. Hepatology. 2008;47(4):1384–93. Wiley Subscription Services, Inc., A Wiley Company.
7. Warnaar N, Molenaar IQ, Colquhoun SD, Slooff MJH, Sherwani S, de Wolf AM, et al. Intraoperative pulmonary embolism and intracardiac thrombosis complicating liver transplantation: a systematic review. J Thromb Haemost. 2008;6(2):297–302. Blackwell Publishing Ltd.
8. Søgaard KK, Horváth-Puhó E, Grønbaek H, Jepsen P, Vilstrup H, Sørensen HT. Risk of venous thromboembolism in patients with liver disease: a nationwide population-based case-control study. Am J Gastroenterol. 2009;104(1):96–101.
9. Caldwell SH, Hoffman M, Lisman T, Macik BG, Northup PG, Reddy KR, et al. Coagulation disorders and hemostasis in liver disease: pathophysiology and critical assessment of current management. Hepatology. 2006;44(4):1039–46. Wiley Subscription Services, Inc., A Wiley Company.
10. Lisman T, Leebeek FWG. Hemostatic alterations in liver disease: a review on pathophysiology, clinical consequences, and treatment. Dig Surg. 2007;24(4):250–8. Karger Publishers.
11. Mannucci PM. Abnormal hemostasis tests and bleeding in chronic liver disease: are they related? No. J Thromb Haemost. 2006;4(4):721–3. Blackwell Science Inc.
12. Tripodi A, Mannucci PM. Abnormalities of hemostasis in chronic liver disease: reappraisal of their clinical significance and need for clinical and laboratory research. J Hepatol. 2007;46(4):727–33.
13. Pereira SP, Rowbotham D, Fitt S, Shearer MJ, Wendon J, Williams R. Pharmacokinetics and efficacy of oral versus intravenous mixed-micellar phylloquinone (vitamin K1) in severe acute liver disease. J Hepatol. 2005;42(3):365–70.
14. Langley PG, Williams R. Physiological inhibitors of coagulation in fulminant hepatic failure. Blood Coagul Fibrinolysis. 1992;3(3):243–7.
15. Hollestelle MJ, Loots CM, Squizzato A, Renné T, Bouma BJ, De Groot PG, et al. Decreased active von Willebrand factor level owing to shear stress in aortic stenosis patients. J Thromb Haemost. 2011;9(5):953–8.
16. Turner N, Nolasco L, Tao Z, Dong J-F, Moake J. Human endothelial cells synthesize and release ADAMTS-13. J Thromb Haemost. 2006;4(6):1396–404.
17. Uemura M, Fujimura Y, Matsumoto M, Ishizashi H, Kato S, Matsuyama T, et al. Comprehensive analysis of ADAMTS13 in patients with liver cirrhosis. Thromb Haemost. 2008;99(6):1019–29.
18. Kerr R, Newsome P, Germain L, Thomson E, Dawson P, Stirling D, et al. Effects of acute liver injury on blood coagulation. J Thromb Haemost. 2003;1(4):754–9.
19. Peck-Radosavljevic M, Wichlas M, Zacherl J, Stiegler G, Stohlawetz P, Fuchsjäger M, et al. Thrombopoietin induces rapid resolution of thrombocytopenia after orthotopic liver transplantation through increased platelet production. Blood. 2000;95(3):795–801.
20. García-Suárez J, Burgaleta C, Hernanz N, Albarran F, Tobaruela P, Alvarez-Mon M. HCV-associated thrombocytopenia: clinical characteristics and platelet response after recombinant alpha2b-interferon therapy. Br J Haematol. 2000;110(1):98–103.
21. Ballard HS. Hematological complications of alcoholism. Alcohol Clin Exp Res. 1989;13(5):706–20.
22. Nagamine T, Ohtuka T, Takehara K, Arai T, Takagi H, Mori M. Thrombocytopenia associated with hepatitis C viral infection. J Hepatol. 1996;24(2):135–40.
23. Feistauer SM, Penner E, Mayr WR, Panzer S. Target platelet antigens of autoantibodies in patients with primary biliary cirrhosis. Hepatology. 1997;25(6):1343–5. Wiley Subscription Services, Inc. A Wiley Company.
24. Afdhal N, McHutchison J, Brown R, Jacobson I, Manns M, Poordad F, et al. Thrombocytopenia associated with chronic liver disease. J Hepatol. 2008;48(6):1000–7.

25. Lisman T, Bongers TN, Janssen HLA, de Maat MPM, de Groot PG, Leebeek FWG. Elevated levels of von Willebrand factor in cirrhosis support platelet adhesion despite reduced functional capacity. Hepatology. 2006;44(1):53–61.
26. Hugenholtz GCG, Adelmeijer J, Meijers JCM, Porte RJ, Stravitz RT, Lisman T. An unbalance between von Willebrand factor and ADAMTS13 in acute liver failure: implications for hemostasis and clinical outcome. Hepatology. 2013;58(2):752–61.
27. Reuken PA, Kussmann A, Kiehntopf M, Budde U, Stallmach A, Claus RA, et al. Imbalance of von Willebrand factor and its cleaving protease ADAMTS13 during systemic inflammation superimposed on advanced cirrhosis. Liver Int. 2015;35(1):37–45.
28. Robson SC, Kahn D, Kruskal J, Bird AR, Kirsch RE. Disordered hemostasis in extrahepatic portal hypertension. Hepatology. 1993;18(4):853–7.
29. Rubin MH, Weston MJ, Bullock G, Roberts J, Langley PG, White YS, et al. Abnormal platelet function and ultrastructure in fulminant hepatic failure. Q J Med. 1977;46(183):339–52.
30. Escolar G, Cases A, Viñas M, Pino M, Calls J, Cirera I, et al. Evaluation of acquired platelet dysfunctions in uremic and cirrhotic patients using the platelet function analyzer (PFA-100): influence of hematocrit elevation. Haematologica. 1999;84(7):614–9.
31. Lisman T, Adelmeijer J, De Groot PG, HLA J, FWG L. No evidence for an intrinsic platelet defect in patients with liver cirrhosis – studies under flow conditions. J Thromb Haemost. 2006;4(9):2070–2. Blackwell Publishing Ltd.
32. Pihusch R, Rank A, Göhring P, Pihusch M, Hiller E, Beuers U. Platelet function rather than plasmatic coagulation explains hypercoagulable state in cholestatic liver disease. J Hepatol. 2002;37(5):548–55.
33. Wolberg AS. Thrombin generation and fibrin clot structure. Blood Rev. 2007;21(3):131–42.
34. Wolberg AS. Plasma and cellular contributions to fibrin network formation, structure and stability. Blood. 2010;16 Suppl 3(Suppl. 1):7–12. Blackwell Publishing Ltd.
35. Segal H, Cottam S, Potter D, Hunt BJ. Coagulation and fibrinolysis in primary biliary cirrhosis compared with other liver disease and during orthotopic liver transplantation. Hepatology. 1997;25(3):683–8. Wiley Subscription Services, Inc. A Wiley Company.
36. Senzolo M, Burra P, Cholongitas E, Burroughs AK. New insights into the coagulopathy of liver disease and liver transplantation. World J Gastroenterol. 2006;12(48):7725–36. Baishideng Publishing Group Inc.
37. Martinez J, MacDonald KA, Palascak JE. The role of sialic acid in the dysfibrinogenemia associated with liver disease: distribution of sialic acid on the constituent chains. Blood. 1983;61(6):1196–202.
38. Huber K, Kirchheimer JC, Korninger C, Binder BR. Hepatic synthesis and clearance of components of the fibrinolytic system in healthy volunteers and in patients with different stages of liver cirrhosis. Thromb Res. 1991;62(5):491–500.
39. Agarwal S, Joyner KA, Swaim MW. Ascites fluid as a possible origin for hyperfibrinolysis in advanced liver disease. Am J Gastroenterol. 2000;95(11):3218–24.
40. Pernambuco JR, Langley PG, Hughes RD, Izumi S, Williams R. Activation of the fibrinolytic system in patients with fulminant liver failure. Hepatology. 1993;18(6):1350–6.
41. Lisman T, Bakhtiari K, Adelmeijer J, Meijers JCM, Porte RJ, Stravitz RT. Intact thrombin generation and decreased fibrinolytic capacity in patients with acute liver injury or acute liver failure. J Thromb Haemost. 2012;10(7):1312–9.
42. Lisman T, Leebeek FW, Mosnier LO, Bouma BN, Meijers JC, Janssen HL, et al. Thrombin-activatable fibrinolysis inhibitor deficiency in cirrhosis is not associated with increased plasma fibrinolysis. Gastroenterology. 2001;121(1):131–9.
43. Haas T, Spielmann N, Mauch J, Madjdpour C, Speer O, Schmugge M, et al. Comparison of thromboelastometry (ROTEM(R)) with standard plasmatic coagulation testing in paediatric surgery. Br J Anaesth. 2011;108(1):36–41.
44. Davenport R, Manson J, De'Ath H, Platton S, Coates A, Allard S, et al. Functional definition and characterization of acute traumatic coagulopathy. Crit Care Med. 2011;39(12):2652–8.
45. Toulon P, Ozier Y, Ankri A, Fléron M-H, Leroux G, Samama C-M. Point-of-care versus central laboratory coagulation testing during haemorrhagic surgery. A Multicenter Study. Thromb Haemost. 2009;101(2):394–401.

46. Haas T, Fries D, Tanaka KA, Asmis L, Curry NS, Schöchl H. Usefulness of standard plasma coagulation tests in the management of perioperative coagulopathic bleeding: is there any evidence? Br J Anaesth. 2015;114(2):217–24. Oxford University Press
47. American Society of Anesthesiologists Task Force on Perioperative Blood Management. Practice guidelines for perioperative blood management: an updated report by the American Society of Anesthesiologists Task Force on Perioperative Blood Management. Anesthesiology. 2015;122:241–75.
48. Rossaint R, Bouillon B, Cerny V, Coats TJ, Duranteau J, Fernández-Mondéjar E, et al. The European guideline on management of major bleeding and coagulopathy following trauma: fourth edition. Crit Care. 2016;20(1):1–55.
49. PA O, Aas K. The control of dicumarol therapy and the quantitative determination of prothrombin and proconvertin. Scand J Clin Lab Invest. 1951;3(3):201–8.
50. Ewe K. Bleeding after liver biopsy does not correlate with indices of peripheral coagulation. Dig Dis Sci. 1981;26(5):388–93.
51. Massicotte L, Thibeault L, Roy A. Classical notions of coagulation revisited in relation with blood losses, transfusion rate for 700 consecutive liver transplantations. Semin Thromb Hemost. 2015;41(5):538–46. Thieme Medical Publishers.
52. Kamath PS, Wiesner RH, Malinchoc M, Kremers W, Therneau TM, Kosberg CL, et al. A model to predict survival in patients with end-stage liver disease. Hepatology. 2001;33(2):464–70. WB Saunders.
53. Kitchens CS. To bleed or not to bleed? Is that the question for the PTT? J Thromb Haemost. 2005;3(12):2607–11. Blackwell Science Inc.
54. BOWYER A, KITCHEN S, Makris M. The responsiveness of different APTT reagents to mild factor VIII, IX and XI deficiencies. Int Jnl Lab Hem. 2010;33(2):154–8.
55. Mitsuguro M, Okamoto A, Shironouchi Y, Sano M, Miyata S, Neki R, et al. Effects of factor VIII levels on the APTT and anti-Xa activity under a therapeutic dose of heparin. Int J Hematol. 2014;101(2):119–25.
56. Ng VL. Prothrombin time and partial thromboplastin time assay considerations. Clin Lab Med. 2009;29(2):253–63.
57. Palascak JE, Martinez J. Dysfibrinogenemia associated with liver disease. J Clin Invest. 1977;60(1):89–95. American Society for Clinical Investigation.
58. de Maat MPM, Nieuwenhuizen W, Knot EAR, van Buuren HR, Swart GR. Measuring plasma fibrinogen levels in patients with liver cirrhosis. The occurrence of proteolytic fibrin(ogen) degradation products and their influence on several fibrinogen assays. Thromb Res. 1995;78(4):353–62.
59. Thakrar SV, Mallett SV. Thrombocytopenia in cirrhosis: impact of fibrinogen on bleeding risk. World J Hepatol. 2017;9(6):318–9.
60. Dötsch TM, Dirkmann D, Bezinover D, Hartmann M, Treckmann JW, Paul A, et al. Assessment of standard laboratory tests and rotational thromboelastometry for the prediction of postoperative bleeding in liver transplantation. Br J Anaesth. 2017;119(3):402–10.
61. Blasi A, Beltran J, Pereira A, Martinez-Palli G, Torrents A, Balust J, et al. An assessment of thromboelastometry to monitor blood coagulation and guide transfusion support in liver transplantation. Transfusion. 2012;52(9):1989–98. Blackwell Publishing Inc.
62. Lancé MD. A general review of major global coagulation assays: thrombelastography, thrombin generation test and clot waveform analysis. Thromb J. 2015;13(1):2607–6.
63. Hemker HC, Dicri Al R, Béguin S. Thrombin generation assays: accruing clinical relevance. Curr Opin Hematol. 2004;11(3):170–5.
64. Tripodi A, Mannucci PM. The coagulopathy of chronic liver disease. N Engl J Med. 2011;365(2):147–56.
65. Gatt A, Riddell A, Calvaruso V, Tuddenham EG, Makris M, Burroughs AK. Enhanced thrombin generation in patients with cirrhosis-induced coagulopathy. J Thromb Haemost. 2010;8(9):1994–2000. Blackwell Publishing Ltd.
66. Tripodi A, Legnani C, Lemma L, Cosmi B, Palareti G, Chantarangkul V, et al. Abnormal Protac-induced coagulation inhibition chromogenic assay results are associated with an increased risk of recurrent venous thromboembolism. J Thromb Thrombolysis. 2010;30(2):215–9. Springer US.

67. Tripodi A, Primignani M, Lemma L, Chantarangkul V, Mannucci PM. Evidence that low protein C contributes to the procoagulant imbalance in cirrhosis. J Hepatol. 2013;59:265.
68. Tripodi A, Primignani M, Chantarangkul V, Clerici M, Dell'era A, Fabris F, et al. Thrombin generation in patients with cirrhosis: the role of platelets. Hepatology. 2006;44(2):440–5. Wiley Subscription Services, Inc., A Wiley Company.
69. Tripodi A, Cappellini MD, Chantarangkul V, Padovan L, Fasulo MR, Marcon A, et al. Hypercoagulability in splenectomized thalassemic patients detected by whole-blood thromboelastometry, but not by thrombin generation in platelet-poor plasma. Haematologica. 2009;94(11):1520–7.
70. Tripodi A, Primignani M, Chantarangkul V, Lemma L, Jovani M, Rebulla P, et al. Global hemostasis tests in patients with cirrhosis before and after prophylactic platelet transfusion. Liver Int. 2012;33(3):362–7.
71. Mosnier LO. Platelet factor 4 inhibits Thrombomodulin-dependent activation of thrombin-activatable fibrinolysis inhibitor (TAFI) by thrombin. J Biol Chem. 2010;286(1):502–10.
72. Hartert H. Blutgerunngunsstudien mit dem Thrombelastographen, einem neuen Untersuchungsverfahren. Klin Wochenschr. 1948;26(37/38):577–83.
73. Herbstreit F, Winter EM, Peters J, Hartmann M. Monitoring of haemostasis in liver transplantation: comparison of laboratory based and point of care tests. Anaesthesia. 2010;65(1):44–9.
74. Blasi A, Muñoz G, de Soto I, Mellado R, Taura P, Rios J, et al. Reliability of thromboelastometry for detecting the safe coagulation threshold in patients taking acenocoumarol after elective heart valve replacement. Thromb Res. 2015;136(3):669–72.
75. Larsen OH, Fenger-Eriksen C, Christiansen K, Ingerslev J, Sørensen B. Diagnostic performance and therapeutic consequence of thromboelastometry activated by kaolin versus a panel of specific reagents. Anesthesiology. 2011;115(2):294–302.
76. Sakai T, Matsusaki T, Dai F, Tanaka KA, Donaldson JB, Hilmi IA, et al. Pulmonary thromboembolism during adult liver transplantation: incidence, clinical presentation, outcome, risk factors, and diagnostic predictors. Br J Anaesth. 2012;108(3):469–77.
77. Song J-G, Jeong S-M, Jun I-G, Lee H-M, Hwang G-S. Five-minute parameter of thromboelastometry is sufficient to detect thrombocytopenia and hypofibrinogenaemia in patients undergoing liver transplantation. Br J Anaesth. 2014;112(2):290–7. Oxford University Press.
78. Coakley M, Reddy K, Mackie I, Mallett S. Transfusion triggers in Orthotopic liver transplantation: a comparison of the Thromboelastometry analyzer, the Thromboelastogram, and conventional coagulation tests. J Cardiothorac Vasc Anesth. 2006;20(4):548–53.
79. Kirchner C, Dirkmann D, Treckmann JW, Paul A, Hartmann M, Saner FH, et al. Coagulation management with factor concentrates in liver transplantation: a single-center experience. Transfusion. 2014;54(10 Pt 2):2760–8.
80. Görlinger K. Coagulation management during liver transplantation. Hamostaseologie. 2006;26(3 Suppl 1):64–76.
81. Roullet S, Pillot J, Freyburger G, Biais M, Quinart A, Rault A, et al. Rotation thromboelastometry detects thrombocytopenia and hypofibrinogenaemia during orthotopic liver transplantation. Br J Anaesth. 2010;104(4):422–8. Oxford University Press.
82. Jeong S-M, Song J-G, Seo H, Choi J-H, Jang D-M, Hwang G-S. Quantification of both platelet count and fibrinogen concentration using maximal clot firmness of Thromboelastometry during liver transplantation. Transplant Proc. 2015;47(6):1890–5.
83. Pereboom ITA, de Boer MT, Haagsma EB, Hendriks HGD, Lisman T, Porte RJ. Platelet transfusion during liver transplantation is associated with increased postoperative mortality due to acute lung injury. Anesth Analg. 2009;108(4):1083–91.
84. Görlinger K, Dirkmann D, Solomon C, Hanke AA. Fast interpretation of thromboelastometry in non-cardiac surgery: reliability in patients with hypo-, normo-, and hypercoagulability. Br J Anaesth. 2013;110(2):222–30.
85. Dirkmann D, Görlinger K, Peters J. Assessment of early thromboelastometric variables from extrinsically activated assays with and without aprotinin for rapid detection of fibrinolysis. Anesth Analg. 2014;119(3):533–42.

86. Mallett SV, Armstrong M. Point-of-care monitoring of haemostasis. Anaesthesia. 2015;70 Suppl 1(Suppl 4):73–7, e25–6.
87. Wang S-C, Shieh J-F, Chang K-Y, Chu Y-C, Liu C-S, Loong C-C, et al. Thromboelastography-guided transfusion decreases intraoperative blood transfusion during orthotopic liver transplantation: randomized clinical trial. Transplant Proc. 2010;42(7):2590–3.
88. Kozek-Langenecker SA, Ahmed AB, Afshari A, Albaladejo P, Aldecoa C, Barauskas G, et al. Management of severe perioperative bleeding. Eur J Anaesthesiol. 2017;34(6):332–95.
89. Mallett SV, Chowdary P, Burroughs AK. Clinical utility of viscoelastic tests of coagulation in patients with liver disease. Liver Int. 2013;33(7):961–74.
90. Corredor C, Wasowicz M, Karkouti K, Sharma V. The role of point-of-care platelet function testing in predicting postoperative bleeding following cardiac surgery: a systematic review and meta-analysis. Anaesthesia. 2015;70(6):715–31.
91. Schulte am Esch J, Akyildiz A, Tustas RY, Ganschow R, Schmelzle M, Krieg A, et al. ADP-dependent platelet function prior to and in the early course of pediatric liver transplantation and persisting thrombocytopenia are positively correlated with ischemia/reperfusion injury. Transpl Int. 2010;23(7):745–52.
92. Esch JSA, Jurk K, Knoefel WT, Roeder G, Voss H, Tustas RY, et al. Platelet activation and increased tissue factor expression on monocytes in reperfusion injury following orthotopic liver transplantation. Platelets. 2010;21(5):348–59.
93. Femia EA, Scavone M, Lecchi A, Cattaneo M. Effect of platelet count on platelet aggregation measured with impedance aggregometry (multiplate™ analyzer) and with light transmission aggregometry. J Thromb Haemost. 2013;11(12):2193–6.
94. Kakouros N, Kickler TS, Laws KM, Rade JJ. Hematocrit alters VerifyNow P2Y12 assay results independently of intrinsic platelet reactivity and clopidogrel responsiveness. J Thromb Haemost. 2013;11(10):1814–22.
95. Janssen PWA, Bergmeijer TO, Godschalk TC, Le TTD, Breet NJ, Kelder JC, et al. The effect of correcting VerifyNow P2Y12 assay results for hematocrit in patients undergoing percutaneous coronary interventions. J Thromb Haemost. 2017;15(4):618–23.
96. Le Quellec S, Bordet JC, Negrier C, Dargaud Y. Comparison of current platelet functional tests for the assessment of aspirin and clopidogrel response. Thromb Haemost. 2016;116(4):638–50. Schattauer Publishers.
97. Karon BS, Tolan NV, Koch CD, Wockenfus AM, Miller RS, Lingineni RK, et al. Precision and reliability of 5 platelet function tests in healthy volunteers and donors on daily antiplatelet agent therapy. Clin Chem. 2014;60(12):1524–31.
98. Saner FH, Abeysundara L, Hartmann M, Mallett SV. Rational approach to transfusion in liver transplantation. Minerva Anestesiol. 2018;84(3):378–88.
99. Giannini EG, Stravitz RT, Caldwell SH. Correction of hemostatic abnormalities and portal pressure variations in patients with cirrhosis. Hepatology. 2014;60:1442.
100. Sarani B, Dunkman WJ, Dean L, Sonnad S, Rohrbach JI, Gracias VH. Transfusion of fresh frozen plasma in critically ill surgical patients is associated with an increased risk of infection. Crit Care Med. 2008;36:1114–8.
101. Abdel-Wahab OI, Healy B, Dzik WH. Effect of fresh-frozen plasma transfusion on prothrombin time and bleeding in patients with mild coagulation abnormalities. Transfusion. 2006;46:1279–85.
102. Abuelkasem E, Hasan S, Mazzeffi MA, Planinsic RM, Sakai T, Tanaka KA. Reduced requirement for prothrombin complex concentrate for the restoration of thrombin generation in plasma from liver transplant recipients. Anesth Analg. 2017;125:609–15.
103. De Pietri L, Bianchini M, Montalti R, et al. Thrombelastography-guided blood product use before invasive procedures in cirrhosis with severe coagulopathy: a randomized, controlled trial. Hepatology. 2016;63:566–73.
104. Leon-Justel A, Noval-Padillo JA, Alvarez-Rios AI, et al. Point-of-care haemostasis monitoring during liver transplantation reduces transfusion requirements and improves patient outcome. Clin Chim Acta. 2015;446:277–83.

105. Hofmann M, Schumann C, Zimmer G, Henzel K, Locher U, Leuschner U. LUV's lipid composition modulates diffusion of bile acids. Chem Phys Lipids. 2001;110:165–71.
106. Scherer R, Gille A, Erhard J, Paar D, Kox WJ. The effect of substitution with AT III- and PPSB-concentrates in patients with terminal liver insufficiency. Anaesthesist. 1994;43:178–82.
107. Saner FH, Kirchner C. Monitoring and treatment of coagulation disorders in end-stage liver disease. Visc Med. 2016;32:241–8.
108. Solomon C, Pichlmaier U, Schoechl H, et al. Recovery of fibrinogen after administration of fibrinogen concentrate to patients with severe bleeding after cardiopulmonary bypass surgery. Br J Anaesth. 2010;104:555–62.
109. Tanaka KA, Bader SO, Gorlinger K. Novel approaches in management of perioperative coagulopathy. Curr Opin Anaesthesiol. 2014;27:72–80.
110. Poon KS, Chen CC, Thorat A, et al. Fibrinolysis after reperfusion of liver graft. Acta Anaesthesiol Taiwanica. 2015;53:41–3.
111. Villa E, Cammà C, Marietta M, Luongo M, Critelli R, Colopi S, et al. Enoxaparin prevents portal vein thrombosis and liver decompensation in patients with advanced cirrhosis. Gastroenterology. 2012;143(5):1253–60.e1–4. Elsevier.
112. Bechmann LP, Sichau M, Wichert M, Gerken G, Kröger K, Hilgard P. Low-molecular-weight heparin in patients with advanced cirrhosis. Liver Int. 2011;31(1):75–82.
113. Maruyama H, Takahashi M, Shimada T, Yokosuka O. Emergency anticoagulation treatment for cirrhosis patients with portal vein thrombosis and acute variceal bleeding. Scand J Gastroenterol. 2012;47(6):686–91.
114. Hall TC, Garcea G, Metcalfe M, Bilk D, Rajesh A, Dennison A. Impact of anticoagulation on outcomes in acute non-cirrhotic and non- malignant portal vein thrombosis: a retrospective observational study. Hepato-Gastroenterology. 2013;60(122):311–7.
115. Beiderlinden M, Treschan TA, Görlinger K, Peters J. Argatroban anticoagulation in critically ill patients. Ann Pharmacother. 2007;41(5):749–54. SAGE Publications Sage CA: Los Angeles, CA.
116. Doepker B, Mount KL, Ryder LJ, Gerlach AT, Murphy CV, Philips GS. Bleeding risk factors associated with argatroban therapy in the critically ill. J Thromb Thrombolysis. 2012;34(4):491–8.

Chapter 8
Management of Thrombosis in the Liver Transplant Candidate

Alberto Zanetto and Marco Senzolo

Coagulopathy in Cirrhosis

Liver cirrhosis is characterized by profound and complex hemostatic alterations that can lead to bleeding or thrombotic complications. Patients usually have pro-hemorrhagic alterations including thrombocytopenia and reduced plasma levels of coagulation factors. Vitamin K deficiency is also frequently found in for these patients and is usually associated with malabsorption/malnutrition. Concurrently, they also have pro-thrombotic abnormalities due to decreased concentrations of anticoagulant factors and increased concentrations of prothrombotic factor VIII (FVIII) and von Willebrand factor (vWF). Dysfibrinogenemia, enhanced fibrinolysis, impaired clearance of activated clotting factors, plasminogen activators, and fibrinogen degradation products contribute to the final hemostatic state in end-stage liver disease [1, 2].

Whereas vWF is synthesized by the endothelium [3] and FVIII is synthesized by hepatic sinusoidal cells and the endothelium, the liver is the site of synthesis for fibrinogen and factors II, V, VII, IX, X, XI, and XII [4, 5]. Thus, the plasma concentration of FVIII does not decrease with liver disease, and may even be elevated due to profound endothelial dysfunction [6]. This leads to an increase in endothelial synthesis and a reduced clearance via low-density lipoprotein receptor-related protein [3] of vWF. The level of vWF is subsequently increased but with reduced biological activity of the synthetized vWF [7].

Vitamin K is an essential cofactor for the production of biologically active forms of the coagulation factors II, VII, IX, and X, enhancing hepatic post-ribosomal conversion of specific glutamic acid residues in the protein precursors to γ-carboxyglutamic acid (Gla). These active forms of the clotting factors chelate calcium at the Gla site, resulting in effective hemostatic function. When γ-carboxylation is impaired

A. Zanetto · M. Senzolo (✉)
Multivisceral Transplant Unit, Gastroenterology, Department of Surgery, Oncology and Gastroenterology, Padua University Hospital, Padua, Italy

D. Bezinover, F. Saner (eds.), *Critical Care for Potential Liver Transplant Candidates*,
https://doi.org/10.1007/978-3-319-92934-7_8

due to a deficiency or antagonism of vitamin K, inert precursors are synthetized (known as "proteins induced by vitamin K absence (PIVKA)") and released into the bloodstream [8]. However, the clinical significance of these modified precursors is not clear. In cholestasis, the reduction of vitamin K absorption from the small intestine due to decreased bile salt production can be countered with parenteral administration of vitamin K at 10 mg daily for 24–48 h. However, in parenchymal liver disease, decreased levels of coagulation factors are due to decreased synthesis, so no improvement can be achieved with vitamin K administration. About 25% of patients with acute liver injury have a subclinical deficit of vitamin K. These patients may benefit from parenteral administration with corresponding improvement of their international normalized ratio (INR).

Antithrombin III (ATIII) is a non-vitamin K-dependent glycoprotein synthesized in the liver as well in the endothelium. Its concentration is reduced in patients with liver disease, due to reduced synthesis and/or increased consumption in the case of hyperfibrinolysis [9].

Proteins C and S are vitamin K-dependent glycoproteins synthesized mainly by hepatocytes [10]. During acute or chronic liver disease, their concentrations can be decreased concomitantly with the other coagulation factors, but rarely below 20% of normal values [11]. However, in the case of severe liver disease, plasma levels may be very low. Excluding a coexistent genetic deficiency can be difficult [12]. A concomitant finding of a normal level of FII and protein C/FVII ratio can help to confirm a coexistent genetic deficit. In acquired deficiency of vitamin K, a defective protein C lacking γ-carboxyl (PIVKA) is produced [13].

A rebalanced hemostatic status in chronic liver disease can easily tip toward bleeding or thrombotic complications. Patients with cirrhosis are not "auto-anticoagulated," as previously thought, but actually have a greater risk than their non-cirrhotic counterparts of developing thrombotic complications [2, 14].

In patients with significant liver disease, both pro- and anti-coagulation factors are affected, but routine coagulation tests usually demonstrate a bleeding tendency and unfortunately do not reflect hypercoagulability.

Global coagulation tests such as the thrombin generation test [TG] [15], rotational thromboelastometry (ROTEM), and thromboelastography (TEG) are able to detect the overall coagulation state in cirrhosis.

The TG assay has shown that not only is the amount of thrombin in cirrhotic patients similar to that of healthy subjects, but also that the balance may tend toward hypercoagulability, especially in patients with more severe liver disease (Child C). In a study performed on 40 healthy controls and 10 patients undergoing liver transplantation for end-stage liver disease, Lisman and collaborators demonstrated that total TG in plasma from healthy volunteers substantially decreased upon the addition of soluble thrombomodulin (ETP without TM (thrombomodulin), 1752 nM min, range [987–2665]; however, mean ETP with TM, 761 [125–1766], $p < 0.0001$), TG was only minimally reduced after the addition of TM in cirrhotic patients [16].

Whole blood ROTEM and TEG are viscoelastic global tests (VETs) that evaluate clot formation and stability as the result of the interplay between plasma coagulation factors and platelets (aggregation, clot strengthening, fibrin cross-linking, and fibrinolysis) [17].

VETs make it possible to monitor changes that occur in clotting blood in an environment that mimics in vivo conditions and can show composite results of the interaction between plasma, blood cells, and platelets and are, therefore, very appropriate laboratory tools for investigating cirrhosis.

It has been shown that VETs can be used to identify cirrhotic patients at higher risk of bleeding to optimize transfusion therapy [18] and patients at higher risk of developing thrombotic complications to optimize anticoagulant therapy [19].

Portal Vein Thrombosis

Epidemiology

Portal vein thrombosis (PVT) represents the most common thrombotic complication occurring in patients with cirrhosis. The 1-year incidence ranges from 7.4% to 11% in prospective studies [19–27]. The prevalence varies in different investigations and depends on the type of diagnostic approach used and on the inclusion or exclusion of patients with hepatocellular carcinoma (HCC) due to the higher risk of thrombotic complications in cancer patients [19]. In a published series of LT candidates without HCC, PVT was shown as ranging from 2.1% to 23.3% [28]. In an autopsy study representing 84% of all inhospital deaths in Malmo (Sweden), the lifetime cumulative prevalence of PVT was found to be 1.0%, and patients with both cirrhosis and HCC had the highest PVT risk (OR 17.1; 95% CI 11.1–26.4) [29]. In a single-center prospective study including 41 HCC patients, the 1-year incidence of non-neoplastic PVT was 24.4% [19].

Pathophysiology and Risk Factors

The pathogenesis of PVT is likely to be multifactorial, and both the local and systemic factors can be responsible for thromboses [30].

The occurrence of pathological thrombosis is determined by an alteration in the equilibrium that regulates both coagulation and anticoagulation. The rebalanced hemostatic status in liver cirrhosis, unlike under physiological conditions, is not able to accommodate dynamic changes, especially in cases of exogenous stimuli. Any shifts in one or more of the coagulation components may result in thrombosis.

Even though cirrhotic patients are exposed to a higher risk of non-splanchnic thrombotic complications than is the case for the general population, the most frequent site of thrombosis is the portal vein. This suggests that local factors are involved in the development of PVT [31]. In patients with end-stage liver disease (ESLD), splanchnic vasodilatation and architectural derangement are responsible for venous stasis. In a prospective study evaluating a cohort of 73 cirrhotic patients, reduced portal flow velocity below 15 cm/s was the only independent variable that correlated with the risk of developing PVT at 1 year follow-up [21].

The risk of PVT has been demonstrated to be independently associated with both the severity of liver disease and portal hypertension (PH). Previous procedures to treat PH including sclerotherapy, transjugular intrahepatic portosystemic shunt (TIPS), shunt surgery, and previous splenectomy, as well as Child-Pugh C cirrhosis are factors that have been found to be significantly associated with an increased risk of PVT [32].

One of the main determinants of in vitro hypercoagulability that occurs in cirrhosis seems to be an intrinsic resistance to the anticoagulant action of thrombomodulin (TM). Whether this is truly representative of in vivo hypercoagulability remains to be fully established. In a recent retrospective study, La Mura et al. demonstrated a significant correlation between resistance to TM and the risk of de novo PVT [33].

The possible role of inherited thrombophilic abnormalities has been advocated in several cross-sectional studies reporting a thrombophilic genotype in up to 9% of cirrhotic patients with PVT. In this scenario, the G20210A prothrombin gene variant is the most common abnormality associated with PVT [34–36]. Despite these findings, screening for thrombophilic conditions is not routinely recommended in cirrhosis [37].

Finally, despite the scarcity of HCC-related hypercoagulability data, it has been demonstrated that plasma fibrinogen is overproduced by HCC and the hypercoagulability in HCC patients is associated with an increased risk of PVT, even in patients with well-compensated liver disease (Child A patients) [19].

Natural History, Clinical Manifestations, and Treatment

PVT can resolve without treatment. Spontaneous recanalization has been described in up to 40% of cases (mainly in cases of partial PVT) [26, 38]. Progression of thrombosis has been reported in 48% to 70% of patients at 2-year follow-up [38, 39].

PVT in cirrhotic patients is often asymptomatic and detected at follow-up ultrasound evaluation. In other instances, PVT is diagnosed at the time of liver decompensation. In a study of 79 cirrhotic patients with newly diagnosed PVT, 39% presented with gastrointestinal bleeding (from varices or portal hypertensive gastropathy) and 18% had abdominal pain. From this subpopulation, 70% had intestinal infarction due to the extension of the thrombus into the mesenteric vein [35]. Luca et al. reported increased mortality in patients who had stable or progressive thrombus (39.1%) versus those who improved (15.8%) [38].

PVT itself increases PH and consequently elevates the risk of variceal bleeding. PVT was independently associated with the risk of failure to control acute variceal bleeding and re-bleeding in a multi-center prospective cohort study in which over 450 cirrhotic patients with upper gastrointestinal bleeding (OR 3.18; $P = 0.002$) were analyzed [40].

Whether PVT itself has any impact on liver function is still a matter of debate. In their prospective multi-center study, Nery et al. analyzed data from ultrasound screening for HCC (at 3 and 6 months) to evaluate the clinical impact of PVT on disease progression. The 5-year cumulative incidence of PVT was 9.23%. PVT was mostly partial (73%) and varied over time. Indeed, during the 80 months of follow-up, 70% of patients had spontaneous complete recanalization of the portal vein. Disease progression was not associated with the prior development of PVT, and decompensation episodes were not related to PVT occurrence [26]. However, the available data are conflicting and sparse. Prospective studies taking into account both the severity of liver disease and the characteristics of thrombosis are needed [41].

If liver disease deteriorates and a patient becomes a candidate for LT, preoperative PVT can affect the perioperative course.

Complete PVT at the time of surgery is a risk factor for early mortality, especially if the thrombosis extends to the splenomesenteric confluence and requires a vascular reconstruction in the recipient.

Several authors have classified PVT according to its extent and severity. However, the most widely used and recommended classification in the setting of LT is proposed by Yerdel et al. [32]. The classification is based on the extent of the thrombosis and the presence/adequacy of collaterals that can potentially be used for extra-anatomic reconstructions to establish portal venous flow. This classification is considered to be the most accurate because it correlates the extent of the thrombosis with the surgical technique and with the outcome. In a systematic review performed by Rodriguez et al., the authors demonstrated that when PVT is complete (Grade III according to Yerdel's classification), 30-day and 1-year posttransplant survival rates are compromised (HR 5.65 [95% CI, 2–15.96], $p = 0.001$ and HR 2.48 [95% CI, 0.99–6.17], respectively) [28]. In fact, in the case of complete obstruction of the portal vein with extension into the superior mesenteric vein, venous jump graft reconstruction or arterialization of the portal vein needs to be performed. Non-anatomic solutions, particularly portacaval hemi-transposition (PCHT), do not solve PH, which complicates the postoperative course of these patients and compromises quality of life in most cases [42, 43]. In a series evaluating posttransplant patients with PCHT, all of them developed temporary ascites and renal insufficiency. Twenty percent of the patients faced recurrent gastroesophageal bleeding. Overall 1-year mortality was 40% (4/11). In a more recent case series of six patients by Ravaioli et al. [44], 100% of them developed renal failure and/or ascites during the postoperative period. Ceulemans et al. [45] reported a good outcome of five patients with operatively confirmed complete splanchnic thrombosis transplanted with the PCHT technique. Graft and patient survival rates were 100% at 3 months after LT and 60% survived 1 year.

Based on the above considerations, a patient should not be refused LT, as long as an acceptable surgical risk based on comorbidities is present and an adequate transplant benefit is expected. Considering the challenging management of complications related to residual PH, the potential transplant benefit to these patients must be discussed.

Published data about the rate of thrombosis progression in patients awaiting LT have demonstrated that PVT should be treated as early as possible, as stated in the European Association for the Study of the Liver (EASL) Clinical Practice Guidelines for the management of vascular liver diseases [37].

The aim of anticoagulation therapy should be the recanalization of the vessel or reduction of the thrombosis in order to ensure anatomical reconstruction. Recurrence after the withdrawal of anticoagulation therapy is high, and prolonged anticoagulation should be performed until the transplant can be performed [46].

Adequate pretransplant screening for thromboses with subsequent prompt treatment is mandatory, and the risk-benefit ratio of anticoagulation prior to LT should be assessed in every case.

Anticoagulant Treatment in Portal Vein Thrombosis

Evidence from several studies has shown the safety and efficacy of anticoagulation for the treatment of PVT in patients with liver cirrhosis. Ageno et al. [47] recently reported the results of a multi-center prospective cohort including 604 consecutive patients (149 cirrhotics) with splanchnic vein thrombosis (SVT). Anticoagulant treatment was safe and effective and was associated with a reduced risk of recurrent splanchnic thrombosis (8.2 95%CI, 4.1–16.5 vs. 14.1 95%CI, 7.6–26.2 in non-treated patients). Furthermore, most of the documented bleeding events occurred in the absence of anticoagulation therapy including two fatal events in untreated high-risk patients with liver cirrhosis and esophageal varices. The results of the multivariable analysis suggested a benefit of anticoagulant treatment in this patient population, with a low risk of major bleeding and vascular events. Although it is likely that the patients who received anticoagulation therapy represented a population at lower risk, the rates of hemorrhage in patients who received anticoagulants were no higher than in those who did not receive anticoagulants, and the fatality rate for major bleeding events in patients receiving anticoagulation treatment was 0%.

Unfortunately, no randomized controlled trials have been conducted yet, and the evidence for the effectiveness of anticoagulation therapy for PVT treatment is based on case series. Different treatment strategies have been adopted in cirrhotic patients with PVT, including the use of low molecular weight heparin (LMWH), vitamin K antagonist (VKA), or different drugs in succession.

To date, data on the efficacy and safety of medical anticoagulation to treat PVT come from seven cohort studies that taken together included 258 patients, most with partial PVT (143/200, 71.5%) (Table 8.1) [20, 39, 46, 48–51]. Globally, the recanalization rate ranged from 56% to 76%.

Among the various published cohorts, pretreatment predictive factors of anticoagulant treatment efficacy were analyzed in six studies, demonstrating a relatively strong correlation between early anticoagulation and the likelihood of recanalization. In fact, beginning anticoagulation treatment less than 6 months after PVT diagnosis is the most important factor for a positive response to therapy [37]. Other factors, such as the involvement of mesenteric veins and/or the severity of baseline liver disease, have been also advocated as possible predictive factors [48, 49].

Table 8.1 Published cohorts of cirrhotic patients with PVT treated with LMWH and/or VKA

Author, year (ref.)	N°	Type of anticoagulation	Dose	EBL	Duration of anticoagulation	PVT (total/partial)	Extension to splanchnic vessels	Portal cavernoma	Repermeation/stabilization/progression of thrombosis	Mean time to repermeation	Complications
Francoz, 2005 [20]	19	Vitamin K antagonist	Target INR (2–3)	Yes, Number NA	Mean 8.1 months	18/1	NA	None	8/0/1	NA	Variceal bleeding following EBL
Amitrano, 2010 [46]	28	Enoxaparin	200 UI/kg/die	7 for previous variceal bleeding	6 months in responders and nonresponders, until the end of follow-up in partial responders	5/23	20	None	21/5/2	6.5 months	Mild anemia in portal hypertensive gastropathy in 2
Delgrado, 2012 [50]	55	47 LWMH (21VKA) 8 VKA	NA, target INR close to 2.0	NA	89% > 3 months 67% > 6 months	14/41	27	None	15/12/0 Among 27 with follow-up	NA	Lower GI, dental, obscure GI, vaginal, surgical wound
Senzolo, 2012 [39]	33	Nadroparin	95 anti-Xa (U/kg) td	12/33 primary prophylaxis	6 months after repermeation; until the end of follow-up in other patients	11/24	14	4	21/7/5	5.5 months	One epistaxis, one hematuria, and one cerebral hemorrhage
Werner, 2013 [51]	28	Vitamin K antagonist	Target INR (2–3)	14/28 primary prophylaxis	302 days (range 54–1,213 days)	NA	15	NA	23/5	NA	One vaginal hemorrhage
Cui, 2015 [49]	65	Enoxaparin	1 mg/kg to 1.5 mg/kg	Secondary prophylaxis	6 months	11/54	NA	NA	51/8/6	NA	10 injection sites, epistaxis hematuria
Chen, 2016 [48]	30	Vitamin K antagonist	Target INR (2–3)	Secondary prophylaxis	7.6 months	NA	20	18	16/4/3	NA	Hematemesis/melena [4]; epistaxis, dental

LMWH low molecular weight heparin, *VKA* vitamin K antagonist, *EBL* esophageal band ligation, *PVT* portal vein thrombosis, *GI* gastrointestinal, *NA* not available

When anticoagulation is withdrawn, thrombosis frequently recurs. In a study by Amitrano et al. [46], patients were followed up for more than 24 months, and re-thrombosis was reported in 3/11 (27%) of cases after the withdrawal of anticoagulation. Similarly, in a study by Delgado et al. [50], 38% (5/13) of the patients experienced recurrence during follow-up.

This suggests that prolonging anticoagulation treatment after recanalization of the PV may be important in order to prevent re-thrombosis. In a prospective study performed by Senzolo et al., patients received anticoagulation prophylactically for 6 months after recanalization achieving a relatively low risk of recurrence (1/14 patients) [39]. The anticoagulant treatment was not associated with a significant risk of bleeding. Overall, bleeding complications were seen in only 19/230 (8.2%) patients, and correlated with PH in three cases (variceal bleeding after esophageal bend ligation in one patient and mild anemia in portal hypertensive gastropathy in two patients). In patients treated with LMWH only, the rate of bleeding complications was even lower (3/78, 3.85%). In a single study, among patients treated with VKA, patients with platelet counts lower than 50.000/uL were at greater risk for bleeding [50].

Transjugular Intrahepatic Portosystemic Shunt (TIPS) for the Treatment of Portal Vein Thrombosis

In cirrhotic patients, TIPS can be considered to treat PVT in cases of an absolute contraindication to anticoagulation or in cases of no response after a maximum of 6 months of anticoagulation treatment. In LT candidates, the indications to TIPS placement are identical to those recommended for non-listed patients. A specific aim of TIPS in listed patients is to guarantee the patency of the portal vein, if the risk of occlusion is high [37, 52].

The largest study published so far on this topic is a single-center study including 75 cirrhotic patients with PVT who underwent TIPS for complications related to PH (48 bleeding, 18 ascites, or hydrothorax) [53]. After TIPS, the portal vein system recanalized completely in 57% of patients, there was a marked decrease in thrombosis in 30% of patients, and no improvement in 13% of patients. Overall, 95% of patients with complete recanalization after TIPS placement subsequently maintained patency of the portal vein.

Patency of intrahepatic portal vein branches, partial and single (main trunk) vein involvement, de novo diagnosis of PVT, and absence of gastroesophageal varices have been found to be positive prognostic factors for technical success [53], whereas the thrombotic occlusion of the intrahepatic portal vein branches and cavernoma transformation, even if not considered as absolute contraindications, have been described as risk factors for technical failure [54]. More specifically, the presence of portal cavernoma in the older series was associated with up to 100% technical failures, whereas in the more recent study, the risk of failure is reported to be between 17% and 46% [55].

Budd-Chiari Syndrome

Epidemiology, Classification, Etiology, and Diagnosis

Budd-Chiari syndrome (BCS) is defined as the obstruction of hepatic venous outflow that can occur from the small hepatic venules up to the entrance of the inferior vena cava (IVC) into the right atrium, in the absence of right-heart failure and constrictive pericarditis [56]. It is a rare disease that occurs in 0.2 per million per year with a prevalence ranging from 1/1.000.000 of the general population in the East up to 1/100.000 in Nepal [57–59].

Primary BCS is caused by thrombosis in the absence of compression by space-occupying lesions or invasion by malignancy or parasites. Secondary BCS is due to other causes.

In primary BCS, 75% of all patients have at least one pro-coagulative disorder and 25% of patients have multiple disorders [60]. This means that identification of one causal factor does not exclude other causes.

Myeloproliferative diseases (MPDs) are the main cause in 20% [61] of patients using standard diagnostic criteria and up to 50% if spontaneous erythroid colony formation is diagnosed [62]. A recent diagnostic advance has been made with the identification of a mutation (V617F) in the Janus tyrosine kinase-2 (JAK2) gene in myeloid cells [63]. JAK2V617F mutation is of major importance in the diagnostic strategy of MPD, and it is present in nearly all patients with polycythemia vera and in about 50% of patients with essential thrombocythemia and primary myelofibrosis. Generally, it has been reported in about 40% of BCS patients and in 80% of BCS patients with MPD. Given the importance of JAK2V617F, screening for it should be performed as part of the standard diagnostic work-up, as stated in EASL guidelines [37].

Recently, the importance of mutations in the calreticulin (CALR) gene has been advocated, too [64]. CALR mutations are absent in polycythemia vera patients but occur in up to 80% of patients with JAK2-negative essential thrombocythemia and primary myelofibrosis. Two recent studies found that CALR mutations are associated with splanchnic vein thrombosis with an incidence of between 0.7% and 1.9%. The incidence was even higher when only patients with CALR and MPD were considered (2.3% and 5.4%, respectively). Indeed, CALR was found to be positive in 9.1% (1 out of 11 patients) and 30% (4 out of 13 patients) of JAK2-negative MPD [65, 66].

When all the published cohorts of BCS are pooled, the prevalence of CALR mutation in BCS patients is 0.9% (5/557 patients). Poisson et al. recently proposed that CALR mutation be considered for patients with SVT without JAK-2 mutation, especially in patients with spleen height ≥ 16 cm and platelet count > 200 ×109 /L [67]. Furthermore, it may also be important in terms of prognosis. That is, as patients with an SVT mutation or a CALR mutation have a significant disease predisposition, they may derive some benefit from JAK inhibitors such as hydroxyurea and ruxolitinib.

Among other acquired thrombophilic conditions is Behcet's disease, which can lead to BCS in the endemic areas. Other conditions associated with hypercoagulability include paroxysmal nocturnal hemoglobinuria (very rare but fairly aggressive), antiphospholipid syndrome, and thrombophilic disorders (i.e., factor V Leiden mutation, G20210A prothrombin gene mutation, and protein C and S deficiency). Use of an oral contraceptive (particularly with high estrogen content) is a risk factor for BCS and is related to heterozygosity or homozygosity for thrombophilic defects [68]. BCS in pregnancy (usually postpartum) is associated with estrogen changes, IVC compression, and physiologic hyperfibrinogenemia.

The clinical presentation of BCS varies from fulminant liver failure to asymptomatic forms and depends on several factors such as the rapidity of the disease onset, the severity of liver dysfunction, and the anatomical sites of thrombosis and etiology.

BCS can be classified anatomically into four types according to the site of the venous obstruction and presence of PVT [69]: (1) hepatic vein obstruction/thrombosis without IVC obstruction/compression, (2) hepatic vein obstruction/thrombosis with IVC obstruction (as a result of compensatory caudate lobe hypertrophy or IVC thrombosis), (3) isolated hepatic webs, and (4) isolated IVC webs. In Western countries, pure hepatic vein thrombosis is the most common presentation, whereas in Asia pure IVC or combined IVC/hepatic vein obstruction predominates.

PVT occurs in about 15% of patients with BCS [70] and affects short- and long- term survival (mean survival is 1 month in BCS patients with PTV compared with 6.3 years in BCS patients without PVT). Similarly, 5-year survival was reported to be 85% in non-PVT BCS patients versus 58% in BCS patients with PVT [71].

There are several diagnostic modalities for BCS. Color and pulsed Doppler ultrasound has a diagnostic sensitivity of almost 75% and is the recommended first-line investigation [72]. Computed tomography or magnetic resonance demonstrates the typical (but not pathognomonic) pattern of multiple small nodules in the hepatic parenchyma, which is characteristic of all diseases involving perfusion defects of the liver. Importantly, further investigation is necessary to confirm the diagnosis as well as to define the extent of the thrombus [73]. Imaging studies have demonstrated hepatic nodules in 60–80% of patients with BCS. These nodules are, however, usually benign and are the result of perfusion disturbances. The nodules are small (in most cases under 4 cm in diameter), multiple (frequently more than 10 lesions), hyper-vascularized, and disseminated throughout the liver.

Finally, although noninvasive studies are sufficient for diagnosis, hepatic venography is still useful to determine the extent of thrombosis, as well as to measure caval pressures.

In BCS patients, liver histology has two aims. Firstly, if imaging has failed to demonstrate obstruction of large veins, it can be used to assess the presence of small hepatic vein thrombosis, which characterizes a very rare but well-recognized form of BCS. Secondly, it is important to estimate liver reserve and the potential reversibility of the liver injury when TIPS is being considered [37].

Clinical Manifestation and Prognosis

The typical patient with BCS is female, about 35 years old, with underlying thrombophilia, often taking oral contraception [58, 59]. In a multi-center prospective study evaluation of patients with BCS, ascites was present in 83% of patients, hepatomegaly in 67%, abdominal pain in 61%, esophageal varices in 58%, and gastrointestinal bleeding in 5% [70].

Depending on clinical presentation, BCS can be hyperacute (5%), acute (20%), or subacute/chronic (60%). However, the prognostic value of this classification has not been prospectively validated, and several authors no longer recommend its use for predicting mortality [74–76].

In clinical practice, BCS should be suspected in patients with acute abdominal pain, an enlarged liver (particularly in patients with known thrombophilic disorders), or alternatively when fulminant liver failure is associated with ascites [77]. Conversely, chronic BCS should be excluded in the presence of refractory ascites, particularly if liver function tests are abnormal [78]. Lower limb edema and venous collaterals on the trunk indicate IVC compression/thrombosis [79]. Asymptomatic presentation (15% of cases) is often associated with the presence of large hepatic venous collaterals [78].

Mortality rates associated with BCS have decreased over time. Five-year survival before 1985 was reported to be 50% compared with 75% thereafter due to a change in treatment strategies [78, 80]. Mortality is highest within 2 years of diagnosis (and independent of treatment in one study), with 77%, 65%, and 57% of patients surviving at 1, 6, and 10 years, respectively [80]. In the largest cohort of 237 patients with BCS, the severity of encephalopathy, ascites, serum prothrombin time, and bilirubin were found to be independent predictive factors for survival. Based on the distribution of these factors, three groups (classes I, II, and III) with statistically different 5-year survival rates of 89%, 74%, and 42%, respectively, were identified [81].

Hepatocellular carcinoma appears to complicate BCS with a cumulative incidence of 4% (11/97 patients) after a median follow-up of 5 years in a recent published cohort [82]. Of note, in patients with membranous IVC obstruction, the incidence of HCC is reported to be significantly higher than 4% (from 25% to 47.5%) [83].

Treatment

Management of BCS is based on a stepwise therapeutic algorithm derived from large, multi-center, prospective series of BCS patients [84, 85] treated with anticoagulant therapy (as first line). In the case of an inadequate response, angioplasty/stenting/thrombolysis can be used as the second-line treatment (in patients with stenosis of short duration not responding to medical therapy). In patients who have not responded to medical therapy or for whom stenoses for angioplasty/stenting/thrombolysis are not suitable, TIPS placement can be performed. Finally, if TIPS is not effective or in the case of hyperacute presentation, LT as the last resort can be considered.

Of note, patients with BCS often require therapy for ascites and varices, and their management should follow the same treatment recommendations as for ascites and PH in cirrhosis [37]. Finally, the underlying prothrombotic cause (for instance, MPDs) should be addressed.

All patients should receive anticoagulation, unless contraindicated, starting with intravenous heparin and then warfarin, to maintain an INR of at least 2.5 [37]. This treatment will be sufficient to control the disease in 10% of cases when the form of disorder is mild [84] and to prevent progression of thrombosis [78, 80].

Experience is very limited in regard to correcting hepatic venous outflow obstruction with thrombolysis. Good results have been reported only in patients with recent and incomplete thrombosis treated with local and early infusion of a thrombolytic agent combined with angioplasty or stenting [86, 87]. In patients with acute BCS, early thrombolytic therapy (i.e., within 2 weeks) administered within 72 h from the time of diagnosis [88] has had variable success when infused directly into the thrombosed hepatic vein for about 24 h [89].

The results of 80 patients who underwent local thrombolysis combined with other endovascular procedures for the treatment of hepatic vein obstruction have demonstrated a rate of technical success of between 82% and 100% [86, 90–94]. However, re-intervention is frequently needed, and, importantly, the procedure can be associated with significant complications such as pulmonary embolism, cerebral hemorrhage, and cardiac tamponade [90]. In cases of short-segment obstruction or webs in hepatic veins or the IVC, balloon dilatation or intravascular stents can be used. In a single-center study conducted by Eapen et al., survival in BCS patients with mild disease and treated only by radiological intervention was 94% and 87% at 1 and 5 years, respectively [95]. When thrombosis of the hepatic vein was more diffuse, angioplasty alone was successful in only 56% of patients, even with additional local thrombolytic therapy. If a combination of angioplasty and stent placement was used, long-term patency rates reached 80–90%. Further re-intervention, however, was performed in 50% of cases in diffuse venous thrombosis [96].

Failure of thrombolysis or angioplasty and the presence of a thrombosis of more than one hepatic vein are indications for shunting. The therapeutic principle of portosystemic shunting is to convert the portal vein into an outflow tract (reversed portal flow), thus decompressing the sinusoids. A side-to-side portal caval shunt (or meso-caval shunt) not only decompresses the liver but also relieves ascites and removes the risk of variceal bleeding.

Even though surgical interventions are important in the treatment algorithm of BCS, they are generally not the first-line of therapy, and the most used treatment for BCS nonresponsive to medical therapy is TIPS (with LT used as a rescue therapy) [84, 85].

In a series published by Orloff et al. including 60 patients who underwent surgical shunting and with a follow-up of between 3.5 and 27 years [97], 95% survival with complete resolution of ascites and no encephalopathy was demonstrated. No technical failures and one operative death were reported. However, other authors were not able to demonstrate comparable outcomes [93, 98]. Furthermore, in most of the reported series, patients with acute liver failure were not considered for the placement of a surgical shunt but for LT. The use of a surgical shunt has been associated with rapid decompensation with in-hospital mortality as high as 25%, primarily because of the patients' poor condition [98]. In fact, acute hepatic decompensation remedied only by emergency salvage liver transplantation has been reported. Surgical shunting is an option in liver transplantation centers where rescue therapy can be performed [37].

TIPS has improved the management of BCS (Table 8.2) [99–110]. It has major advantages compared to surgical shunts: (1) it avoids laparotomy, overcoming caudate lobe compression and occlusion of the IVC, with less perioperative mortality (particularly in patients with poor liver function); (2) it does not preclude subsequent surgical shunting or liver transplantation; and (3) it can also be placed in patients with PVT.

Since Rossle's description in 1989 of the first procedure on human patients [111], TIPS has been widely accepted as a noninvasive technique to manage complications of PH. In the past, most of the studies were based on the use of bare stents and were associated with a high incidence of shunt failure. Patients required several revisions during follow-up. After the introduction of polytetrafluoroethylene (PTFE)-covered stent grafts, this problem was completely solved, eliminating repeated interventions and significantly improving patients' quality of life [112]. The patency rate of TIPS at 1 year is up to 70% [103]. In a recent multi-center European study, long-term data on TIPS treatment for 147 BCS patients not responding to medical treatment or recanalization showed a 10-year survival rate of 69%. TIPS was successful in 124 BCS patients, who were then followed for a median of 36.7 months. The main complication was hepatic encephalopathy in 21% of the cases. Five-year survival in high-risk patients after TIPS placement was significantly higher than estimated by the Rotterdam BCS index (71 vs. 42%) [101].

Several single-center studies have confirmed an excellent outcome after TIPS in the hyperacute setting. A recent report demonstrated that for five patients with fulminant hepatic failure, TIPS allowed resolution of the disease in one and acted as a bridge to liver transplantation within 1 month in three other patients [99].

TIPS with PTFE-covered stents should be considered as the first-line therapy in BCS patients with signs of PH both in acute and chronic presentations and also in patients with hyperacute BCS, if a liver donor is not available within 2–3 days [37].

Although most patients with BCS can be treated medically or by interventional radiological procedures, some patients progress to chronic liver failure with subsequent need for LT. After TIPS placement, the percentage of patients who will require LT has been reported to be between 7% [85] and 38% [84] in two different large cohorts. Pre-identified prognostic factors proposed in the BCS-TIPS index by Garcia-Pagan et al. include age, bilirubin, and INR [101].

LT is indicated in hyperacute BCS. It is associated with a large area of necrosis, even with early shunting (surgical or TIPS). Patient selection plays a dominant

Table 8.2 Published cohorts of BCS patients treated by TIPS

Author, year (ref.)	Patients who underwent TIPS	Mean age (range)	Most frequent C-P class	Presentation acute/chronic	Type of stent	Success (%)	Mean follow-up	Death (%)	LT (%)
Perello, 2002 [106]	13	36 (17–67)	B	4/6	NA	92	4 years	10	15
Mancuso, 2003 [104]	15	39.5 (20–73)	C	9/6	1 covered 13 uncovered 1 NA	93	24 months	30	0
Rossle, 2004 [109]	35	43 (12–74)	B	12/29	13 uncovered 6 self-expandable uncovered 8 covered 8 NA	100	37 months	9	0
Hernandez-Guerra, 2004 [103]	21	40 (17–54)	B	NA	9 covered 12 uncovered	70	20 months	0	0
Attwell, 2004 [99]	17	50 (16–68)	MELD 21 (4–55)	5/12	NA	100	5.9 years	23	29
Plessier, 2006 [84]	25	34 (25–47)	B	NA	11 covered	83	35 months	8	12
Garcia-Pagan, 2008 [101]	133	38 (35–40)	B	85/39	48 covered 61 uncovered 15 both	93	37 months	13	24
Seijo, 2013 [85]	62	37 (16–83)[a]	B	28/43	NA	100	50 months	16	6
Qi, 2014 [107]	51	36.5 (16–74)	B	29/10 (12 NA)	35 covered 16 uncovered	100	732 days	23.5	0
Tripathi, 2014 [110]	67	40 (NA)	B	6/61	40 covered 8 uncovered covered 19 uncovered	100	82 months	25	3
Rosenqvist, 2016 [108]	13	36 (16–63)	B	10/3	Covered	100	36 months	7.7	8
Fan, 2016 [100]	33	39 (NA)	B	NA	Covered	100	82 months	3[b]	0
Mo, 2017 [105]	27	42 (21–76)	MELD 14 (7–28)	NA	Covered	100	59 months	22[c]	0
Hayek, 2017 [102]	54	36 (15–67)	B	13/41	Covered	93	56 months	17	13

TIPS transjugular intrahepatic portosystemic shunt, *LT* liver transplant, *NA* not available
[a]Entire cohort
[b]Two patients among the whole cohort of 60 patients (33 who underwent TIPS and 27 angioplasties)
[c]Two patients (7.4% died from non-liver-related causes)

prognostic role in the treatment of BCS. Venous decompression and LT should both be integrated in a common therapeutic concept, and the decision regarding which approach to use in each individual case should be based on the leading clinical syndrome, i.e., PH or liver failure, together with an assessment of the reversibility of hepatic damage and the potential for curing the underlying disease.

Short- and medium-term follow-up data of BCS after LT have been published by several groups, and survival data of the largest cohort are published yearly by the European transplant registry. There are 12 published series with 316 transplanted patients in total, with reported long-term survival rates (5 years) between 50% (in the older series) and 98% (in the more recent series) (Table 8.3) [70, 98, 113–122]. A recent retrospective analysis of series from the USA [15] and Europe [123] demonstrated a 5-year survival rate of 80%.

Although almost all genetic thrombophilic disorders are cured by transplantation, thrombosis still occurs and routine anticoagulation therapy is necessary [124]. Recurrence of venous thrombosis or BCS occurred in about 10% of patients, confirming the need for lifelong anticoagulation [37]. When MPD is present, treatment aimed at decreasing platelet production may be needed to further decrease the use of thrombotic complications of posttransplantation. Melear et al. [125] reported on 17 patients who had undergone transplantation for BCS; all the patients with an underlying MPD [12] received a vitamin K antagonist, aspirin, and oncocarbide to prevent thrombotic complications. Only one patient developed recurrent thrombosis, and this occurred more than 10 years after the original transplant.

Deep Vein Thrombosis and Pulmonary Embolism

The association between liver cirrhosis and the risk of pulmonary thromboembolism (PE) or deep vein thrombosis (DVT) among hospitalized patients with cirrhosis has been evaluated in retrospective case-control studies and is between 0.8% and 7%.

These patients do not demonstrate a reduced risk of PE/DVT when compared to patients without cirrhosis [126, 127], and, importantly, a prolonged INR does not negate a risk of venous thromboembolism (VTE) [128]. In a case-control Danish population-based study of 99,444 patients with thromboembolic disease, patients with cirrhosis had a 1.7-fold increased relative risk of venous thrombosis compared to the general population [129]. In a retrospective case-control study by Northup et al. [127], liver cirrhosis was recognized, for the first time, as a thrombophilic condition. One hundred and thirteen hospitalized cirrhotic patients with a documented new VTE were included in the analysis and compared to controls. Of the 113 events, 74 (65.5%) involved a DVT only, 22 (19.5%) involved a PE only, and 17 (15%) involved both a PE and DVT. Traditional markers of coagulation impairment in liver disease (such as INR and platelet count) were not predictive of VTE. The multivariate analysis demonstrated that low serum albumin remained independently predictive of VTE, with an odds ratio of 0.25 (95% CI 0.10–0.56), possibly

Table 8.3 Liver transplantation for Budd-Chiari syndrome

Author, year (ref.)	Patients (years)	Mean age (years)	MPD (*n*)	Time interval between diagnosis and LT	Mean follow-up	Survival rate (time)	Thrombotic complications (*n*)	Hemorrhagic complications (*n*)
Campbell, 1988 [113]	17	28	NA	NA	28 months	88% (3 years)	3	7
Halff, 1989 [115]	23 (1974–1988)	30	5	2.3 years	46 months	44.7% (5 years)	3	0
Jamieson, 1991 [116]	26 (1976–1990)	36	6	NA	20 months	69% (3 years) 50% (5 years)	NA	NA
Shaked, 1992 [120]	14	32	NA	NA	2 months–5 years (range 1)	85% (end of follow-up)	2	3
Sakai, 1994 [119]	11	36	NA	2 days (fulminant) 650 days (chronic)	60 months	64% (5 years)	0	0
Ringe, 1995 [98]	43 (1981–1993)	33	7	NA	49.4 months	69% (10 years)	0	2
Srinivasan, 2002 [121]	19 (1988–1999)	32	8	NA	89 months	84% (end of follow-up)	2 (BCS recurrence → re.LT)	2 (re-LT)
Cruz, 2005 [114]	11 (1988–2002)	48	6	1–18 months	4–7 years	65% (5 years) 65% (10 years)	3 (1 BCS recurrence)	4
Ulrich, 2008 [122]	39 (1988–2006)	35	13	37 days (acute) 174 (subacute) 740 (chronic)	96 months	5y: 89.4% 10y: 83.3%	3 (re-LT)	3
Darwish Murrad, 2009 [70]	20 (2003–2005)	38	NA	NA	19 months	90% (end of follow-up)	1	0
Ołdakowska-Jedynak, 2014 [117]	25 (2000–2009)	29	21	NA	58.8 months	84% (end of follow-up)	5	5
Raza, 2017 [118]	68[a] (1993–2016)	31	NA	NA	78 months	89% (5 years)	1 BCS recurrence	0

MPD myeloproliferative diseases, *LT* liver transplant, *BCS* Budd-Chiari syndrome, *NA* not available
[a]Including three living donor liver transplantations

Table 8.4 Deep vein thrombosis in patients with cirrhosis

Author, year (ref.)	Type of study	Patients with liver disease (*n*)	Deep vein thrombosis (*n*)	Deep vein thrombosis prevalence (%)
Northup, 2006 [127]	Case control	21,000	74	0.35
Garcia Fuster, 2008 [133]	Retrospective	2074	11	0.8
Lesmana, 2010 [135]	Retrospective	256	12	4.7
Ali, 2010 [132]	Retrospective	449,798	4,335	0.9
Aldawood, 2011 [131]	Retrospective	226	6	2.7
Girleanu, 2012 [134]	Retrospective	3,108	31	0.99
Shah, 2012 [136]	Retrospective	85	6	7
Al-Dorzi, 2013 [130]	Retrospective	75	2	2.7

reflecting the low level of endogenous anticoagulants typically found in cirrhosis coagulopathy. The importance of a low level of albumin in predicting the risk of VTE in liver cirrhosis has been confirmed by Gulley et al. [126] in 963 cirrhotics. Multivariate analysis showed that prolonged PTT and low serum albumin are independent predictors of DVT/PE.

A number of published studies specifically looked at the risk of DVT in patients with cirrhosis (Table 8.4) [127, 130–136].

Validated risk stratification scores that predict VTE within a general population of hospitalized patients also appear to accurately predict VTE among hospitalized patients specifically with chronic liver disease, i.e., the Padua Predictor Score, and can be used to decide if antithrombotic prophylaxis should be started [137].

Several studies investigated the role of anticoagulation in preventing thromboembolic disease in patients with chronic liver disease. Current guidelines do not recognize the thromboembolic risk associated with chronic liver disease and do not make specific recommendations for the prophylaxis or treatment of thromboembolic disease in this special population [138]. The reported use of prophylactic anticoagulation for VTE in patients with chronic liver disease (21–25%) remains significantly lower than in other inpatient groups (30–70%) [139]. One of the problems is that the studies investigating the relationship between the use of prophylactic anticoagulation in patients with cirrhosis and the risk of VTE have demonstrated contradictory results. The vast majority of these investigations are retrospective studies with differences in coding and/or defining cases of chronic liver disease. More specifically, some investigations failed to demonstrate a significant difference in the incidence of VTE in people with chronic liver disease given prophylactic anticoagulation compared to those who were not given this treatment [128], or observed no significant difference between the incidence of VTE in patients treated with pharmacological, mechanical, or no prophylaxis. In contrast, Barclay et al. found a decreased incidence of VTE in patients with chronic liver disease given pharmacological prophylaxis [140].

Further prospective studies are required to determine not only if cirrhotic patients may benefit from receiving prophylactic doses of anticoagulant therapy in preventing VTE but also to determine which prophylactic regimen is most appropriate. The interim suggestion is that VTE prophylaxis is considered on a case-by-case basis in hospitalized cirrhotic patients, based on risk factor assessment for VTE (particularly, the likelihood of prolonged immobilization). If anticoagulation is contraindicated (e.g., because of the potential risk of bleeding), then mechanical prophylaxis should be considered [141].

Anticoagulation in Cirrhosis

The decision to use anticoagulation in cirrhosis patients requires a careful assessment of the perceived risks and benefits of anticoagulation.

Initial studies in patients with cirrhosis revealed that traditional therapeutic and prophylactic anticoagulation therapies with LMWH or VKA are potentially safe in stable cirrhotic patients [20, 39, 46, 48–51]. However, these studies are generally small and retrospective, with considerable variation in study design.

One major concern regarding the use of LMWH in chronic liver failure is the reduction of antithrombin in patients with advanced liver disease, owing to the fact that LMWH requires antithrombin to exert its anticoagulant function. Furthermore, a superimposed condition of renal failure, which frequently occurs in cirrhotic patients, can critically influence the catabolism of heparin. Finally, LMWH is administered as a subcutaneous injection, and this can be cumbersome for some patients. In vitro studies demonstrated conflicting results. The anti-Xa assay cannot be used to monitor LMWH activity in cirrhotic patients. Bechmann et al. [142] demonstrated that after LMWH administration, anti-Xa activity was lower in cirrhotics than in controls, correlating with the degree of disease severity. This finding suggests the need to increase the LMWH dose in cirrhotics. However, Lisman et al. demonstrated in vitro that the anti-Xa assay underestimates LMWH plasma levels in these patients [143]. The measured anti-Xa activity does not reflect the functional anticoagulation effects of LMWH but is a surrogate for LMWH concentration in the patient's blood. Anti-Xa is quantified by a chromogenic assay, in which a given amount of activated factor Xa as well as a chromogenic substrate is added to the undiluted plasma sample of a patient. Abundant LMWH will bind to AT in the plasma sample. When LMWH and AT are bound together, two competing reactions occur simultaneously: firstly, the externally added factor Xa is inhibited by the AT-LMWH complex; secondly, the non-inhibited factor Xa reacts with the chromogenic substrate, which resembles the natural substrate of factor Xa, resulting in the cleavage of p-nitroaniline (pNA), which is inversely proportional to the LMWH level in the sample. AT-deficient plasma, such as that observed in cirrhosis, has been documented to yield false anti-Xa determinations, possibly as a result of a decrease in the accuracy of classical anti-Xa assays [144].

This has been confirmed by an in vitro study using thrombin generation (TG) to evaluate the effect of LMWH on endogenous thrombin potential (ETP) in 30 cirrhotic patients (10 Child A, 10 Child B, and 10 Child C) [145]. It was demonstrated that, after the addition of LMWH, the ETP ratio was significantly lower in the cirrhotic patients than in the controls. Importantly, the reduction correlated with the severity of the liver disease, in spite of the concomitant decrease in AT activity. The role of TG in monitoring anticoagulant therapy was recently evaluated by Tripodi et al. in a prospective study including 23 cirrhotic patients treated with LMWH followed by vitamin K antagonist [146]. Among the different tools for monitoring the anticoagulant therapy that were tested, only ETP accurately reflected the antithrombotic action elicited by these drugs.

While VKAs are desirable for their low cost and oral administration, close monitoring of the international normalized ratio (INR) is necessary to determine therapeutic range. Dosing of VKA in cirrhosis patients is particularly challenging due to preexisting elevations of the INR. As the vitamin K-dependent anticoagulant factor protein C (also inhibited by VKA) is low in cirrhosis, VKA may not be a particularly desirable agent. A cohort study evaluating 29.000 INR measurements during a period of 6 months demonstrated that underlying liver disease or alcohol abuse was independently correlated with a risk of excessive anticoagulation (INR > 6) [147].

Direct Oral Anticoagulants

Recently, several direct-acting oral anticoagulants (DOACs) have been approved, and a small case series reported the use of these agents in cirrhosis. DOACs are especially attractive considering the problems posed by traditional anticoagulants in this clinical setting. Advantages of these medications include quick onset of action, oral use, and no need for routine monitoring of drug levels or effects. However, each agent has distinctive properties requiring particular attention to dosing, absorption, and clearance. Similar to LMWH, careful consideration of the use of DOACs in patients with cirrhosis and renal impairment is essential, as DOACs are all dependent on renal clearance to varying degrees. Large trials to establish the safety and efficacy of these medications excluded patients with liver disease, and consequently, clinical experience is very limited. A theoretical risk of excessive anticoagulation exists when using DOACs in cirrhotic patients. However, conflicting laboratory data have been published, and no conclusions can be drawn yet, as a wide variation in TG response has been observed between different classes of DOACs.

Potze et al. recently demonstrated a decreased in vitro anticoagulant effect of rivaroxaban in cirrhotic patients by using TG. On the other hand, a significantly increased anticoagulant response to dabigatran was found. Interestingly, the enhanced effect of dabigatran on TG was proportional to the severity of the liver disease [148]. The same group examined the in vitro anticoagulant potency of apixaban [149]. Twenty-five ng/mL of apixaban or 50 ng/mL of rivaroxaban were added to the plasma samples of 11 healthy individuals and 14 cirrhotic patients (nine Child B and five Child C). Whereas a fixed dose of the drugs decreased total TG in healthy volunteers by 55 ± 6% (rivaroxaban) and 51 ± 4% (apixaban), the mean decrease in TG in patients was significantly lower (30 ± 9% for rivaroxaban, $P < 0.0001$; 32 ± 10% for apixaban, $P < 0.0001$).

In the clinical setting, rivaroxaban and apixaban (oral factor Xa inhibitors) have been used for PVT treatment; only a few of these patients, however, had compensated liver disease [150, 151]. Intagliata et al. [150] compared rates of bleeding complications in patients treated with apixaban and rivaroxaban to those of cirrhotic patients treated with VKA and LMWH. For 39 patients (only Child A and B) who received anticoagulation therapy over a 3-year period (20 patients on FXa inhibitors and 19 patients on traditional anticoagulation), there were three documented bleeding events in the traditional anticoagulation group (two major events) and four bleeding events in the DOAC group (one major event). In another multi-center cohort of 36 cirrhotic patients (Child A and B patients), 22 (61%) receiving anticoagulation treatment for PVT were followed up for a median duration of 15 months. Most of the patients (83%) received rivaroxaban, whereas dabigatran and apixaban were used in 11% and 6% of the cases, respectively. Adverse events occurred in 17% of patients including five cases of bleeding [151].

In conclusion, even though some data are now emerging supporting the use of DOACs in well-compensated cirrhosis patients, larger studies are needed to improve our understanding of the pharmacologic properties of these medications and their safety in this special population [37].

Key Points

1. Patients with end-stage liver disease (ESLD) are not auto-anticoagulated.
2. Viscoelastic tests enable optimal transfusion management and identification of patients at risk for thrombotic events.
3. The aim of anticoagulation therapy in PVT should be to recanalize the vessel or reduce the thrombosis in order to ensure anatomical reconstruction.
4. Budd-Chiari syndrome may need anticoagulation, portal venous decompression, or liver transplantation depending on clinical presentation.
5. VTE prophylaxis should be considered on a case-by-case basis in hospitalized cirrhotic patients.
6. More research is needed to determine whether DOACs are safe in ESLD.

References

1. Caldwell SH, Hoffman M, Lisman T, Macik BG, Northup PG, Reddy KR, et al. Coagulation disorders and hemostasis in liver disease: pathophysiology and critical assessment of current management. Hepatology. 2006;44:1039.
2. Lisman T, Caldwell SH, Burroughs AK, Northup PG, Senzolo M, Stravitz RT, et al. Hemostasis and thrombosis in patients with liver disease: the ups and downs. J Hepatol. 2010;53:362.
3. Ferro D, Quintarelli C, Lattuada A, Leo R, Alessandroni M, Mannucci PM, et al. High plasma levels of von Willebrand factor as a marker of endothelial perturbation in cirrhosis: relationship to endotoxemia. Hepatology. 1996;23:1377.

4. Hollestelle MJ, Geertzen HG, Straatsburg IH, van Gulik TM, van Mourik JA. Factor VIII expression in liver disease. Thromb Haemost. 2004;91:267.
5. Kelly DA, Summerfield JA. Hemostasis in liver disease. Semin Liver Dis. 1987;7:182.
6. Kerr R. New insights into haemostasis in liver failure. Blood Coagul Fibrinolysis. 2003;14(Suppl 1):S43.
7. Maisonneuve P, Sultan Y. Modification of factor VIII complex properties in patients with liver disease. J Clin Pathol. 1977;30:221.
8. Blanchard RA, Furie BC, Jorgensen M, Kruger SF, Furie B. Acquired vitamin K-dependent carboxylation deficiency in liver disease. N Engl J Med. 1981;305:242.
9. Liebman HA, McGehee WG, Patch MJ, Feinstein DI. Severe depression of antithrombin III associated with disseminated intravascular coagulation in women with fatty liver of pregnancy. Ann Intern Med. 1983;98:330.
10. Fair DS, Marlar RA. Biosynthesis and secretion of factor VII, protein C, protein S, and the protein C inhibitor from a human hepatoma cell line. Blood. 1986;67:64.
11. Mannucci PM, Vigano S. Deficiencies of protein C, an inhibitor of blood coagulation. Lancet. 1982;2:463.
12. Senzolo M, Cholongitas EC, Patch D, Burroughs AK. Update on the classification, assessment of prognosis and therapy of Budd-Chiari syndrome. Nat Clin Pract Gastroenterol Hepatol. 2005;2:182.
13. Lisman T, Leebeek FW, de Groot PG. Haemostatic abnormalities in patients with liver disease. J Hepatol. 2002;37:280.
14. Lisman T, Leebeek FW. Hemostatic alterations in liver disease: a review on pathophysiology, clinical consequences, and treatment. Dig Surg. 2007;24:250.
15. Segev DL, Nguyen GC, Locke JE, Simpkins CE, Montgomery RA, Maley WR, et al. Twenty years of liver transplantation for Budd-Chiari syndrome: a national registry analysis. Liver Transpl. 2007;13:1285.
16. Lisman T, Bakhtiari K, Pereboom IT, Hendriks HG, Meijers JC, Porte RJ. Normal to increased thrombin generation in patients undergoing liver transplantation despite prolonged conventional coagulation tests. J Hepatol. 2010;52:355.
17. Rossetto V, Spiezia L, Senzolo M, Rodriguez-Castro KI, Maggiolo S, Simioni P. Whole blood rotation thromboelastometry (ROTEM(R)) profiles in subjects with non-neoplastic portal vein thrombosis. Thromb Res. 2013;132:e131.
18. Debernardi Venon W, Ponzo P, Sacco M, Mengozzi G, Raso S, Valpreda A, et al. Usefulness of thromboelastometry in predicting the risk of bleeding in cirrhotics who undergo invasive procedures. Eur J Gastroenterol Hepatol. 2015;27:1313.
19. Zanetto A, Senzolo M, Vitale A, Cillo U, Radu C, Sartorello F, et al. Thromboelastometry hypercoagulable profiles and portal vein thrombosis in cirrhotic patients with hepatocellular carcinoma. Dig Liver Dis. 2017;49:440.
20. Francoz C, Belghiti J, Vilgrain V, Sommacale D, Paradis V, Condat B, et al. Splanchnic vein thrombosis in candidates for liver transplantation: usefulness of screening and anticoagulation. Gut. 2005;54:691.
21. Zocco MA, Di Stasio E, De Cristofaro R, Novi M, Ainora ME, Ponziani F, et al. Thrombotic risk factors in patients with liver cirrhosis: correlation with MELD scoring system and portal vein thrombosis development. J Hepatol. 2009;51:682.
22. Abdel-Razik A, Mousa N, Elhelaly R, Tawfik A. De-novo portal vein thrombosis in liver cirrhosis: risk factors and correlation with the Model for End-stage Liver Disease scoring system. Eur J Gastroenterol Hepatol. 2015;27:585.
23. Amitrano L, Brancaccio V, Guardascione MA, Margaglione M, Sacco M, Martino R, et al. Portal vein thrombosis after variceal endoscopic sclerotherapy in cirrhotic patients: role of genetic thrombophilia. Endoscopy. 2002;34:535.
24. John BV, Konjeti R, Aggarwal A, Lopez R, Atreja A, Miller C, et al. Impact of untreated portal vein thrombosis on pre and post liver transplant outcomes in cirrhosis. Ann Hepatol. 2013;12:952.

25. Maruyama H, Okugawa H, Takahashi M, Yokosuka O. De novo portal vein thrombosis in virus-related cirrhosis: predictive factors and long-term outcomes. Am J Gastroenterol. 2013;108:568.
26. Nery F, Chevret S, Condat B, de Raucourt E, Boudaoud L, Rautou PE, et al. Causes and consequences of portal vein thrombosis in 1,243 patients with cirrhosis: results of a longitudinal study. Hepatology. 2015;61:660.
27. Villa E, Camma C, Marietta M, Luongo M, Critelli R, Colopi S, et al. Enoxaparin prevents portal vein thrombosis and liver decompensation in patients with advanced cirrhosis. Gastroenterology. 2012;143:1253.
28. Rodriguez-Castro KI, Porte RJ, Nadal E, Germani G, Burra P, Senzolo M. Management of nonneoplastic portal vein thrombosis in the setting of liver transplantation: a systematic review. Transplantation. 2012;94:1145.
29. Ogren M, Bergqvist D, Bjorck M, Acosta S, Eriksson H, Sternby NH. Portal vein thrombosis: prevalence, patient characteristics and lifetime risk: a population study based on 23,796 consecutive autopsies. World J Gastroenterol. 2006;12:2115.
30. Senzolo M, Caldwell S. Portal vein thrombosis in cirrhosis: ignore, prevent, or treat? Gastroenterology. 2013;144:e19.
31. Tsochatzis EA, Senzolo M, Germani G, Gatt A, Burroughs AK. Systematic review: portal vein thrombosis in cirrhosis. Aliment Pharmacol Ther. 2010;31:366.
32. Yerdel MA, Gunson B, Mirza D, Karayalcin K, Olliff S, Buckels J, et al. Portal vein thrombosis in adults undergoing liver transplantation: risk factors, screening, management, and outcome. Transplantation. 2000;69:1873.
33. La Mura V, Tripodi A, Tosetti G, Cavallaro F, Chantarangkul V, Colombo M, et al. Resistance to thrombomodulin is associated with de novo portal vein thrombosis and low survival in patients with cirrhosis. Liver Int. 2016;36:1322.
34. Amitrano L, Brancaccio V, Guardascione MA, Margaglione M, Iannaccone L, D'Andrea G, et al. Inherited coagulation disorders in cirrhotic patients with portal vein thrombosis. Hepatology. 2000;31:345.
35. Amitrano L, Guardascione MA, Brancaccio V, Margaglione M, Manguso F, Iannaccone L, et al. Risk factors and clinical presentation of portal vein thrombosis in patients with liver cirrhosis. J Hepatol. 2004;40:736.
36. Mangia A, Villani MR, Cappucci G, Santoro R, Ricciardi R, Facciorusso D, et al. Causes of portal venous thrombosis in cirrhotic patients: the role of genetic and acquired factors. Eur J Gastroenterol Hepatol. 2005;17:745.
37. European Association for the Study of the Liver. Electronic address eee. EASL clinical practice guidelines: vascular diseases of the liver. J Hepatol. 2016;64:179.
38. Luca A, Caruso S, Milazzo M, Marrone G, Mamone G, Crino F, et al. Natural course of extrahepatic nonmalignant partial portal vein thrombosis in patients with cirrhosis. Radiology. 2012;265:124.
39. Senzolo M, T MS, Rossetto V, Burra P, Cillo U, Boccagni P, et al. Prospective evaluation of anticoagulation and transjugular intrahepatic portosystemic shunt for the management of portal vein thrombosis in cirrhosis. Liver Int. 2012;32:919.
40. D'Amico G, De Franchis R, Cooperative Study G. Upper digestive bleeding in cirrhosis. Post-therapeutic outcome and prognostic indicators. Hepatology. 2003;38:599.
41. Senzolo M. Liver: PVT in cirrhosis, not always an innocent bystander. Nat Rev Gastroenterol Hepatol. 2015;12:11.
42. Olausson M, Norrby J, Mjornstedt L, Liden H, Friman S. Liver transplantation using cavoportal hemitransposition- a life-saving procedure in the presence of extensive portal vein thrombosis. Transplant Proc. 2001;33:1327.
43. Pinna AD, Nery J, Kato T, Levi D, Nishida S, Tzakis AG. Liver transplant with portocaval hemitransposition: experience at the University of Miami. Transplant Proc. 2001; 33:1329.
44. Ravaioli M, Zanello M, Grazi GL, Ercolani G, Cescon M, Del Gaudio M, et al. Portal vein thrombosis and liver transplantation: evolution during 10 years of experience at the University of Bologna. Ann Surg. 2011;253:378.

45. Ceulemans B, Aerts R, Monbaliu D, Coosemans W, Verslype C, Van Steenbergen W, et al. Liver transplantation using cavoportal transposition: an effective treatment in patients with complete splanchnic venous thrombosis. Transplant Proc. 2005;37:1112.
46. Amitrano L, Guardascione MA, Menchise A, Martino R, Scaglione M, Giovine S, et al. Safety and efficacy of anticoagulation therapy with low molecular weight heparin for portal vein thrombosis in patients with liver cirrhosis. J Clin Gastroenterol. 2010;44:448.
47. Ageno W, Riva N, Schulman S, Beyer-Westendorf J, Bang SM, Senzolo M, et al. Long-term clinical outcomes of splanchnic vein thrombosis: results of an international registry. JAMA Intern Med. 2015;175:1474.
48. Chen H, Liu L, Qi X, He C, Wu F, Fan D, et al. Efficacy and safety of anticoagulation in more advanced portal vein thrombosis in patients with liver cirrhosis. Eur J Gastroenterol Hepatol. 2016;28:82.
49. Cui SB, Shu RH, Yan SP, Wu H, Chen Y, Wang L, et al. Efficacy and safety of anticoagulation therapy with different doses of enoxaparin for portal vein thrombosis in cirrhotic patients with hepatitis B. Eur J Gastroenterol Hepatol. 2015;27:914.
50. Delgado MG, Seijo S, Yepes I, Achecar L, Catalina MV, Garcia-Criado A, et al. Efficacy and safety of anticoagulation on patients with cirrhosis and portal vein thrombosis. Clin Gastroenterol Hepatol. 2012;10:776.
51. Werner KT, Sando S, Carey EJ, Vargas HE, Byrne TJ, Douglas DD, et al. Portal vein thrombosis in patients with end stage liver disease awaiting liver transplantation: outcome of anticoagulation. Dig Dis Sci. 2013;58:1776.
52. Fagiuoli S, Bruno R, Debernardi Venon W, Schepis F, Vizzutti F, Toniutto P, et al. Consensus conference on TIPS management: techniques, indications, contraindications. Dig Liver Dis. 2017;49:121.
53. Luca A, Miraglia R, Caruso S, Milazzo M, Sapere C, Maruzzelli L, et al. Short- and long-term effects of the transjugular intrahepatic portosystemic shunt on portal vein thrombosis in patients with cirrhosis. Gut. 2011;60:846.
54. Senzolo M, Burra P, Patch D, Burroughs AK. Tips for portal vein thrombosis (pvt) in cirrhosis: not only unblocking a pipe. J Hepatol. 2011;55:945.
55. Rossle M. TIPS: 25 years later. J Hepatol. 2013;59:1081.
56. Okuda K, Kage M, Shrestha SM. Proposal of a new nomenclature for Budd-Chiari syndrome: hepatic vein thrombosis versus thrombosis of the inferior vena cava at its hepatic portion. Hepatology. 1998;28:1191.
57. Okuda H, Yamagata H, Obata H, Iwata H, Sasaki R, Imai F, et al. Epidemiological and clinical features of Budd-Chiari syndrome in Japan. J Hepatol. 1995;22:1.
58. Valla DC. The diagnosis and management of the Budd-Chiari syndrome: consensus and controversies. Hepatology. 2003;38:793.
59. Valla DC. Primary Budd-Chiari syndrome. J Hepatol. 2009;50:195.
60. Denninger MH, Beldjord K, Durand F, Denie C, Valla D, Guillin MC. Budd-Chiari syndrome and factor V Leiden mutation. Lancet. 1995;345:525.
61. Janssen HL, Meinardi JR, Vleggaar FP, van Uum SH, Haagsma EB, van Der Meer FJ, et al. Factor V Leiden mutation, prothrombin gene mutation, and deficiencies in coagulation inhibitors associated with Budd-Chiari syndrome and portal vein thrombosis: results of a case-control study. Blood. 2000;96:2364.
62. Hirshberg B, Shouval D, Fibach E, Friedman G, Ben-Yehuda D. Flow cytometric analysis of autonomous growth of erythroid precursors in liquid culture detects occult polycythemia vera in the Budd-Chiari syndrome. J Hepatol. 2000;32:574.
63. James C, Ugo V, Le Couedic JP, Staerk J, Delhommeau F, Lacout C, et al. A unique clonal JAK2 mutation leading to constitutive signalling causes polycythaemia vera. Nature. 2005;434:1144.
64. Abhinav J, Pratik T, Akash S. Calreticulin mutations and their importance in Budd-Chiari syndrome. J Hepatol. 2017;67(5):1111–2.
65. Plompen EP, Valk PJ, Chu I, Darwish Murad SD, Plessier A, Turon F, et al. Somatic calreticulin mutations in patients with Budd-Chiari syndrome and portal vein thrombosis. Haematologica. 2015;100:e226.

66. Turon F, Cervantes F, Colomer D, Baiges A, Hernandez-Gea V, Garcia-Pagan JC. Role of calreticulin mutations in the aetiological diagnosis of splanchnic vein thrombosis. J Hepatol. 2015;62:72.
67. Poisson J, Plessier A, Kiladjian JJ, Turon F, Cassinat B, Andreoli A, et al. Selective testing for calreticulin gene mutations in patients with splanchnic vein thrombosis: a prospective cohort study. J Hepatol. 2017;67:501.
68. Minnema MC, Janssen HL, Niermeijer P, de Man RA. Budd-Chiari syndrome: combination of genetic defects and the use of oral contraceptives leading to hypercoagulability. J Hepatol. 2000;33:509.
69. Gupta S, Barter S, Phillips GW, Gibson RN, Hodgson HJ. Comparison of ultrasonography, computed tomography and 99mTc liver scan in diagnosis of Budd-Chiari syndrome. Gut. 1987;28:242.
70. Darwish Murad S, Plessier A, Hernandez-Guerra M, Fabris F, Eapen CE, Bahr MJ, et al. Etiology, management, and outcome of the Budd-Chiari syndrome. Ann Intern Med. 2009;151:167.
71. Darwish Murad S, Valla DC, de Groen PC, Zeitoun G, Haagsma EB, Kuipers EJ, et al. Pathogenesis and treatment of Budd-Chiari syndrome combined with portal vein thrombosis. Am J Gastroenterol. 2006;101:83.
72. Ohta M, Hashizume M, Tomikawa M, Ueno K, Tanoue K, Sugimachi K. Analysis of hepatic vein waveform by Doppler ultrasonography in 100 patients with portal hypertension. Am J Gastroenterol. 1994;89:170.
73. Erden A, Erden I, Karayalcin S, Yurdaydin C. Budd-Chiari syndrome: evaluation with multiphase contrast-enhanced three-dimensional MR angiography. AJR Am J Roentgenol. 2002;179:1287.
74. Langlet P, Escolano S, Valla D, Coste-Zeitoun D, Denie C, Mallet A, et al. Clinicopathological forms and prognostic index in Budd-Chiari syndrome. J Hepatol. 2003;39:496.
75. Singh V, Sinha SK, Nain CK, Bambery P, Kaur U, Verma S, et al. Budd-Chiari syndrome: our experience of 71 patients. J Gastroenterol Hepatol. 2000;15:550.
76. Tang TJ, Batts KP, de Groen PC, van Hoek B, Haagsma EB, Hop WC, et al. The prognostic value of histology in the assessment of patients with Budd-Chiari syndrome. J Hepatol. 2001;35:338.
77. Janssen HL, Garcia-Pagan JC, Elias E, Mentha G, Hadengue A, Valla DC, et al. Budd-Chiari syndrome: a review by an expert panel. J Hepatol. 2003;38:364.
78. Hadengue A, Poliquin M, Vilgrain V, Belghiti J, Degott C, Erlinger S, et al. The changing scene of hepatic vein thrombosis: recognition of asymptomatic cases. Gastroenterology. 1994;106:1042.
79. Okuda K. Inferior vena cava thrombosis at its hepatic portion (obliterative hepatocavopathy). Semin Liver Dis. 2002;22:15.
80. Zeitoun G, Escolano S, Hadengue A, Azar N, El Younsi M, Mallet A, et al. Outcome of Budd-Chiari syndrome: a multivariate analysis of factors related to survival including surgical portosystemic shunting. Hepatology. 1999;30:84.
81. Darwish Murad S, Valla DC, de Groen PC, Zeitoun G, Hopmans JA, Haagsma EB, et al. Determinants of survival and the effect of portosystemic shunting in patients with Budd-Chiari syndrome. Hepatology. 2004;39:500.
82. Moucari R, Rautou PE, Cazals-Hatem D, Geara A, Bureau C, Consigny Y, et al. Hepatocellular carcinoma in Budd-Chiari syndrome: characteristics and risk factors. Gut. 2008;57:828.
83. Shrestha SM, Okuda K, Uchida T, Maharjan KG, Shrestha S, Joshi BL, et al. Endemicity and clinical picture of liver disease due to obstruction of the hepatic portion of the inferior vena cava in Nepal. J Gastroenterol Hepatol. 1996;11:170.
84. Plessier A, Sibert A, Consigny Y, Hakime A, Zappa M, Denninger MH, et al. Aiming at minimal invasiveness as a therapeutic strategy for Budd-Chiari syndrome. Hepatology. 2006;44:1308.
85. Seijo S, Plessier A, Hoekstra J, Dell'era A, Mandair D, Rifai K, et al. Good long-term outcome of Budd-Chiari syndrome with a step-wise management. Hepatology. 2013;57:1962.

86. Sharma S, Texeira A, Texeira P, Elias E, Wilde J, Olliff SP. Pharmacological thrombolysis in Budd Chiari syndrome: a single centre experience and review of the literature. J Hepatol. 2004;40:172.
87. Smalberg JH, Spaander MV, Jie KS, Pattynama PM, van Buuren HR, van den Berg B, et al. Risks and benefits of transcatheter thrombolytic therapy in patients with splanchnic venous thrombosis. Thromb Haemost. 2008;100:1084.
88. Frank JW, Kamath PS, Stanson AW. Budd-Chiari syndrome: early intervention with angioplasty and thrombolytic therapy. Mayo Clin Proc. 1994;69:877.
89. Raju GS, Felver M, Olin JW, Satti SD. Thrombolysis for acute Budd-Chiari syndrome: case report and literature review. Am J Gastroenterol. 1996;91:1262.
90. Griffith JF, Mahmoud AE, Cooper S, Elias E, West RJ, Olliff SP. Radiological intervention in Budd-Chiari syndrome: techniques and outcome in 18 patients. Clin Radiol. 1996;51:775.
91. Kuo GP, Brodsky RA, Kim HS. Catheter-directed thrombolysis and thrombectomy for the Budd-Chiari syndrome in paroxysmal nocturnal hemoglobinuria in three patients. J Vasc Interv Radiol. 2006;17:383.
92. Sang HF, Li XQ. Endovascular treatment of Budd-Chiari syndrome with hepatic vein obstruction in China. J Laparoendosc Adv Surg Tech A. 2014;24:846.
93. Slakey DP, Klein AS, Venbrux AC, Cameron JL. Budd-Chiari syndrome: current management options. Ann Surg. 2001;233:522.
94. Zhang Q, Xu H, Zu M, Gu Y, Wei N, Wang W, et al. Catheter-directed thrombolytic therapy combined with angioplasty for hepatic vein obstruction in Budd-Chiari syndrome complicated by thrombosis. Exp Ther Med. 2013;6:1015.
95. Eapen CE, Velissaris D, Heydtmann M, Gunson B, Olliff S, Elias E. Favourable medium term outcome following hepatic vein recanalisation and/or transjugular intrahepatic portosystemic shunt for Budd Chiari syndrome. Gut. 2006;55:878.
96. Zhang CQ, Fu LN, Xu L, Zhang GQ, Jia T, Liu JY, et al. Long-term effect of stent placement in 115 patients with Budd-Chiari syndrome. World J Gastroenterol. 2003;9:2587.
97. Orloff MJ, Daily PO, Orloff SL, Girard B, Orloff MS. A 27-year experience with surgical treatment of Budd-Chiari syndrome. Ann Surg. 2000;232:340.
98. Ringe B, Lang H, Oldhafer KJ, Gebel M, Flemming P, Georgii A, et al. Which is the best surgery for Budd-Chiari syndrome: venous decompression or liver transplantation? A single-center experience with 50 patients. Hepatology. 1995;21:1337.
99. Attwell A, Ludkowski M, Nash R, Kugelmas M. Treatment of Budd-Chiari syndrome in a liver transplant unit, the role of transjugular intrahepatic porto-systemic shunt and liver transplantation. Aliment Pharmacol Ther. 2004;20:867.
100. Fan X, Liu K, Che Y, Wang S, Wu X, Cao J, et al. Good clinical outcomes in Budd-Chiari syndrome with hepatic vein occlusion. Dig Dis Sci. 2016;61:3054.
101. Garcia-Pagan JC, Heydtmann M, Raffa S, Plessier A, Murad S, Fabris F, et al. TIPS for Budd-Chiari syndrome: long-term results and prognostics factors in 124 patients. Gastroenterology. 2008;135:808.
102. Hayek G, Ronot M, Plessier A, Sibert A, Abdel-Rehim M, Zappa M, et al. Long-term outcome and analysis of dysfunction of transjugular intrahepatic portosystemic shunt placement in chronic primary Budd-Chiari syndrome. Radiology. 2017;283:280.
103. Hernandez-Guerra M, Turnes J, Rubinstein P, Olliff S, Elias E, Bosch J, et al. PTFE-covered stents improve TIPS patency in Budd-Chiari syndrome. Hepatology. 2004;40:1197.
104. Mancuso A, Fung K, Mela M, Tibballs J, Watkinson A, Burroughs AK, et al. TIPS for acute and chronic Budd-Chiari syndrome: a single-centre experience. J Hepatol. 2003;38:751.
105. Mo A, Testro A, French J, Robertson M, Angus P, Grigg A. Early radiological intervention and haematology screening is associated with excellent outcomes in Budd Chiari syndrome. Intern Med J. 2017;47:1361.
106. Perello A, Garcia-Pagan JC, Gilabert R, Suarez Y, Moitinho E, Cervantes F, et al. TIPS is a useful long-term derivative therapy for patients with Budd-Chiari syndrome uncontrolled by medical therapy. Hepatology. 2002;35:132.

107. Qi X, Guo W, He C, Zhang W, Wu F, Yin Z, et al. Transjugular intrahepatic portosystemic shunt for Budd-Chiari syndrome: techniques, indications and results on 51 Chinese patients from a single centre. Liver Int. 2014;34:1164.
108. Rosenqvist K, Sheikhi R, Eriksson LG, Rajani R, Rorsman F, Sangfelt P, et al. Endovascular treatment of symptomatic Budd-Chiari syndrome – in favour of early transjugular intrahepatic portosystemic shunt. Eur J Gastroenterol Hepatol. 2016;28:656.
109. Rossle M, Olschewski M, Siegerstetter V, Berger E, Kurz K, Grandt D. The Budd-Chiari syndrome: outcome after treatment with the transjugular intrahepatic portosystemic shunt. Surgery. 2004;135:394.
110. Tripathi D, Macnicholas R, Kothari C, Sunderraj L, Al-Hilou H, Rangarajan B, et al. Good clinical outcomes following transjugular intrahepatic portosystemic stent-shunts in Budd-Chiari syndrome. Aliment Pharmacol Ther. 2014;39:864.
111. Rossle M, Richter GM, Noldge G, Palmaz JC, Wenz W, Gerok W. New non-operative treatment for variceal haemorrhage. Lancet. 1989;2:153.
112. Keller FS, Farsad K, Rosch J. The transjugular intrahepatic portosystemic shunt: technique and instruments. Tech Vasc Interv Radiol. 2016;19:2.
113. Campbell DA Jr, Rolles K, Jamieson N, O'Grady J, Wight D, Williams R, et al. Hepatic transplantation with perioperative and long term anticoagulation as treatment for Budd-Chiari syndrome. Surg Gynecol Obstet. 1988;166:511.
114. Cruz E, Ascher NL, Roberts JP, Bass NM, Yao FY. High incidence of recurrence and hematologic events following liver transplantation for Budd-Chiari syndrome. Clin Transpl. 2005;19:501.
115. Halff G, Todo S, Tzakis AG, Gordon RD, Starzl TE. Liver transplantation for the Budd-Chiari syndrome. Ann Surg. 1990;211:43.
116. Jamieson NV, Williams R, Calne RY. Liver transplantation for Budd-Chiari syndrome, 1976-1990. Ann Chir. 1991;45:362.
117. Oldakowska-Jedynak U, Ziarkiewicz M, Ziarkiewicz-Wroblewska B, Dwilewicz-Trojaczek J, Gornicka B, Nyckowski P, et al. Myeloproliferative neoplasms and recurrent thrombotic events in patients undergoing liver transplantation for Budd-Chiari syndrome: a single-center experience. Ann Transplant. 2014;19:591.
118. Raza SM, Zainab S, Shamsaeefar AR, Nikeghbalian S, Malek Hosseini SA. Experience of liver transplant in patients diagnosed with Budd-Chiari syndrome. Exp Clin Transplant. 2018;16(2):177–81.
119. Sakai Y, Wall WJ. Liver transplantation for Budd-Chiari syndrome: a retrospective study. Surg Today. 1994;24:49.
120. Shaked A, Goldstein RM, Klintmalm GB, Drazan K, Husberg B, Busuttil RW. Portosystemic shunt versus orthotopic liver transplantation for the Budd-Chiari syndrome. Surg Gynecol Obstet. 1992;174:453.
121. Srinivasan P, Rela M, Prachalias A, Muiesan P, Portmann B, Mufti GJ, et al. Liver transplantation for Budd-Chiari syndrome. Transplantation. 2002;73:973.
122. Ulrich F, Pratschke J, Neumann U, Pascher A, Puhl G, Fellmer P, et al. Eighteen years of liver transplantation experience in patients with advanced Budd-Chiari syndrome. Liver Transpl. 2008;14:144.
123. Mentha G, Giostra E, Majno PE, Bechstein WO, Neuhaus P, O'Grady J, et al. Liver transplantation for Budd-Chiari syndrome: a European study on 248 patients from 51 centres. J Hepatol. 2006;44:520.
124. Klein AS, Molmenti EP. Surgical treatment of Budd-Chiari syndrome. Liver Transpl. 2003;9:891.
125. Melear JM, Goldstein RM, Levy MF, Molmenti EP, Cooper B, Netto GJ, et al. Hematologic aspects of liver transplantation for Budd-Chiari syndrome with special reference to myeloproliferative disorders. Transplantation. 2002;74:1090.
126. Gulley D, Teal E, Suvannasankha A, Chalasani N, Liangpunsakul S. Deep vein thrombosis and pulmonary embolism in cirrhosis patients. Dig Dis Sci. 2008;53:3012.

127. Northup PG, McMahon MM, Ruhl AP, Altschuler SE, Volk-Bednarz A, Caldwell SH, et al. Coagulopathy does not fully protect hospitalized cirrhosis patients from peripheral venous thromboembolism. Am J Gastroenterol. 2006;101:1524.
128. Dabbagh O, Oza A, Prakash S, Sunna R, Saettele TM. Coagulopathy does not protect against venous thromboembolism in hospitalized patients with chronic liver disease. Chest. 2010;137:1145.
129. Huerta C, Johansson S, Wallander MA, Garcia Rodriguez LA. Risk factors and short-term mortality of venous thromboembolism diagnosed in the primary care setting in the United Kingdom. Arch Intern Med. 2007;167:935.
130. Al-Dorzi HM, Tamim HM, Aldawood AS, Arabi YM. Venous thromboembolism in critically ill cirrhotic patients: practices of prophylaxis and incidence. Thrombosis. 2013; 2013:807526.
131. Aldawood A, Arabi Y, Aljumah A, Alsaadi A, Rishu A, Aldorzi H, et al. The incidence of venous thromboembolism and practice of deep venous thrombosis prophylaxis in hospitalized cirrhotic patients. Thromb J. 2011;9:1.
132. Ali M, Ananthakrishnan AN, McGinley EL, Saeian K. Deep vein thrombosis and pulmonary embolism in hospitalized patients with cirrhosis: a nationwide analysis. Dig Dis Sci. 2011;56:2152.
133. Garcia-Fuster MJ, Abdilla N, Fabia MJ, Fernandez C, Oliver V, Forner MJ. Venous thromboembolism and liver cirrhosisRev Esp Enferm Dig. 2008;100:259.
134. Girleanu I, Trifan A, Cojocariu C, Singeap AM, Sfarti C, Stanciu C. The risk of thrombotic events in patients with liver cirrhosis. Rev Med Chir Soc Med Nat Iasi. 2012;116:991.
135. Lesmana CR, Inggriani S, Cahyadinata L, Lesmana LA. Deep vein thrombosis in patients with advanced liver cirrhosis: a rare condition? Hepatol Int. 2010;4:433.
136. Shah NL, Northup PG, Caldwell SH. A clinical survey of bleeding, thrombosis, and blood product use in decompensated cirrhosis patients. Ann Hepatol. 2012;11:686.
137. Bogari H, Patanwala AE, Cosgrove R, Katz M. Risk-assessment and pharmacological prophylaxis of venous thromboembolism in hospitalized patients with chronic liver disease. Thromb Res. 2014;134:1220.
138. Excellence NIfHaC. Venous thromboembolism: reducing the risk for patients in hospital (update 2015). http://www.nice.org.uk/CG092. 2015.
139. Cohen AT, Tapson VF, Bergmann JF, Goldhaber SZ, Kakkar AK, Deslandes B, et al. Venous thromboembolism risk and prophylaxis in the acute hospital care setting (ENDORSE study): a multinational cross-sectional study. Lancet. 2008;371:387.
140. Barclay SM, Jeffres MN, Nguyen K, Nguyen T. Evaluation of pharmacologic prophylaxis for venous thromboembolism in patients with chronic liver disease. Pharmacotherapy. 2013;33:375.
141. Pincus KJ, Tata AL, Watson K. Risk of venous thromboembolism in patients with chronic liver disease and the utility of venous thromboembolism prophylaxis. Ann Pharmacother. 2012;46:873.
142. Bechmann LP, Wichert M, Kroger K, Hilgard P. Dosing and monitoring of low-molecular-weight heparin in cirrhotic patients. Liver Int. 2011;31:1064.
143. Lisman T, Porte RJ. Towards a rational use of low-molecular-weight heparin in patients with cirrhosis. Liver Int. 2011;31:1063.
144. Lehman CM, Rettmann JA, Wilson LW, Markewitz BA. Comparative performance of three anti-factor Xa heparin assays in patients in a medical intensive care unit receiving intravenous, unfractionated heparin. Am J Clin Pathol. 2006;126:416.
145. Senzolo M, Rodriguez-Castro KI, Rossetto V, Radu C, Gavasso S, Carraro P, et al. Increased anticoagulant response to low-molecular-weight heparin in plasma from patients with advanced cirrhosis. J Thromb Haemost. 2012;10:1823.
146. Tripodi A, Primignani M, Braham S, Chantarangkul V, Clerici M, Moia M, et al. Coagulation parameters in patients with cirrhosis and portal vein thrombosis treated sequentially with low molecular weight heparin and vitamin K antagonists. Dig Liver Dis. 2016;48:1208.

147. Brigden ML, Kay C, Le A, Graydon C, McLeod B. Audit of the frequency and clinical response to excessive oral anticoagulation in an out-patient population. Am J Hematol. 1998;59:22.
148. Potze W, Arshad F, Adelmeijer J, Blokzijl H, van den Berg AP, Meijers JC, et al. Differential in vitro inhibition of thrombin generation by anticoagulant drugs in plasma from patients with cirrhosis. PLoS One. 2014;9:e88390.
149. Potze W, Adelmeijer J, Lisman T. Decreased in vitro anticoagulant potency of Rivaroxaban and Apixaban in plasma from patients with cirrhosis. Hepatology. 2015;61:1435.
150. Intagliata NM, Henry ZH, Maitland H, Shah NL, Argo CK, Northup PG, et al. Direct oral anticoagulants in cirrhosis patients pose similar risks of bleeding when compared to traditional anticoagulation. Dig Dis Sci. 2016;61:1721.
151. De Gottardi A, Trebicka J, Klinger C, Plessier A, Seijo S, Terziroli B, et al. Antithrombotic treatment with direct-acting oral anticoagulants in patients with splanchnic vein thrombosis and cirrhosis. Liver Int. 2017;37:694.

Chapter 9
Acute Kidney Injury and Hepatorenal Syndrome

Salvatore Piano and Paolo Angeli

Introduction

Patients with liver cirrhosis have a higher risk of developing acute kidney injury (AKI) [1]. AKI is characterized by a wide spectrum of renal dysfunction, which may involve both a reduction in the glomerular filtration rate (GFR) and some degree of parenchymal kidney damage. AKI in patients with cirrhosis is associated with high morbidity and mortality, and prompt diagnosis and treatment of AKI is crucial in these patients. Type 1 hepatorenal syndrome (HRS-AKI) is a particular form of AKI characterized by severe renal vasoconstriction and associated with a poor prognosis.

Definition and Types of AKI in Patients with Cirrhosis

The definition of AKI requires four components: (a) a biomarker of renal function, (b) a baseline value for this biomarker, (c) a range of changes in this biomarker, and (d) a timeframe of when these changes occur. Serum creatinine (sCR) is still the most frequently used biomarker of renal function in patients with cirrhosis [2], and the definition of AKI is based on changes in sCR [3]. Previously, an increase in sCR of at least 50% from the baseline to a final value above 1.5 mg/dl has been used to define AKI in this patient population and has been shown to be a strong predictor of mortality [4–6]. However, more recently, new criteria have been proposed and validated in the general population, namely, the Kidney Disease Improving Global Outcomes (KDIGO) criteria [7]. These criteria define AKI as an absolute increase

S. Piano · P. Angeli (✉)
Unit of Internal Medicine and Hepatology, Department of Medicine,
University of Padova, Padova, Italy
e-mail: pangeli@unipd.it

D. Bezinover, F. Saner (eds.), *Critical Care for Potential Liver Transplant Candidates*,
https://doi.org/10.1007/978-3-319-92934-7_9

Table 9.1 International Club of Ascites definitions of acute kidney injury in cirrhosis

Subject	Definition
Baseline sCR	A value of sCR obtained in the previous 3 months, when available, can be used as a baseline sCR. In patients with more than one value within the previous 3 months, the value closest to the admission time to the hospital should be used. In patients without a previous sCR value, the sCR on admission should be used as baseline.
Definition of AKI	Increase in sCR ≥ 0.3 mg/dL (≥ 26.5 mmol/L) within 48 h; or a percentage increase sCR ≥ 50% from a baseline that is known, or presumed, to have occurred within the prior 7 days.
Staging of AKI	*Stage 1*: Increase in sCR ≥ 0.3 mg/dL (26.5 mmol/L) or an increase in sCR ≥ 1.5-fold to 2-fold from baseline *Stage 2*: Increase in sCR > 2- to 3-fold from baseline *Stage 3*: Increase of sCR > 3-fold from baseline or sCR ≥4.0 mg/dL (353.6 mmol/L) with an acute increase ≥ 0.3 mg/dL (26.5 mmol/L) or initiation of renal replacement therapy

sCR serum creatinine, *AKI* acute kidney injury

of sCR ≥ 0.3 mg/dl in 48 h or a percentage increase ≥ 50% that occurred (or is presumed to have occurred) in the previous 7 days. The KDIGO criteria also introduced urinary output criteria; however, their applicability in patients with cirrhosis has been questioned due to the avid fluid and sodium retention and oliguria observed in patients with advanced cirrhosis and ascites. Nonetheless, despite these changes, renal function may remain adequate [3]. The KDIGO criteria also provided a staging of AKI according to the increase in sCR: (i) stage 1, an increase in sCR of between 1.5- and 2-fold from baseline; (ii) stage 2, an increase in sCR from 2- to 3-fold from baseline; and (iii) stage 3, an increase in sCR above 3-fold or an increase above 4 mg/dl. The mortality rate increased in a stepwise manner according to the AKI stages. Finally, the progression of AKI to a higher stage was associated with an even worse survival rate [8, 9]. The potential benefit of the new criteria is early diagnosis of AKI to enable prompt treatment and reduce the risk of AKI progression, which is associated with a worse prognosis [8, 9]. Several studies have validated the KDIGO criteria based on sCR in patients with cirrhosis [8–14].

The new International Club of Ascites (ICA) AKI criteria proposed the use of modified KDIGO criteria to diagnose AKI in patients with cirrhosis (Table 9.1) [3]. The ICA also based the definition of AKI on the sCR value: the last available preadmission value of sCR obtained in the 3 months before admission. In cases for which no preadmission value of sCR is available, the admission value should be used as a baseline, as other strategies may lead to relevant bias [15]. The staging of the ICA-AKI criteria was similar to that provided by the KDIGO criteria (Table 9.1).

Traditionally, three types of AKI have been considered: (a) prerenal AKI, (b) intrinsic AKI, and (c) post renal AKI [1]. Hypovolemia and hepatorenal syndrome (HRS-AKI) are the two main types of prerenal AKI, whereas acute tubular necrosis (ATN-AKI) is the most common type of intrinsic AKI.

Hypovolemia is the most common type of AKI in patients with cirrhosis followed by ATN-AKI and HRS-AKI. Post renal AKI is rare in patients with cirrhosis.

AKI associated with bacterial infections can show characteristics of hypovolemia, HRS-AKI, or ATN-AKI according to the clinical scenario [16].

HRS-AKI is the most life-threatening type of AKI and requires prompt diagnosis and treatment [17]. It is characterized by a severe vasoconstriction of renal arterioles not responding to fluid administration [18, 19]. The incidence of HRS in the natural history of cirrhosis is estimated to be 18% after 1 year and 39% after 5 years [20]. Classically, two clinical types of HRS can be identified [18, 19]:

1. Type 1 HRS, characterized by a rapidly progressive reduction of renal function, is classically defined by a doubling of the initial serum creatinine (sCR) concentration to more than 226 mmol/l (2.5 mg/dl) in less than 2 weeks
2. Type 2 HRS, moderate renal failure (sCR from 133 to 226 mmol/l or from 1.5 to 2.5 mg/dl), with a steady or slowly progressive course, is usually associated with refractory ascites

With the adoption of the ICA-AKI criteria, the cutoff of 2.5 mg/dl required for the diagnosis of type 1 HRS was removed, and it is now defined as HRS-AKI [3]. Conversely, type 2 HRS has been considered to be a form of chronic kidney disease, although this definition is still a matter of debate [21].

Pathophysiology of AKI and HRS in Patients with Cirrhosis

The following factors render patients with cirrhosis susceptible to the development of AKI and HRS-AKI (Fig. 9.1):

(a) Severe splanchnic arterial vasodilation
(b) Reduction in cardiac output
(c) Systemic inflammation

The "peripheral arterial vasodilation hypothesis" has been considered for several years as the main pathophysiological mechanism of renal dysfunction in patients with cirrhosis [22]. Portal hypertension causes the release of vasodilators in the splanchnic circulation such as nitric oxide (NO), carbon monoxide (CO), adenomedullin, glucagon, and prostacyclin. The splanchnic arterial vasodilation causes a reduction in the effective circulating volume with subsequent stimulation of baroreceptors and, thus, activation of vasoconstrictor systems including production of catecholamine, activation of the renin-angiotensin-aldosterone system, and nonosmotic release of arginine vasopressin. This results in increased heart rate and cardiac output, with the development of a hyperdynamic circulation, as well as in the retention of sodium and water in the kidney (which causes the development of ascites and peripheral edema). Vasoconstrictor systems ensure the restoration of effective circulating volume. However, in the advanced stages of liver disease, the further increase of splanchnic vasodilation cannot be compensated by an increase in vasoconstrictor system activity. At this time, further water and sodium retention causes the formation of ascites and/or the development of dilutional hyponatremia. In the most

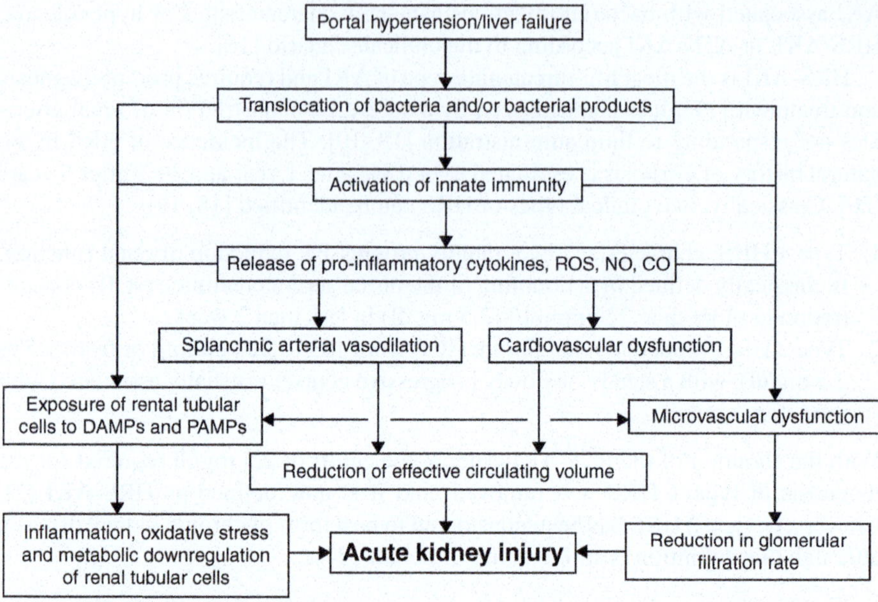

Fig. 9.1 Pathophysiology of acute kidney injury in cirrhosis. *ROS* reactive oxygen species, *NO* nitric oxide, *CO* carbon monoxide, *DAMPs* danger-associated molecular patterns, *PAMPs* pathogen-associated molecular patterns

advanced stages, the maximal activity of the vasoconstrictor systems leads to severe renal vasoconstriction, which is the cause of HRS. A precipitating event that can further worsen splanchnic vasodilation, such as a bacterial infection, or the administration of some medications, including nonsteroidal anti-inflammatory drugs (NSAIDs) or angiotensin-converting enzyme inhibitors, can trigger the development of AKI [12, 23–26].

In the early years of the twenty-first century, a new hypothesis was added to the splanchnic arterial vasodilation hypothesis. In fact, three hemodynamic studies demonstrated reduced cardiac output in patients who develop HRS-AKI. The first study compared the baseline characteristics of patients who developed HRS after an episode of SBP with those of patients who did not do so [27]. Patients with HRS had significantly higher levels of plasma renin activity and lower cardiac output as compared with patients who did not develop HRS. It is interesting that the concentrations of tumor necrosis factor alpha (TNF-α) were significantly higher in patients who developed HRS, highlighting the role of inflammation. The second study was performed in patients with cirrhosis, ascites, and normal renal function. Significantly lower cardiac output and mean arterial pressure and significantly higher plasma renin activity levels were found in patients who had developed HRS vs. those who had not developed HRS [28]. Furthermore, when HRS occurred, a further reduction in cardiac output was observed, suggesting that HRS is the result of a decrease in cardiac output in the setting of severe arterial vasodilation. In the third study, again, a reduction in the cardiac index was found to be a strong predictor of HRS development [29]. The mechanism of cardiac alterations in patients with cirrhosis is still unclear, but specific cardiac abnormalities including systolic and diastolic dysfunction, changes in electrophysiological repolarization, and enlargement of cardiac chambers were found in affected patients. Overall, these abnormalities are commonly referred to as "cirrhotic cardiomyopathy" [30].

New data suggest that systemic inflammation is likely to play a central role in both promoting splanchnic arterial vasodilation and reducing cardiac output. In patients with cirrhosis, the main driver of chronic inflammation is the translocation of bacteria from intestinal lumen to systemic circulation [31]. This pathological process is the result of increased gut permeability, intestinal bacterial overgrowth, and changes in microbiome. The translocation of bacteria or bacterial products (pathogen-associated molecular patterns [PAMPs]) stimulates pattern recognition receptors (PRRs) such as toll-like receptors (TLRs) on immune cells, thereby stimulating the production of inflammatory cytokines including TNF-alpha, interleukin-6 (IL-6), and interleukin-1beta (IL-1beta). Studies performed on an experimental model of cirrhosis suggest that these proinflammatory mediators cause oxidative stress and stimulate the synthesis of NO, further enhancing splanchnic arterial vasodilation [32]. Intestinal decontamination with norfloxacin administration leads to a reduction in the inflammatory mediator plasma concentration as well as a decrease in NO synthesis. This suggests that bacterial translocation is the cause of the inflammatory response. Proinflammatory cytokines are also involved in the pathogenesis of cardiac dysfunction in cirrhosis. In fact, TNF-alpha stimulates the production of NO in the cardiac tissue of cirrhotic rats by exerting a negative inotropic effect [33]. Interestingly, TNF-alpha knockout mice and those treated with anti-TNF-alpha antibodies demonstrated restored cardiac contractility. Finally, it has recently been shown that PAMPs may directly cause renal damage due to the activation of TLR-4 and local inflammation. The latter was demonstrated in both experimental and clinical studies [34, 35]. All these data have led experts in this field to introduce a new hypothesis for the development of AKI and other organ failures in patients with cirrhosis: the "systemic inflammation hypothesis" [36]. According to this hypothesis, systemic inflammation is the main driver of AKI. A superimposed precipitating event, such as a bacterial infection, can cause systemic inflammation with a subsequent further increase in splanchnic arterial vasodilation, a depression of cardiac contractility, and a reduction of the effective circulating volume, resulting in renal hypoperfusion. Systemic inflammation can also damage the kidney directly due to the action of inflammatory mediators [16].

Epidemiology and Clinical Features of AKI in Patients with Cirrhosis

The prevalence of AKI in hospitalized patients with cirrhosis is variable according to the criteria used, and ranges from 20 to 50% [1, 13]. About two-thirds of episodes are community-acquired, whereas the remaining are nosocomial [13]. Most of the cases are diagnosed while in stage 1, and progression of AKI occurs in 20–50% of patients [8–10]. AKI occurs more frequently in patients with ascites and bacterial infections (the most common precipitating event of AKI) [23, 24]. Of the infections, spontaneous bacterial peritonitis (SBP) is the one most frequently associated with the development of AKI and HRS-AKI. Other predisposing factors are less common and include gastrointestinal bleeding or acute alcohol consumption. However, AKI has a significant negative prognostic impact on these subgroups of patients [37, 38]. The spectrum of clinical manifestations of AKI may be very different, and sometimes the precipitating event (bacterial infection, GI bleeding, etc.) is the main clinical manifestation. However, sometimes, oliguria and a worsening of ascites may be the trigger. Finally, it should be remembered that hepatic encephalopathy may be the first manifestation of AKI.

Management and Differential Diagnosis of AKI in Cirrhosis

AKI should be managed according to the algorithm provided by the ICA [3] (Fig. 9.2). This algorithm differentiates between the management of patients according to two groups: those with AKI stage 1 and those with AKI stage 2 or 3.

In both groups, the first steps are to identify and treat potential precipitating factors. Thus, diuretics should be tapered or withdrawn, and a precise diagnostic workup for infection should be performed (paracentesis to rule out SBP, chest X-ray, urinalysis, and blood, urine and ascitic fluid cultures). All potential nephrotoxic drugs (NSAIDs, vasodilators, angiotensin-converting enzyme inhibitors, etc.) should be withdrawn. In patients with AKI stage 1, volume expansion should be administered with crystalloids in cases of dehydration (diarrhea or overdiuresis), packed red blood cells in cases of GI bleeding, and albumin in patients with SBP (1.5 g/kg on day 1 and 1 g/kg on day 3) [4]. In cases of progression to a higher stage, patients should receive the treatment provided for patients with AKI stage > 1. Diuretics should be withdrawn, and albumin should be administered at a dose of 1 g/kg per day for 2 days. In cases in which there is no response, the main differential diagnosis is between HRS-AKI and ATN-AKI (other types of AKI are quite rare). Patients with ascites, and without several pathological factors including signs of shock, the use of a nephrotoxic drug, and macroscopic signs of kidney parenchymal damage (normal renal ultrasound, no sign of proteinuria, no sign of hematuria) meet the criteria for HRS-AKI (Table 9.2). It should be highlighted that new biomarkers of renal tubular damage have recently become available. Among these biomarkers, urinary neutrophil gelatinase-associated lipocalin (NGAL) is the most investigated in patients with cirrhosis. Urinary NGAL was found to be significantly higher in patients with ATN-AKI than in those with HRS-AKI, with the lowest levels demonstrated in patients with hypovolemic AKI [39]. More recently, it has been suggested that a combination of several urinary biomarkers such as kidney injury molecule 1, interleukin-18, liver fatty acid-binding protein, and albumin may improve the differential diagnosis among ATN-AKI and other types of AKI. Further studies are needed before urinary biomarkers are included in a diagnostic algorithm of AKI; however, this diagnostic approach is very promising.

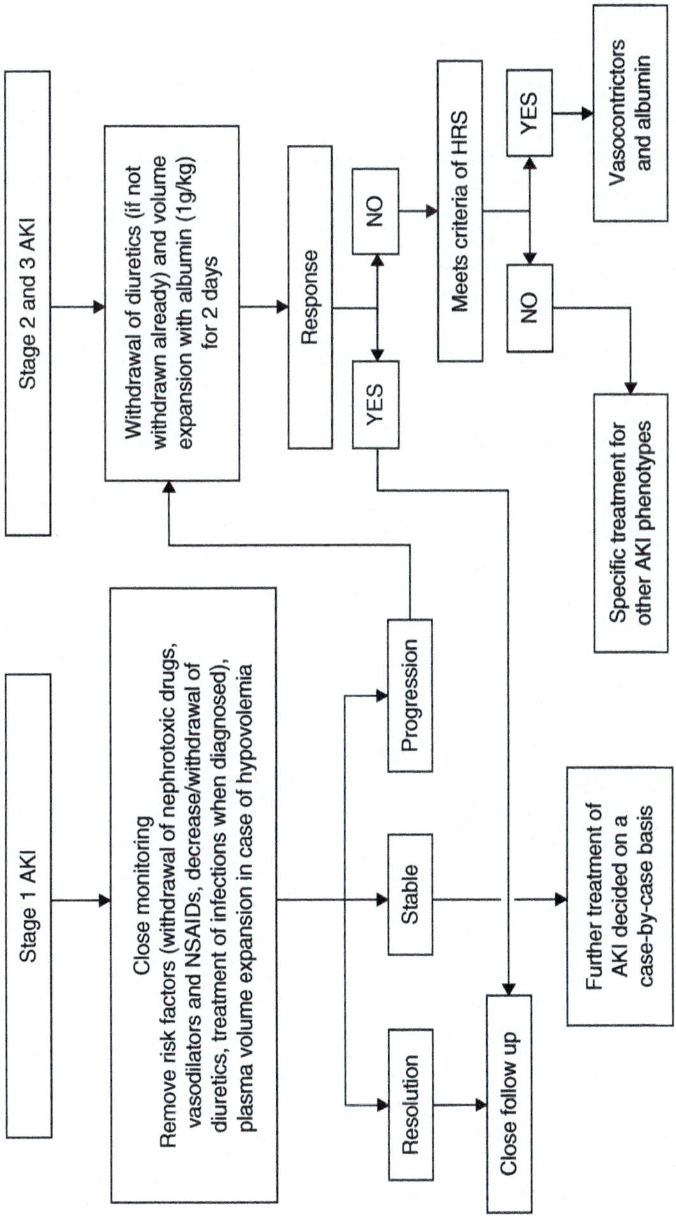

Fig. 9.2 Management of acute kidney injury in cirrhosis. (Modified from Ref. [3]). *AKI* acute kidney injury, *NSAIDs* nonsteroidal anti-inflammatory drugs, *HRS* hepatorenal syndrome

Table 9.2 Diagnostic criteria of hepatorenal syndrome acute kidney injury (HRS-AKI) according to International Club of Ascites (ICA) criteria

HRS-AKI
Diagnosis of cirrhosis and ascites
Diagnosis of acute kidney injury
No response after 2 consecutive days of diuretic withdrawal and plasma volume expansion with albumin 1 g per kg of body weight
Absence of shock
No current or recent use of nephrotoxic drugs (NSAIDs, aminoglycosides, iodinated contrast media, etc.)
No macroscopic signs of structural kidney injury, defined as: Absence of proteinuria (> 500 mg/day) Absence of microhematuria (> 50 RBCs per high-power field) Normal findings on renal ultrasonography

Modified from [3, 19]

ICA International Club of Ascites, *NSAIDs* nonsteroidal anti-inflammatory drugs, *RBC* red blood cells

Management of HRS-AKI

General management of HRS-AKI should include monitoring the patient's parameters, such as fluid balance, arterial pressure, and vital signs. Treatment of bacterial infections should be started as soon as possible. There are no data supporting the use of empirical antibiotic treatment for unproven infections. When terlipressin is administered, beta-blockers should be discontinued [40]. Paracentesis with albumin administration can be performed in a patient with HRS and tense ascites, but removing more than 5l per paracentesis is not recommended. The use of diuretics should be avoided, but furosemide may be useful in treating central volume overload. Figure 9.3 summarizes available treatments for patients with HRS according to the pathogenesis of the condition.

Vasoconstrictors Plus Albumin

The combination of arterial vasoconstrictors with albumin is the most effective and investigated treatment for HRS-AKI [41]. The rationale behind the use of vasoconstrictors is to counteract splanchnic arterial vasodilation, while albumin expands the effective blood volume. However, both clinical and experimental studies suggest that the positive effects of albumin are not only mediated by plasma volume expansion. It has been demonstrated that in patients with cirrhosis and SBP, albumin in comparison to hydroxyethyl starch is capable of increasing cardiac stroke volume and systemic vascular resistance [42]. Conversely, no difference was found before and after the administration of hydroxyethyl starch, suggesting that albumin may improve cardiac output and vascular resistance with mechanisms other than plasma expansion. Experimental animal studies demonstrated that albumin is able to restore

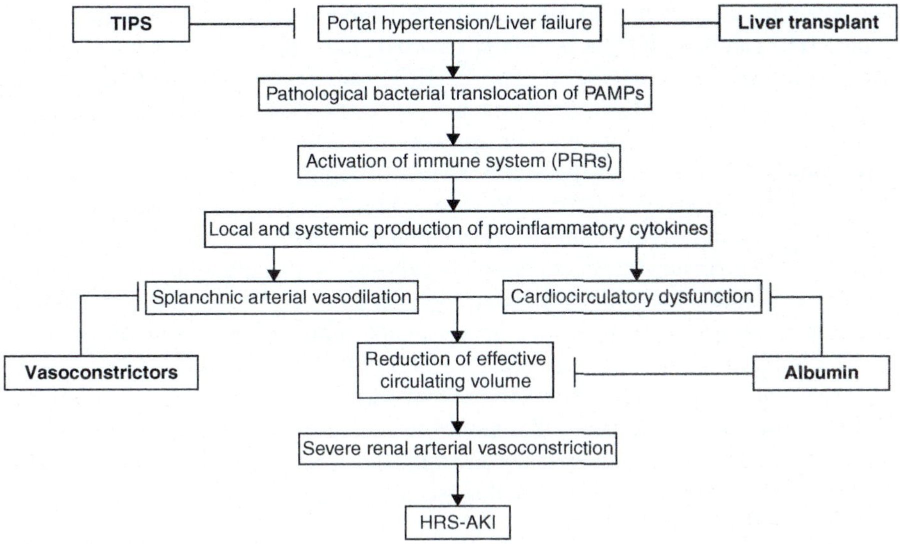

Fig. 9.3 Pathophysiological basis and targets of available treatments for hepatorenal syndrome. *TIPS* transjugular intrahepatic portosystemic shunt, *PAMPs* pathogen-associated molecular patterns, *PRRs* pattern recognition receptors, *HRS-AKI* hepatorenal syndrome acute kidney injury

cardiac contractility in cirrhotic rats and, by a reduction of the TNF-α-induced activation of the NF-κB-iNOS pathway, diminish oxidative stress in the cardiac tissue [43]. In fact, albumin has several non-oncotic properties such as the capacity to bind and inactivate PAMPs, NO, and reactive oxygen species [44]. The importance of the combination of using albumin and vasoconstrictors is supported by a lower rate of positive response when each of these drugs is administered alone [45].

Three types of vasoconstrictors are currently available for the treatment of HRS: terlipressin, noradrenaline, and the combination of midodrine + octreotide.

Terlipressin, a vasopressin analog, is the most investigated vasoconstrictor in this field. Three randomized controlled trials found that the combination of terlipressin plus albumin is more effective than albumin alone in the treatment of HRS [46–48]. The use of terlipressin and albumin in combination for the management of HRS is reported to be successful in 34–54% of cases. Terlipressin can be administered both as intravenous boluses (starting from 0.5–1 mg every 4–6 h to a maximum dose of 2 mg every 4 h) and as a continuous intravenous infusion (starting from 2 mg/day to a maximum dose of 12 mg/day). Continuous intravenous infusion is associated with a significantly lower incidence of side effects than bolus administration [49]. It has also been demonstrated that continuous infusion is effective at a lower dose compared to intravenous boluses. These findings are consistent with the short half-life of terlipressin, lasting 3–4 h [50]. Doses of terlipressin should be increased in a stepwise manner if serum creatinine does not decrease at least 25% after 3 days of treatment [51]. Albumin should be administered at the dose of 20–40 g/day. Usually, full response to treatment occurs within 14 days. After discontinuation of terlipressin and albumin, a recurrence of HRS can be observed in about 20% of patients with type 1 HRS, and retreatment is usually effective. Conversely, recurrence of HRS is quite common in patients with type 2 HRS, and treatment should be reserved for the most severe patients (sCR > 2 mg/dl). Some patients with AKI-HRS may require long-term treatment with terlipressin and albumin [52], and a specific LT allocation policy has been suggested for these patients [53]. Several predicting factors of a positive response to treatment were found, including baseline sCR, bilirubin, and the delta increase in mean arterial pressure on day 3 [54, 55]. Additionally, patients who responded to treatment with terlipressin plus albumin demonstrated a better survival rate than non-responders [49]. In a recent meta-analysis of randomized trials, the use of terlipressin was associated with a trend toward an improvement in survival vs. those treated with placebo [56].

The usual adverse effects of treatment with terlipressin include diarrhea, abdominal cramps, nausea, and headache. Also, some severe side effects, such as angina, cardiac arrhythmia, and intestinal ischemia, have been described. Patients with severe hypertension, ischemic heart disease, and peripheral vascular disease should not be treated with terlipressin.

Midodrine (an α1-agonist drug) combined with octreotide (a somatostatin analog) in combination with albumin infusion has been demonstrated as effective in treating HRS-AKI [57]. Midodrine is administered orally at a dose of 2.5 mg t.i.d., which can be increased to 12.5 mg t.i.d. if there is not a reduction in sCR of at least 25%, compared to baseline at day 3 of treatment. The starting dose of octreotide is 100 mcg t.i.d., and it can be increased to a maximum of 200 mcg t.i.d. The albumin dose is the same as that provided for terlipressin. In a randomized controlled trial, the combination of terlipressin plus albumin was significantly more effective than the combination of midodrine plus octreotide and albumin in treating HRS-AKI (an improvement in renal function of 70 vs. 29%, respectively; $p = 0.01$) [58]. Thus, this treatment should be considered only in patients with contraindications to terlipressin.

The administration of norepinephrine (administered at a dose of 0.5–3 mg/h) plus albumin has been investigated for treatment in HRS-AKI. The efficacy of noradrenaline was similar to that of terlipressin in treating HRS-AKI [59]. Norepinephrine is cheaper than terlipressin. However, it should be administered in a central venous line and under continuous monitoring, such that its use is limited to patients admitted to the intensive care unit. The treatment with vasoconstrictors plus albumin should be continued until sCR reaches a value below 1.5 mg/dl.

Liver Transplantation

Liver transplantation (LT) represents the best treatment for HRS-AKI [60]. Unfortunately, the timing of the transplantation procedure is unpredictable, and liver transplant candidates (LTCs) with HRS-AKI should be treated with vasoconstrictor plus albumin while on the waiting list. In fact, LTCs with HRS-AKI responding to terlipressin and albumin while on the waiting list demonstrated a better posttransplantation course, a shorter period of hospitalization, and less requirement for renal replacement therapy (RRT) after LT [61]. Conversely, in a recent case control study, the use of terlipressin and albumin in patients with type 2 HRS is questioned, as no differences were found in terms of post-LT outcomes between patients treated with terlipressin and those not treated with it [62].

Patients with HRS responding to treatment with vasoconstrictors plus albumin may be penalized by a current organ-distribution model based on MELD. In fact, patients with AKI-HRS have a higher mortality rate than other cirrhotic patients for any point of the MELD score [63]. Furthermore, patients showing continuous recurrence of HRS during any attempt to withdraw vasoconstrictors and albumin may be further disadvantaged [52]. In these two groups of patients, it has been suggested that the peak of sCR be used to estimate the MELD score (for responders to vasoconstrictors) and to compute the MELD score as provided for patients in dialysis (patients on long-term treatment with terlipressin) [53].

Transjugular Intrahepatic Portosystemic Shunt

Transjugular intrahepatic portosystemic shunt (TIPS) is a technique used to create a shunt between the portal and hepatic veins in the liver. TIPS is usually well tolerated; however, some complications can occur, including thrombosis/occlusion of the shunt, fistulae, hemolysis, infections, and, more commonly, hepatic encephalopathy [51].

From a pathophysiological point of view, TIPS is beneficial, because it reduces portal hypertension and increases cardiac output. TIPS improves renal perfusion and water excretion and optimizes sodium and has been reported to reduce serum creatinine in selected patients with HRS [64, 65]. However, the applicability of TIPS in patients with HRS is very limited because many affected patients have contraindications to the use of TIPS. Furthermore, the available data regarding the use of TIPS in patients with HRS-AKI are mainly based on case series. Randomized controlled trials are necessary before TIPS can be implemented in clinical practice for patients with HRS.

Renal Replacement Therapy

The data pertaining to the use of RRT in patients with HRS-AKI are limited. However, if a patient does not respond to vasoconstrictors plus albumin, with volume overload, metabolic acidosis, severe hyperkalemia, and/or hyponatremia, RRT should be considered as an option, particularly for LTCs on the waiting list [56, 66]. No data are available regarding the optimal technique of RRT (intermittent hemodialysis vs. continuous RRT) in these patients. However, it has been suggested that continuous RRT may be the better option given the lower risk of hypotension as compared to the risk with intermittent hemodialysis. In patients who are not eligible for liver transplantation, the decision to perform RRT should be made on a case-by-case basis in order to avoid rendering futile treatment.

Key Points

1. Patients with cirrhosis have a high risk of developing acute kidney injury (AKI), which is associated with a poor prognosis. The higher the stage of AKI, the higher the mortality rate.
2. Bacterial infections (in particular, spontaneous bacterial peritonitis) are the most important trigger of AKI in patients with cirrhosis. Other triggers are an overdose of diuretics, the presence of gastrointestinal bleeding, and the use of nephrotoxic drugs (nonsteroidal anti-inflammatory drugs, ACE inhibitors, aminoglycosides, etc.).
3. Hepatorenal syndrome AKI (HRS-AKI) is a specific type of AKI occurring in patients with cirrhosis and ascites. HRS-AKI is characterized by severe renal vasoconstriction with renal hypoperfusion, without macroscopic signs of intrinsic kidney injury.
4. Liver transplantation is the optimal treatment for HRS-AKI. The use of vasoconstrictors plus albumin is the most effective medical treatment for HRS-AKI, being effective in about 50% of cases.

References

1. Garcia-Tsao G, Parikh CR, Viola A. Acute kidney injury in cirrhosis. Hepatology. 2008;48:2064–77.
2. Piano S, Romano A, Di Pascoli M, Angeli P. Why and how to measure renal function in patients with liver disease. Liver Int. 2017;37:116–22.
3. Angeli P, Gines P, Wong F, Bernardi M, Boyer TD, Gerbes A, et al. Diagnosis and management of acute kidney injury in patients with cirrhosis: revised consensus recommendations of the International Club of Ascites. J Hepatol. 2015;62:968–74.
4. Sort P, Navasa M, Arroyo V, Aldeguer X, Planas R, Ruiz-del-Arbol L, et al. Effect of intravenous albumin on renal impairment and mortality in patients with cirrhosis and spontaneous bacterial peritonitis. N Engl J Med. 1999;341:403–9.
5. Angeli P, Fasolato S, Mazza E, Okolicsanyi L, Maresio G, Velo E, et al. Combined versus sequential diuretic treatment of ascites in non-azotaemic patients with cirrhosis: results of an open randomised clinical trial. Gut. 2010;59:98–104.
6. Ginès A, Fernández-Esparrach G, Monescillo A, Vila C, Domènech E, Abecasis R, et al. Randomized trial comparing albumin, dextran 70, and polygeline in cirrhotic patients with ascites treated by paracentesis. Gastroenterology. 1996;111:1002–10.
7. KDIGO. Clinical practice guideline for acute kidney injury. Kidney Int. 2012;2:1–138.
8. Piano S, Rosi S, Maresio G, Fasolato S, Cavallin M, Romano A, et al. Evaluation of the Acute Kidney Injury Network criteria in hospitalized patients with cirrhosis and ascites. J Hepatol. 2013;59:482–9.

9. Belcher JM, Garcia-Tsao G, Sanyal AJ, Bhogal H, Lim JK, Ansari N, et al. Association of AKI with mortality and complications in hospitalized patients with cirrhosis. Hepatology. 2013;57:753–62.
10. Fagundes C, Barreto R, Guevara M, Garcia E, Solà E, Rodríguez E, et al. A modified acute kidney injury classification for diagnosis and risk stratification of impairment of kidney function in cirrhosis. J Hepatol. 2013;59:474–81.
11. Tsien CD, Rabie R, Wong F. Acute kidney injury in decompensated cirrhosis. Gut. 2013;62:131–7.
12. Wong F, O'Leary JG, Reddy KR, Patton H, Kamath PS, Fallon MB, et al. New consensus definition of acute kidney injury accurately predicts 30-day mortality in patients with cirrhosis and infection. Gastroenterology. 2013;145:1280–8.e1.
13. Huelin P, Piano S, Solà E, Stanco M, Solé C, Moreira R, et al. Validation of a staging system for acute kidney injury in patients with cirrhosis and association with acute on chronic liver failure. Clin Gastroenterol Hepatol. 2017;15:438–45.
14. Angeli P, Rodríguez E, Piano S, Ariza X, Morando F, Solà E, et al. Acute kidney injury and acute-on-chronic liver failure classifications in prognosis assessment of patients with acute decompensation of cirrhosis. Gut. 2015;64:1616–22.
15. Rosi S, Piano S, Frigo AC, Morando F, Fasolato S, Cavallin M, et al. New ICA criteria for the diagnosis of acute kidney injury in cirrhotic patients: can we use an imputed value of serum creatinine? Liver Int. 2015;35:2108–14.
16. Angeli P, Tonon M, Pilutti C, Morando F, Piano S. Sepsis-induced acute kidney injury in patients with cirrhosis. Hepatol Int. 2016;10:115–23.
17. Martin-Llahi M, Guevara M, Torre A, Fagundes C, Restuccia T, Gilabert R, et al. Prognostic importance of the cause of renal failure in patients with cirrhosis. Gastroenterology. 2011;140:488–96.
18. Arroyo V, Ginès P, Gerbes AL, Dudley FJ, Gentilini P, Laffi G, et al. Definition and diagnostic criteria of refractory ascites and hepatorenal syndrome in cirrhosis. Hepatology. 1996;23:164–76.
19. Salerno F, Gerbes A, Gines P, Wong F, Arroyo V. Diagnosis, prevention and treatment of hepatorenal syndrome in cirrhosis. Gut. 2007;56:1310–8.
20. Ginès A, Escorsell A, Ginès P, Saló J, Jiménez W, Inglada L, Navasa M, Clària J, Rimola AAV. Incidence, predictive factors, and prognosis of the hepatorenal syndrome in cirrhosis with ascites. Gastroenterology. 1993;105:229–36.
21. Wong F, Nadim MK, Kellum JA, Salerno F, Bellomo R, Gerbes A, et al. Working party proposal for a revised classification system of renal dysfunction in patients with cirrhosis. Gut. 2011;60:702–9.
22. Schrier RW, Arroyo V, Bernardi M, Epstein M, Henriksen JH, Rodés J. Peripheral arterial vasodilation hypothesis: a proposal for the initiation of renal sodium and water retention in cirrhosis. Hepatology. 1988;8:1151–7.
23. Fasolato S, Angeli P, Dallagnese L, Maresio G, Zola E, Mazza E, et al. Renal failure and bacterial infections in patients with cirrhosis: epidemiology and clinical features. Hepatology. 2007;45:223–9.
24. Terra C, Guevara M, Torre A, Gilabert R, Fernández J, Martín-Llahí M, et al. Renal failure in patients with cirrhosis and sepsis unrelated to spontaneous bacterial peritonitis: value of MELD score. Gastroenterology. 2005;129:1944–53.
25. Ackerman Z, Cominelli F, Reynolds TB. Effect of misoprostol on ibuprofen-induced renal dysfunction in patients with decompensated cirrhosis: results of a double-blind placebo-controlled parallel group study. Am J Gastroenterol. 2002;97:2033–9.
26. Elia C, Graupera I, Barreto R, Solà E, Moreira R, Huelin P, et al. Severe acute kidney injury associated with non-steroidal anti-inflammatory drugs in cirrhosis: a case-control study. J Hepatol. 2015;63:593–600.
27. Ruiz-del-Arbol L, Urman J, Fernández J, González M, Navasa M, Monescillo A, et al. Systemic, renal, and hepatic hemodynamic derangement in cirrhotic patients with spontaneous bacterial peritonitis. Hepatology. 2003;38:1210–8.

28. Ruiz-del-Arbol L, Monescillo A, Arocena C, Valer P, Ginès P, Moreira V, et al. Circulatory function and hepatorenal syndrome in cirrhosis. Hepatology. 2005;42:439–47.
29. Krag A, Bendtsen F, Henriksen JH, Møller S. Low cardiac output predicts development of hepatorenal syndrome and survival in patients with cirrhosis and ascites. Gut. 2009;59:105–10.
30. Wiese S, Hove JD, Bendtsen F, Moller S. Cirrhotic cardiomyopathy: pathogenesis and clinical relevance. Nat Rev Gastroenterol Hepatol. 2014;11:177–86.
31. Wiest R, Lawson M, Geuking M. Pathological bacterial translocation in liver cirrhosis. J Hepatol. 2014;60:197–209.
32. Tazi KA, Moreau R, Hervé P, Dauvergne A, Cazals-Hatem D, Bert F, et al. Norfloxacin reduces aortic NO synthases and proinflammatory cytokine up-regulation in cirrhotic rats: role of Akt signaling. Gastroenterology. 2005;129:303–14.
33. Yang Y-Y, Liu H, Nam SW, Kunos G, Lee SS. Mechanisms of TNFα-induced cardiac dysfunction in cholestatic bile duct-ligated mice: interaction between TNFα and endocannabinoids. J Hepatol. 2010;53:298–306.
34. Shah N, Dhar D, El Zahraa Mohammed F, Habtesion A, Davies NA, Jover-Cobos M, et al. Prevention of acute kidney injury in a rodent model of cirrhosis following selective gut decontamination is associated with reduced renal TLR4 expression. J Hepatol. 2012;56:1047–53.
35. Shah N, Mohamed FE, Jover-Cobos M, Macnaughtan J, Davies N, Moreau R, et al. Increased renal expression and urinary excretion of TLR4 in acute kidney injury associated with cirrhosis. Liver Int. 2013;33:398–409.
36. Bernardi M, Moreau R, Angeli P, Schnabl B, Arroyo V. Mechanisms of decompensation and organ failure in cirrhosis: from peripheral arterial vasodilation to systemic inflammation hypothesis. J Hepatol. 2015;63:1272–84.
37. Cárdenas A, Ginès P, Uriz J, Bessa X, Salmerón JM, Mas A, et al. Renal failure after upper gastrointestinal bleeding in cirrhosis: incidence, clinical course, predictive factors, and short-term prognosis. Hepatology. 2001;34:671–6.
38. Altamirano J, Fagundes C, Dominguez M, García E, Michelena J, Cárdenas A, et al. Acute kidney injury is an early predictor of mortality for patients with alcoholic hepatitis. Clin Gastroenterol Hepatol. 2012;10:65–71.e3.
39. Fagundes C, Pépin MN, Guevara M, Barreto R, Casals G, Solà E, et al. Urinary neutrophil gelatinase-associated lipocalin as biomarker in the differential diagnosis of impairment of kidney function in cirrhosis. J Hepatol. 2012;57:267–73.
40. de Franchis R. Expanding consensus in portal hypertension. J Hepatol. 2015;63:743–52.
41. Cavallin M, Fasolato S, Marenco S, Piano S, Tonon M, Angeli P. The treatment of hepatorenal syndrome. Dig Dis. 2015;33:548–54.
42. Fernández J, Monteagudo J, Bargallo X, Jiménez W, Bosch J, Arroyo V, et al. A randomized unblinded pilot study comparing albumin versus hydroxyethyl starch in spontaneous bacterial peritonitis. Hepatology. 2005;42:627–34.
43. Bortoluzzi A, Ceolotto G, Gola E, Sticca A, Bova S, Morando F, et al. Positive cardiac inotropic effect of albumin infusion in rodents with cirrhosis and ascites: molecular mechanisms. Hepatology. 2013;57:266–76.
44. Arroyo V, García-Martinez R, Salvatella X. Human serum albumin, systemic inflammation, and cirrhosis. J Hepatol. 2014;61:396–407.
45. Ortega R, Ginès P, Uriz J, Cárdenas A, Calahorra B, De Las Heras D, et al. Terlipressin therapy with and without albumin for patients with hepatorenal syndrome: results of a prospective, nonrandomized study. Hepatology. 2002;36:941–8.
46. Sanyal AJ, Boyer T, Garcia-Tsao G, Regenstein F, Rossaro L, Appenrodt B, et al. A randomized, prospective, double-blind, placebo-controlled trial of terlipressin for type 1 hepatorenal syndrome. Gastroenterology. 2008;134:1360–8.
47. Martín-Llahí M, Pépin MN, Guevara M, Díaz F, Torre A, Monescillo A, et al. Terlipressin and albumin vs albumin in patients with cirrhosis and hepatorenal syndrome: a randomized study. Gastroenterology. 2008;134:1352–9.
48. Boyer TD, Sanyal AJ, Wong F, Frederick RT, Lake JR, O'Leary JG, et al. Terlipressin plus albumin is more effective than albumin alone in improving renal function in patients with cirrhosis and hepatorenal syndrome type 1. Gastroenterology. 2016;150:1579–89.e2.

49. Cavallin M, Piano S, Romano A, Fasolato S, Frigo AC, Benetti G, et al. Terlipressin given by continuous intravenous infusion versus intravenous boluses in the treatment of hepatorenal syndrome: a randomized controlled study. Hepatology. 2016;63:983–92.
50. Escorsell À, Bandi JC, Moitinho E, Feu F, García-Pagán JC, Bosch J, et al. Time profile of the haemodynamic effects of terlipressin in portal hypertension. J Hepatol. 1997;26:621–7.
51. European Association for the Study of the Liver. EASL clinical practice guidelines on the management of ascites, spontaneous bacterial peritonitis, and hepatorenal syndrome in cirrhosis. J Hepatol. 2010;53:397–417.
52. Piano S, Morando F, Fasolato S, Cavallin M, Boscato N, Boccagni P, et al. Continuous recurrence of type 1 hepatorenal syndrome and long-term treatment with terlipressin and albumin: a new exception to MELD score in the allocation system to liver transplantation? J Hepatol. 2011;55:491–6.
53. Angeli P, Gines P. Hepatorenal syndrome, MELD score and liver transplantation: an evolving issue with relevant implications for clinical practice. J Hepatol. 2012;57:1135–40.
54. Boyer TD, Sanyal AJ, Garcia-Tsao G, Blei A, Carl D, Bexon AS, et al. Predictors of response to terlipressin plus albumin in hepatorenal syndrome (HRS) type 1: relationship of serum creatinine to hemodynamics. J Hepatol. 2011;55:315–21.
55. Nazar A, Pereira GH, Guevara M, Martín-Llahi M, Pepin MN, Marinelli M, et al. Predictors of response to therapy with terlipressin and albumin in patients with cirrhosis and type 1 hepatorenal syndrome. Hepatology. 2010;51:219–26.
56. Facciorusso A, Chandar AK, Murad MH, Prokop LJ, Muscatiello N, Kamath PS, et al. Comparative efficacy of pharmacological strategies for management of type 1 hepatorenal syndrome: a systematic review and network meta-analysis. Lancet Gastroenterol Hepatol. 2017;2:94–102.
57. Angeli P, Volpin R, Gerunda G, Craighero R, Roner P, Merenda R, et al. Reversal of type 1 hepatorenal syndrome with the administration of midodrine and octreotide. Hepatology. 1999;29:1690–7.
58. Cavallin M, Kamath PS, Merli M, Fasolato S, Toniutto P, Salerno F, et al. Terlipressin plus albumin versus midodrine and octreotide plus albumin in the treatment of hepatorenal syndrome: a randomized trial. Hepatology. 2015;62:567–74.
59. Singh V, Ghosh S, Singh B, Kumar P, Sharma N, Bhalla A, et al. Noradrenaline vs. terlipressin in the treatment of hepatorenal syndrome: a randomized study. J Hepatol. 2012;56:1293–8.
60. Boyer TD, Sanyal AJ, Garcia-Tsao G, Regenstein F, Rossaro L, Appenrodt B, et al. Impact of liver transplantation on the survival of patients treated for hepatorenal syndrome type 1*. Liver Transpl. 2011;17:1328–32.
61. Restuccia T, Ortega R, Guevara M, Ginès P, Alessandria C, Ozdogan O, et al. Effects of treatment of hepatorenal syndrome before transplantation on posttransplantation outcome. A case-control study. J Hepatol. 2004;40:140–6.
62. Rodriguez E, Henrique Pereira G, Solà E, Elia C, Barreto R, Pose E, et al. Treatment of type 2 hepatorenal syndrome in patients awaiting transplantation: effects on kidney function and transplantation outcomes. Liver Transpl. 2015;21:1347–54. https://doi.org/10.1002/lt.24210.
63. Alessandria C, Ozdogan O, Guevara M, Restuccia T, Jiménez W, Arroyo V, et al. MELD score and clinical type predict prognosis in hepatorenal syndrome: relevance to liver transplantation. Hepatology. 2005;41:1282–9.
64. Guevara M, Ginès P, Bandi JC, Gilabert R, Sort P, Jiménez W, et al. Transjugular intrahepatic portosystemic shunt in hepatorenal syndrome: effects on renal function and vasoactive systems. Hepatology. 1998;28:416–22.
65. Wong F, Pantea L, Sniderman K. Midodrine, octreotide, albumin, and TIPS in selected patients with cirrhosis and type 1 hepatorenal syndrome. Hepatology. 2004;40:55–64.
66. Francoz C, Nadim MK, Baron A, Prié D, Antoine C, Belghiti J, et al. Glomerular filtration rate equations for liver-kidney transplantation in patients with cirrhosis: validation of current recommendations. Hepatology. 2014;59:1514–21.

Chapter 10
Management of Upper GI Bleeding in Cirrhotic Patients

Alexander Dechêne

Introduction

Upper gastrointestinal (GI) hemorrhage is a frequent and severe complication of (sinusoidal) portal hypertension (PH) and an important cause of mortality in patients with liver cirrhosis.

With an elevation of the hepatic venous pressure gradient (HVPG) $\geq$ 10 mmHg (defined as clinically significant portal hypertension, CSPH), the risk of hemorrhage from esophageal and/or gastric (gastroesophageal) varices (GEV) is markedly increased [1]. Portal hypertensive gastropathy (PHG) is also a common etiology of acute and chronic bleeding specific to cirrhotic patients. GI ulcers are another cause of upper GI bleeding, but in patients with liver cirrhosis these are less common than variceal bleeding (VB) [2].

Bleeding Sources in Patients with Liver Cirrhosis and Portal Hypertension

The focus of this review is the diagnosis and treatment of upper GI bleeding predominantly from varices developed due to PH.

Varices occur not only in the esophagus and stomach (Figs. 10.1 and 10.2) but also in the small intestinum (duodenum) (Fig. 10.3), the colon, and the rectum (perianal). Esophageal varices are approximately 20 times more frequent than gastric

---

A. Dechêne (✉)
Department of Gastroenterology, Hepatology, Endocrinology and Nutritional Medicine, Paracelsus Medical University, Nuremberg, Germany
e-mail: Alexander.Dechene@klinikum-nuernberg.de

D. Bezinover, F. Saner (eds.), *Critical Care for Potential Liver Transplant Candidates*, https://doi.org/10.1007/978-3-319-92934-7_10

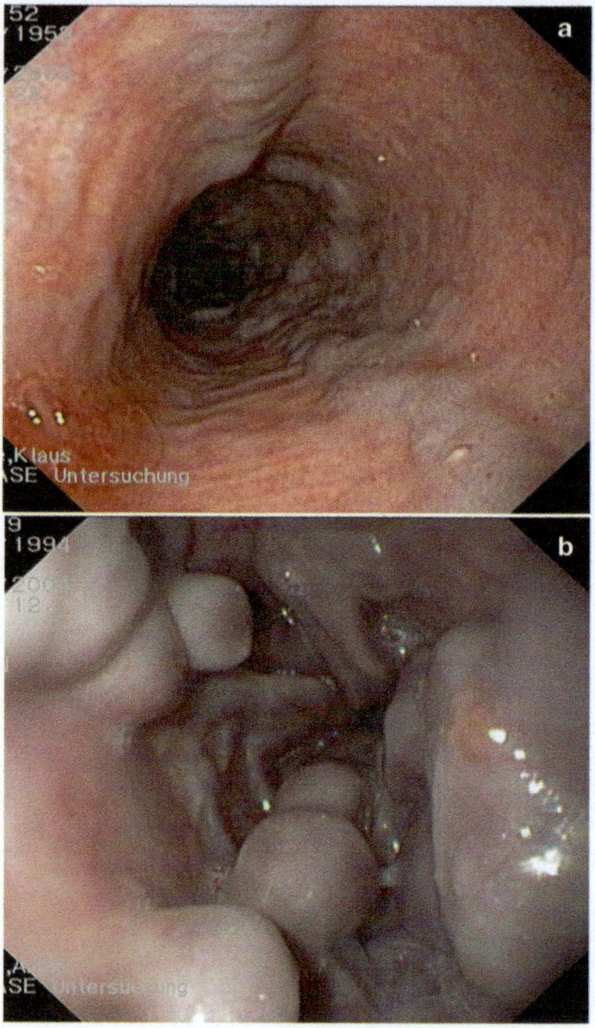

Fig. 10.1 Small (**a**) and large (**b**) esophageal varices without signs of acute bleeding

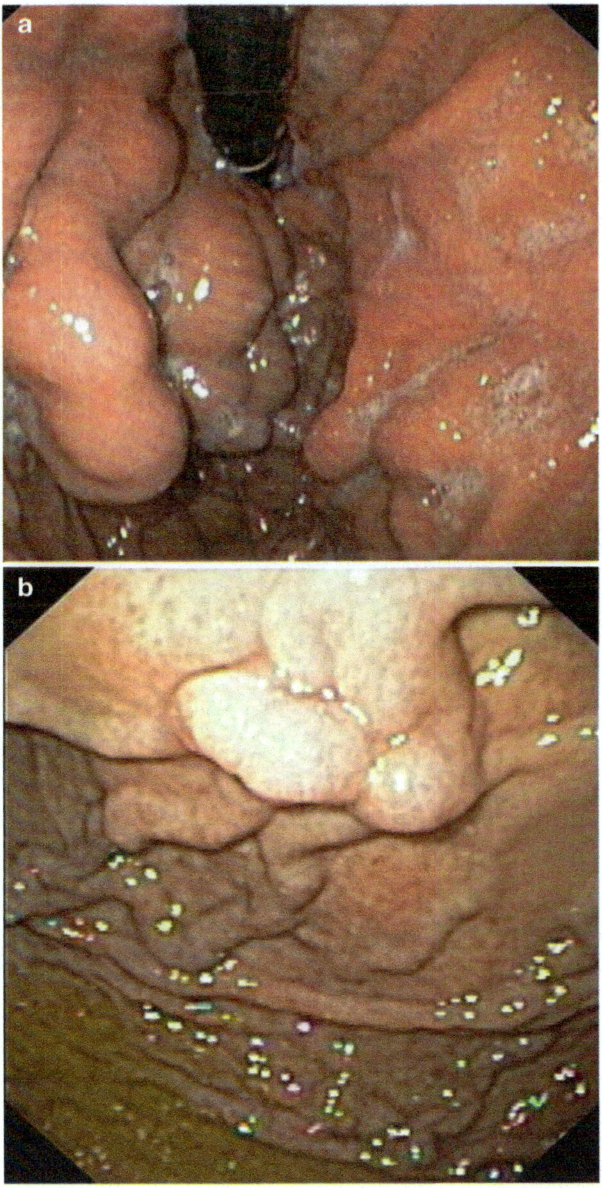

Fig. 10.2 (**a**, **b**) Gastric varices

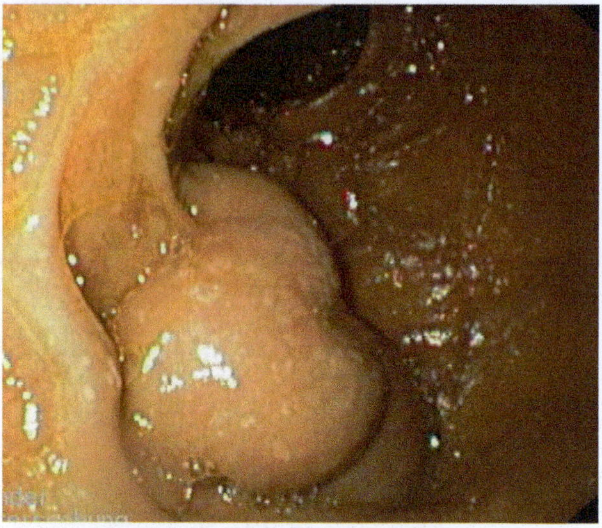

Fig. 10.3 Isolated duodenal varices

varices [3]. Non-variceal bleeding can also be observed in patients with PHG, and this is a common feature of PH found in more than one-third of patients with compensated liver cirrhosis without a history of gastrointestinal bleeding (GIB) [4].

Identification of Patients at Risk for Variceal Bleeding

A number of risk factors can predispose patients to VB. Also, several measurements have been developed to assess bleeding risk.

Clinically significant PH is the main predisposing factor for VB. Noninvasive measurements of liver stiffness (i.e., transient elastography (TE) or similar methods) make it possible to identify patients with chronic liver disease at risk of developing CSPH.

The term "compensated advanced chronic liver disease (cACLD)" has been introduced to characterize patients with either advanced or compensated cirrhosis at risk for VB. A liver biopsy can confirm cACLD, and the invasive HVPG measurement is the gold standard in the diagnosis of PH. If TE is below 10 kPa, cACLD can be practically ruled out. A measurement above 15 kPa is highly suggestive of cACLD [5]. Increased TE in combination with other clinical features, such as elevated liver stiffness spleen-size-to-platelet ratio risk score (LSPS) (liver stiffness × spleen size/platelet count), can be even more predictive of VB [6].

The prevalence of GEV in patients with an established diagnosis of liver cirrhosis is approximately 35–50% and even higher in decompensated cirrhosis. The incidence of GEV is 5–9% per year for cirrhotic patients with no varices at baseline endoscopy.

Less common are gastric varices, which present in approximately 2% of patients with liver cirrhosis [3, 7, 8].

The most sensitive tool for diagnosing GEV is upper gastrointestinal endoscopy (UGI), which is recommended for all patients with a new diagnosis of cACLD, CSPH, or manifest liver cirrhosis. Exemptions can be made for patients with a TE < 20 kPa and a platelet count > 150,000/μl, as their risk of having GEV is very low and annual repetition of TE and platelet count are recommended [9, 10].

Although a combination of endoscopic and pharmacological therapies has been shown to significantly reduce mortality from VB, the risk of death within 6 weeks after VB is as high as 15% [11].

Definitions

- VB is defined as:
    (a) Active bleeding from esophageal or gastric varices.
    (b) Presence of larger varices and luminal blood in the stomach without other sources of bleeding [12].

Hematemesis is the most common symptom of VB, and an endoscopy often reveals an active hemorrhage. Not all patients have both VB signs.

- Blood loss is considered to be significant if the patient requires more than two packed RBCs, in combination with a heart rate above 100 bpm and/or systolic blood pressure of below 100 mmHg at initial presentation.
- The consensus-defined time frame of one episode of acute VB is 5 days or 120 h after the occurrence of the first symptoms. Rebleeding within 5 days is defined as primary failure, and rebleeding later as secondary failure of hemostasis.
- Failure of treatment of an acute episode of VB is defined as either [13]:
    (a) Repeat hematemesis more than 2 h after initiation of treatment (endoscopic or pharmacologic)
    (b) Decline of serum hemoglobin below 3 g/dl (if no transfusions have been performed)
    (c) Development of hypovolemic shock
- If repeat bleeding occurs again after 5 days of treatment, it is considered a failure of secondary prophylaxis, and endoscopic and pharmacologic treatment of acute VB should be restarted [12].

Primary Prophylaxis of Variceal Bleeding

It is important that patients without GEV receive the usual treatment for chronic liver disease. Any specific treatment directed at preventing the formation of de novo varices should not be performed. Nonselective beta-blockers (NSBB) have not been shown to be more effective than placebo treatment in regard to both decreasing the incidence of varices and improving survival in patients with liver cirrhosis. Nor has NSBB been shown to prevent the progression of small varices [8, 14].

Primary prophylaxis of VB is indicated in patients with small varices (< 5 mm) and endoscopic signs of increased risk of bleeding (red spots on varices, red wale signs) and in patients with larger varices (> 5 mm). The goals of primary prophylaxis should be to reduce HVPG to below 12 mmHg or to decrease HVPG by more than 10 mmHg (measured invasively) or alternatively to reduce heart rate to 50–55 bpm (indirect parameter, if no invasive measurements are available).

Effective NSBB treatment (usually propranolol or carvedilol) reduces both the risk of first VB and mortality by approximately 10% [15]. Patients for whom propranolol does not achieve a sufficient reduction in portal pressure can safely and effectively be treated with carvedilol [16].

Endoscopic variceal ligation (EVL) is also effective for primary prophylaxis of GEV bleeding; however, no benefit regarding overall survival or bleeding-related mortality over NSBB treatment has been demonstrated [17]. Consensus guidelines recommend either NSBB treatment or EVL, but not a combination of these for primary bleeding prophylaxis [12].

Diagnosis and Grading of Upper Gastrointestinal Bleeding in Cirrhotic Patients

The risk of bleeding from GEV in individual patients can be predicted by measuring LSPS using noninvasive, ultrasound-based tools such as TE or acoustic radiation force impulse. Upper GI endoscopy is the gold standard for diagnosing, locating, and managing hemorrhage from GEV [2, 18].

The severity (or grade) of upper GIB can usually be estimated by reviewing non-endoscopic parameters. The serum hemoglobin level, in particular, is a well-accepted factor that can rapidly be determined on first contact with a patient with suspected upper GIB [19]. Patients with upper GIB in the setting of liver cirrhosis should be considered as high risk due to high mortality. Hospital admission for these patients is mandatory in almost all cases even in the absence of obvious hemodynamic problems [12]. Patients with manifest hemodynamic instability should be admitted to an intensive care unit.

Pre-endoscopic Management of Cirrhotic Patients with Suspected Bleeding from GEV

If GIB is suspected, a complete physical and laboratory examination should be performed to detect signs of infection, hepatic encephalopathy, and hemodynamic impairment. Continuous monitoring of hemodynamics and recording of oxygen saturation are also recommended [13].

Fluid resuscitation is critical and should be started as soon as possible to preserve tissue perfusion. In the general population, resuscitation using crystalloids rather than colloid solutions/plasma expanders seems to be associated with a lower incidence of renal failure and decreased mortality in critically ill patients. This trend has not been demonstrated specifically in patients with hemorrhage from GEV or with hepatic failure [20]. It is, however, a common practice to use albumin to stabilize cirrhotic patients with hemodynamic impairment because it can effect a more rapid improvement in circulation than can crystalloid solutions given that chronic hypoalbuminemia is very common in this patient population [21].

The threshold of serum hemoglobin for blood replacement therapy in cirrhotic patients is 7 g/dl. Over-transfusion leads to an increase in HVPG and an excessive risk of rebleeding and increased mortality in patients in Child-Pugh stages A and B [22].

If PH in a patient with GIB is suspected, pharmacologic treatment to reduce portal pressure should be immediately initiated even before first (index) endoscopy. Two types of vasoactive drugs are commonly used: vasopressin and somatostatin (and the respective analogues).

Vasopressin reduces portal blood flow and intravariceal pressure at the price of increasing systemic peripheral resistance and decreasing coronary perfusion. Vasopressin administration also reduces the rate of endoscopic treatment failure, but not mortality [23]. On the other hand, the use of terlipressin, a synthetic vasopressin analogue, demonstrated a favorable effect on both endoscopic treatment outcomes and decreased mortality compared to placebo and, therefore, is the treatment of choice at many centers [24].

Somatostatin and its analogue, octreotide, also reduce portal blood flow and intravariceal pressure. The effect of these substances on acute GEV seems to be comparable to that of terlipressin in regard to treatment success, rebleeding rate, and mortality [25]. For dosing and the treatment characteristics of terlipressin, somatostatin, and octreotide, see Table 10.1.

Infections with gram-negative bacteria (e.g., spontaneous bacterial peritonitis) are commonly associated with bleeding from GEV. Intravenous antibiotic treatment should be started on initial suspicion of GIB associated with PH. Early antibiotic therapy results in a reduced infection incidence, less frequent rebleeding, and decreased mortality [26]. Antibiotic therapy can be administered using third-generation cephalosporins (e.g., ceftriaxone 1 g i.v. q.d.) and fluoroquinolones (e.g., ciprofloxa-

Table 10.1 Dosages and outcomes of pharmacological co-treatment of acute variceal bleeding in combination with endoscopic treatment

	Terlipressin	Somatostatin	Octreotide
Bolus dose before endoscopy	2 mg	250 μg	50 μg
Continuous dose	1 mg 4×/day	250 μg/h	25 μg/h
Treatment success after 60 h	86.2%	83.4%	83.8%
Mortality after 60 h	8.0%	8.9%	8.8%

Modified from Seo et al. [25]

cin 250 mg i.v. b.i.d.), depending on local resistance patterns. Antibiotic treatment is recommended for the duration of the acute bleeding episode (usually 5 days).

The motilin-receptor agonist erythromycin is used (off-label) to accelerate gastric removal of fresh blood to prepare and facilitate endoscopic treatment of GEV hemorrhage. A single infusion of 250 mg of erythromycin 60–120 min before therapeutic endoscopy improves the endoscopic view of gastric mucosa and decreases the need for a second endoscopic examination, the likelihood that a transfusion will be required, and the duration of a patient's stay in the hospital [27]. Caution should be taken in patients with a macrolide allergy and QT-time prolongation. The dopamine-receptor antagonist metoclopramide is less studied but can be used as an alternative to activate gastrointestinal tract motility and clear the stomach lumen from the blood in patients who cannot be treated with erythromycin [28].

Proton-pump inhibitors (PPI) are clearly beneficial in non-variceal bleeding (i.e., peptic ulcers). The role of PPI in variceal hemorrhage is not clear. Short-term use seems to be effective; however, there is evidence of a higher incidence of bacterial peritonitis in patients with ascites who have undergone long-term PPI treatment [29].

Location and Timing of Endoscopy

Endoscopic hemostasis is the most effective non-pharmacological treatment of VB. At the same time, sufficient preparation of both the patient and the endoscopy team is essential to achieving an optimal outcome. Especially in patients with hemodynamic impairment and/or hemorrhagic shock, volume resuscitation and stabilization of hemodynamics before endoscopy (which almost always requires sedation) is necessary [13]. Considering that the majority of patients with variceal bleeding have severe liver disease associated with a high mortality rate, treatment should be carried out in either an intensive care unit or an intermediate care unit for hemodynamically stable patients.

Airway management is critical in patients with severe hematemesis. Impaired vigilance due to manifest hepatic encephalopathy can lead to aspiration, and prophylactic intubation should be considered [19]. There are, however, reports describing an increased risk of cardiopulmonary complications during and after airway instrumentation in patients with VB, and the necessity of prophylactic intubation in this patient population should be carefully evaluated [30].

After overall stabilization, therapeutic endoscopy should not be delayed. International consensus guidelines recommend endoscopic treatment within 12 h after the first clinical signs of variceal hemorrhage. In patients with signs of hemorrhagic shock, endoscopic treatment should be started as soon as possible [12]. The management of VB should be performed as a combination of pharmacologic and endoscopic approaches due to the clear advantages of this approach [31].

Endoscopic Therapy of Acute Bleeding

The preferred modality for treating hemorrhage from esophageal varices is endoscopic band ligation (EBL) using a flexible video gastroscope (Fig. 10.4). This method has largely replaced sclerotherapy during the last three decades and is associated with decreased procedure-related complications and reduced mortality [32]. Frequent adverse events of EBL include thoracic pain and minor bleeding episodes from shallow mucosal and submucosal ulcerations after the rubber bands' detachment. Severe complications are not associated with this type of therapy.

In patients with bleeding from gastric varices, EBL is seldom the best treatment modality because the large variceal conglomerates in the stomach cannot be ligated sufficiently. In these cases, an injection of n-butyl-2-cyanoacrylate (a semiliquid glue that hardens rapidly on contact with water and/or blood) and Lipiodol injected into the varices is often the better choice (Fig. 10.5) [33]. Complications after this approach are more frequent than after EBL and include displacement of emboli into the pulmonary vessels, deep ulcerations, and sepsis [34].

Recent data have demonstrated that trans-endoscopic application of hemostatic powders is an effective and relatively simple approach that can be used by an experienced endoscopist to achieve early hemostasis before subsequent definitive endoscopic treatment (i.e., EBL or endoscopic embolization) [35].

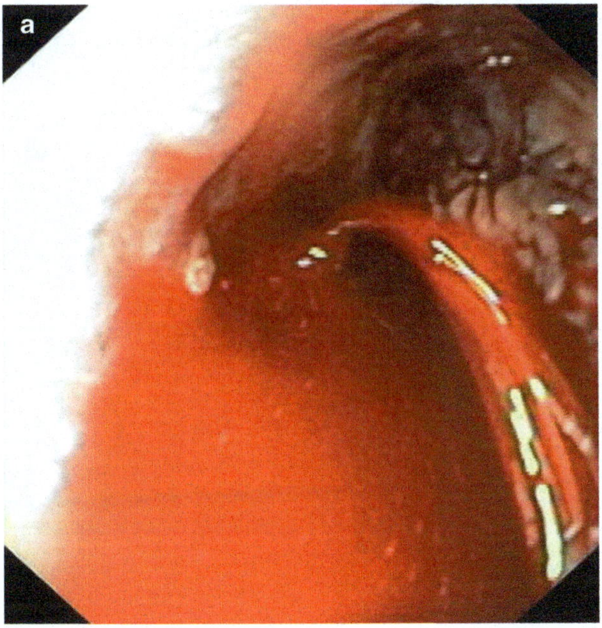

Fig. 10.4 Acute spurting esophageal variceal hemorrhage (**a**), band ligation (**b**), after successful endoscopic hemostasis (**c**)

Fig. 10.4 (continued)

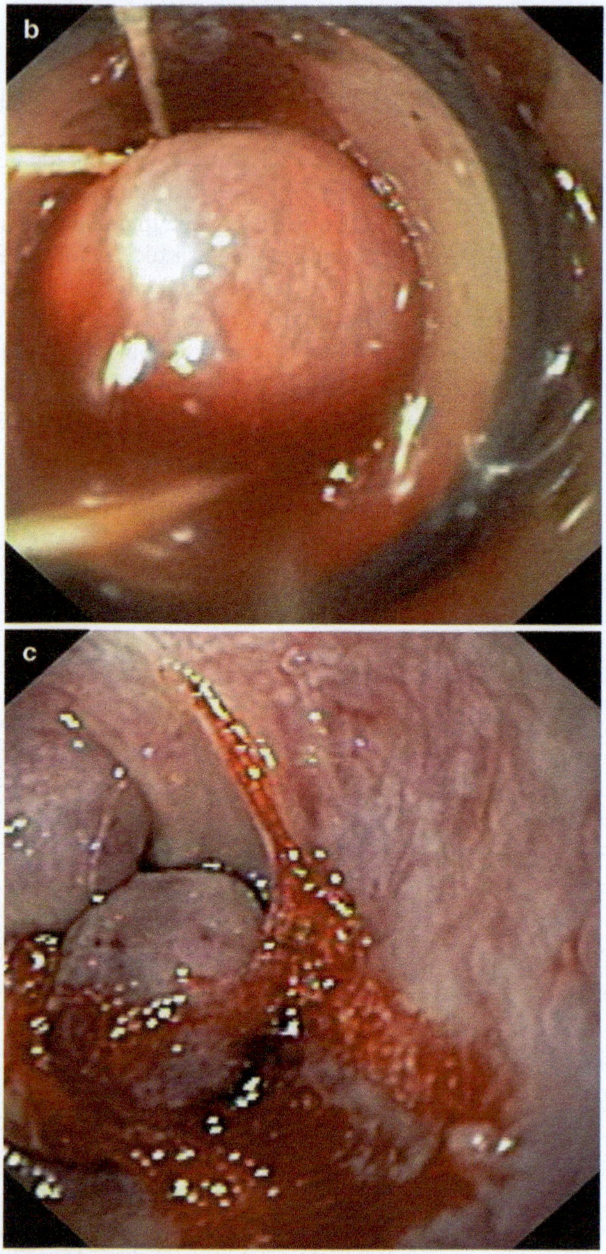

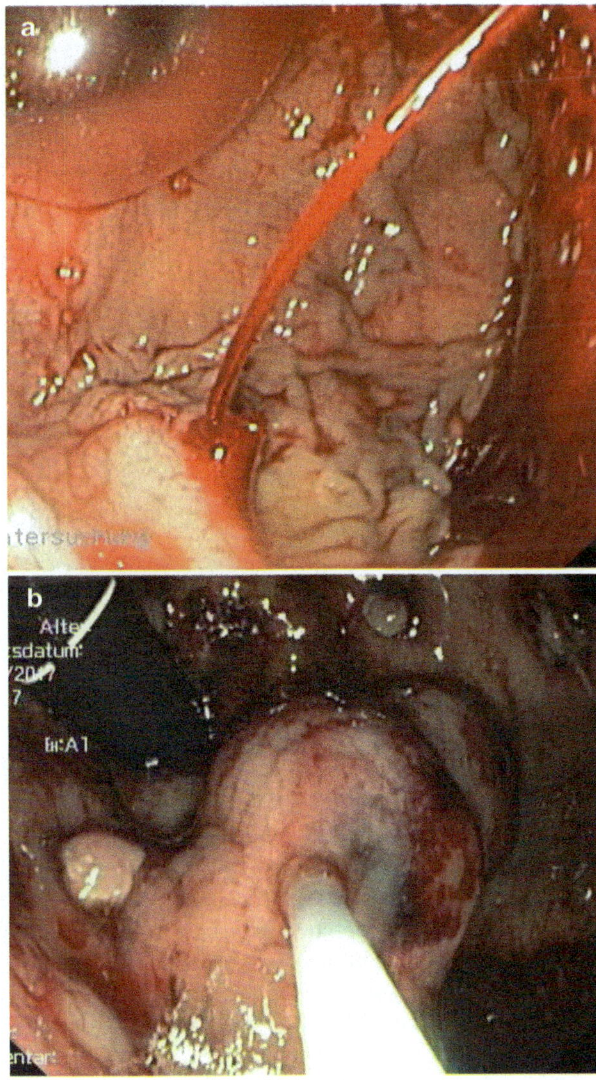

Fig. 10.5 Acute bleeding from gastric varix (**a**), injection therapy (**b**), after injection therapy (**c**)

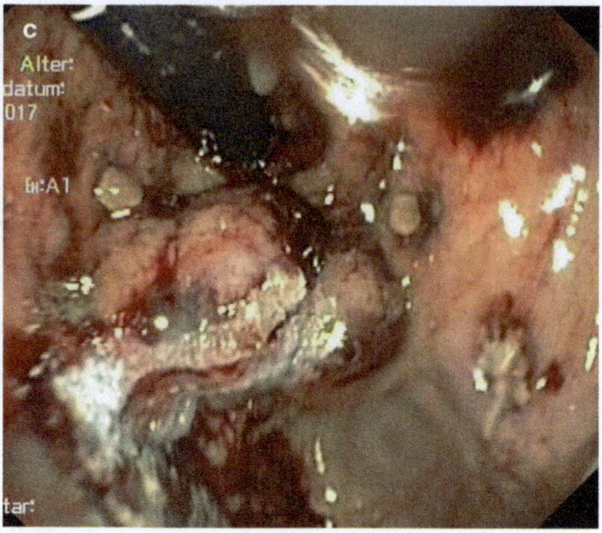

Fig. 10.5 (continued)

Rescue Treatments

Primary treatment failure in GEV hemorrhage is defined as combined pharmacologic and endoscopic treatment not resulting in durable hemostasis or rebleeding occurring within 5 days after the onset of the initial episode. In these cases, the risk of fatal complications is very high.

In patients with an endoscopically confirmed bleeding source in the esophagus, implantation of a designated fully covered self-expanding metal stent (SEMS) in the distal third of the esophagus can help to stop the bleeding by compressing the varices. SEMS has a high success rate and is associated with fewer complications than balloon tamponade [36, 37]. The stents can be left in place for a week or more. During this period, hemodynamic stabilization and treatment of PH must be performed.

Because SEMS is not effective in bleeding sources distal to the gastroesophageal junction, gastric varices can be compressed only by traditional balloon tamponade (via Linton-Nachlas tube). Balloon tamponade is a temporal approach (not longer than 24 h) with high rates of complication.

All patients for whom pharmacologic and endoscopic treatments have failed should be evaluated for implantation of a transjugular intrahepatic portosystemic shunt (TIPS). The use of TIPS for uncontrolled bleeding from GEV is associated with high short-term mortality of up to 75%. All efforts to stop acute bleeding, at least temporarily, should be made before TIPS placement [38].

Secondary Failure to Control Variceal Hemorrhage and Secondary Prevention

Rebleeding that occurs 5 or more days after therapy is defined as secondary treatment failure. Acute treatment in this situation follows the same principles as in the initial bleeding episode: a combination of pharmacologic and endoscopic therapy should be used.

Considering that the risk of rebleeding after hemostasis is up to 60%, with mortality associated with acute variceal bleeding about 30%, secondary prophylaxis of rebleeding is indicated in all patients with clinically relevant PH [39].

The preferred secondary prophylaxis method is a combined treatment with NSBB (or carvedilol) ± nitrates and endoscopic variceal ligation or embolization. This therapy results in a reduction of the recurrent variceal hemorrhage incidence, although the effect on all-cause mortality is not completely clear [40–42]. HVPG measurements can be used to guide the treatment of PH [43]. Additionally, there is some controversy over whether NSBB has a negative effect on the survival of patients with liver cirrhosis and refractory ascites [44, 45]. Recent consensus guidelines recommend monitoring hemodynamic parameters and renal function in patients receiving NSBB therapy. In patients with hypotension, hyponatremia, and/or renal failure, therapy with NSBB should be discontinued [12]. In patients with intolerance of or contraindications to NSBB, EVL alone should be continued. EVL is performed at 2–4 week intervals until all varices of more than the first degree have been eradicated. Endoscopic surveillance is then recommended at 6-month intervals with repeat EVL if the varices increase in size [13].

After bleeding from gastric varices has been treated, secondary prophylaxis follows the same principle: a combination of pharmacologic (NSBB or carvedilol) and endoscopic treatment including an injection of n-butyl-2-cyanoacrylate.

There is growing evidence showing that early TIPS implantation (within 24–72 h after admission) can help to achieve initial hemostasis in patients at high risk of rebleeding. The criteria for a high rebleeding risk include HVPG above 20 mmHg and Child-Pugh stage B in patients with active bleeding at index endoscopy as well as Child-Pugh stage C [46, 47]. In recent studies, early TIPS resulted in a lower risk of treatment failure (rebleeding) and an improved survival rate as compared to combined pharmacologic and endoscopic treatment [48].

The placement of portosystemic stents has also been evaluated as an approach for secondary prophylaxis in patients with a history of GEV hemorrhage. Although overall survival did not increase, rebleeding and hemorrhage-associated mortality were less frequent after TIPS implantation. There was, however, a consistently higher rate of hepatic encephalopathy after TIPS placement compared to endoscopic treatment [49]. Newer data suggest that implanting TIPS with a diameter of less than 10 mm results in less encephalopathy and hepatic dysfunction without compromising the ability of TIPS to prevent bleeding [50].

Whenever TIPS is implanted to treat or prevent VB, transjugular catheterization and subsequent embolization of gastroesophageal collaterals from the portal vein with glue, coils, or plug devices should be evaluated. These measures may improve TIPS function and further reduce rebleeding rates [51].

An alternative to TIPS placement for the treatment of gastric varices, is balloon-occluded retrograde transvenous obliteration (BRTO) via a gastrorenal shunt, accessed through a jugular or femoral vein. This procedure reduces the risk of hepatic encephalopathy associated with TIPS. However, high-quality prospective data on safety and efficacy are lacking so far.

In patients with a contraindication to TIPS placement (e.g., congestive heart failure or splenic vein thrombosis), partial spleen embolization can be performed to reduce blood flow via the spleen and, thus, reduce portal pressure without creating a shunt to systemic circulation [52].

Surgical approaches to target gastric varices and/or PH are currently used less frequently than endoscopic and radiologic treatment. Devascularization of the distal esophagus and proximal stomach and distal splenorenal shunting have been performed for many years and offer good control of variceal bleeding but are associated with a high rate of early mortality [53, 54].

Management of Bleeding from Portal Hypertensive Gastropathy

PHG is represented by macroscopic mucosal changes in the gastric body and fundus. PHG is visible via endoscopy and is accompanied by mucosal and submucosal vascular dilation found in up to 80% of patients with PH (Fig. 10.6) [55, 56]. Stigmata of increased risk of bleeding such as red marks and intramucosal vessel ruptures can also be identified endoscopically.

PHG is a common cause of chronic bleeding leading to anemia. Much less frequently (< 2.5% of cases), PHG is the cause of acute hemorrhage with symptoms such as hemorrhagic shock and hematemesis [57].

Pharmacologic treatment of bleeding from PHG closely follows the same principles as management of hemorrhage from GEV: vasoactive drugs (vasopressin or somatostatin and analogues) followed by NSBB for secondary prophylaxis [58, 59].

TIPS placement as well as surgical shunting may be acceptable options for patients with recurrent severe bleeding. This approach, however, has not been extensively evaluated for isolated PHG.

In the few patients with acute bleeding refractory to pharmacologic treatment and with contraindications to shunt procedures, endoscopic thermal ablation of the main bleeding source and/or application of hemostatic powders may be a less invasive approach but often has only a temporary effect [60, 61].

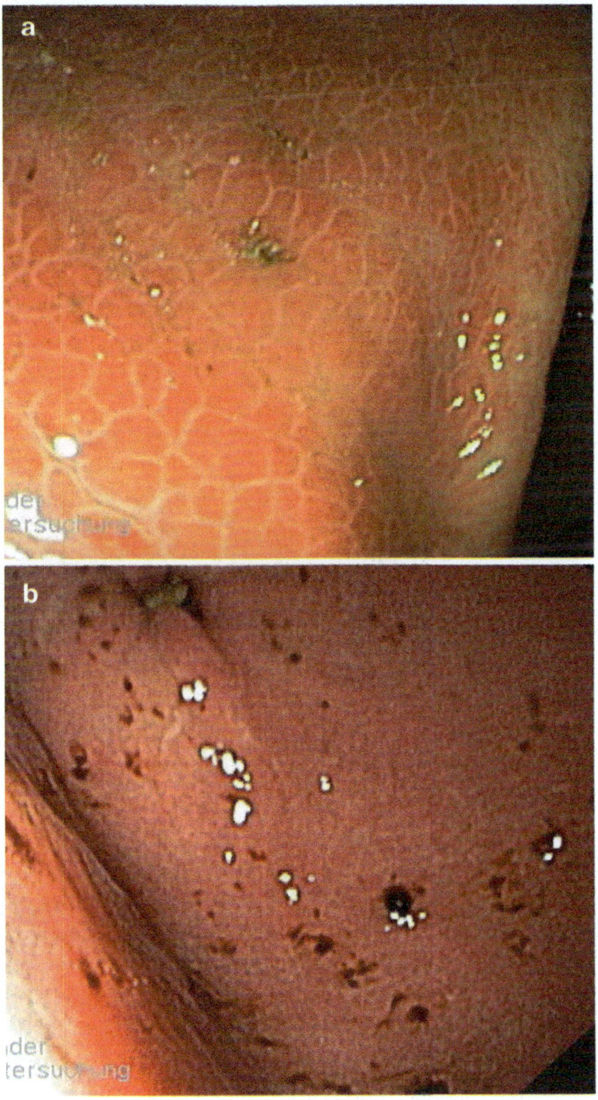

Fig. 10.6 Portal hypertensive gastropathy without bleeding (**a**), with acute bleeding (**b**), with chronic bleeding (**c**)

Fig. 10.6 (continued)

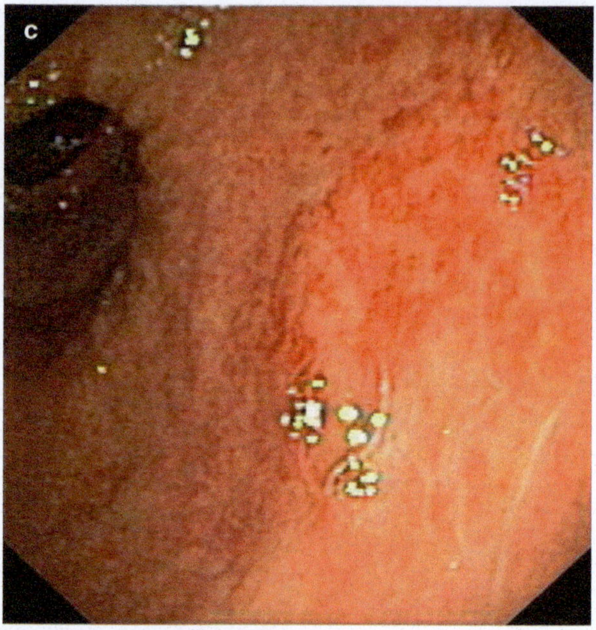

Key Points

1. Upper gastrointestinal bleeding is a frequent cause of mortality in patients with advanced chronic liver disease. The prevalence of esophageal and/or gastric varices in patients with liver cirrhosis is up to 50% and increases with further elevation of portal pressure. The gold standard for the bleeding diagnostic is upper gastrointestinal endoscopy.
2. In patients with esophageal or gastric varices at high bleeding risk, primary prophylaxis (non-selective beta-blockers or endoscopic ligation of varices) reduces the incidence of bleeding episodes.
3. Cirrhotic patients with clinical suspicion of upper gastrointestinal bleeding should be admitted to an intensive care or intermediate care unit for fluid resuscitation and hemodynamic stabilization.
4. Vasopressors (terlipressin, somatostatin, or analogues) and antibiotics should be administered as early as possible if upper gastrointestinal hemorrhage is suspected in cirrhotic patients.
5. The treatment of choice for a hemorrhage associated with esophageal varices is endoscopic band ligation. In the case of gastric varices, endoscopic embolization is a preferable approach.
6. Patients with a high risk of rebleeding could benefit from the early implantation of a transjugular portosystemic stent (TIPS).

References

1. Ripoll C, Groszmann R, Garcia-Tsao G, Grace N, Burroughs A, Planas R, et al. Hepatic venous pressure gradient predicts clinical decompensation in patients with compensated cirrhosis. Gastroenterology. 2007;133:481–8.
2. Rockey DC, Elliott A, Lyles T. Prediction of esophageal varices and variceal hemorrhage in patients with acute upper gastrointestinal bleeding. J Investig Med. 2016;64:745–51.
3. D'Amico G, Pasta L, Morabito A, D'Amico M, Caltagirone M, Malizia G, et al. Competing risks and prognostic stages of cirrhosis: a 25-year inception cohort study of 494 patients. Aliment Pharmacol Ther. 2014;39:1180–93.
4. Fontana RJ, Sanyal AJ, Mehta S, Doherty MC, Neuschwander-Tetri BA, Everson GT, et al. Portal hypertensive gastropathy in chronic hepatitis C patients with bridging fibrosis and compensated cirrhosis: results from the HALT-C trial. Am J Gastroenterol. 2006;101:983–92.
5. Llop E, Lopez M, de la Revilla J, Fernandez N, Trapero M, Hernandez M, et al. Validation of noninvasive methods to predict the presence of gastroesophageal varices in a cohort of patients with compensated advanced chronic liver disease. J Gastroenterol Hepatol. 2017;32:1867–72.
6. Berzigotti A, Seijo S, Arena U, Abraldes JG, Vizzutti F, Garcia-Pagan JC, et al. Elastography, spleen size, and platelet count identify portal hypertension in patients with compensated cirrhosis. Gastroenterology. 2013;144:102–11.e1.
7. Kovalak M, Lake J, Mattek N, Eisen G, Lieberman D, Zaman A. Endoscopic screening for varices in cirrhotic patients: data from a national endoscopic database. Gastrointest Endosc. 2007;65:82–8.
8. Groszmann RJ, Garcia-Tsao G, Bosch J, Grace ND, Burroughs AK, Planas R, et al. Beta-blockers to prevent gastroesophageal varices in patients with cirrhosis. N Engl J Med. 2005;353:2254–61.
9. Abraldes JG, Bureau C, Stefanescu H, Augustin S, Ney M, Blasco H, et al. Noninvasive tools and risk of clinically significant portal hypertension and varices in compensated cirrhosis: the "anticipate" study. Hepatology. 2016;64:2173–84.
10. Maurice JB, Brodkin E, Arnold F, Navaratnam A, Paine H, Khawar S, et al. Validation of the Baveno VI criteria to identify low risk cirrhotic patients not requiring endoscopic surveillance for varices. J Hepatol. 2016;65:899–905.
11. Carbonell N, Pauwels A, Serfaty L, Fourdan O, Levy VG, Poupon R. Improved survival after variceal bleeding in patients with cirrhosis over the past two decades. Hepatology. 2004;40:652–9.
12. de Franchis R, Baveno VIF. Expanding consensus in portal hypertension: report of the Baveno VI consensus workshop: stratifying risk and individualizing care for portal hypertension. J Hepatol. 2015;63:743–52.
13. Tripathi D, Stanley AJ, Hayes PC, Patch D, Millson C, Mehrzad H, et al. U.K. guidelines on the management of variceal haemorrhage in cirrhotic patients. Gut. 2015;64:1680–704.
14. Qi XS, Bao YX, Bai M, Xu WD, Dai JN, Guo XZ. Nonselective beta-blockers in cirrhotic patients with no or small varices: a meta-analysis. World J Gastroenterol. 2015;21:3100–8.
15. Cheng JW, Zhu L, Gu MJ, Song ZM. Meta analysis of propranolol effects on gastrointestinal hemorrhage in cirrhotic patients. World J Gastroenterol. 2003;9:1836–9.
16. Reiberger T, Ulbrich G, Ferlitsch A, Payer BA, Schwabl P, Pinter M, et al. Carvedilol for primary prophylaxis of variceal bleeding in cirrhotic patients with haemodynamic non-response to propranolol. Gut. 2013;62:1634–41.
17. Gluud LL, Krag A. Banding ligation versus beta-blockers for primary prevention in oesophageal varices in adults. Cochrane Database Syst Rev. 2012;(8):CD004544.
18. Takuma Y, Nouso K, Morimoto Y, Tomokuni J, Sahara A, Takabatake H, et al. Prediction of oesophageal variceal bleeding by measuring spleen stiffness in patients with liver cirrhosis. Gut. 2016;65:354–5.

19. Gralnek IM, Dumonceau JM, Kuipers EJ, Lanas A, Sanders DS, Kurien M, et al. Diagnosis and management of nonvariceal upper gastrointestinal hemorrhage: European Society of Gastrointestinal Endoscopy (ESGE) Guideline. Endoscopy. 2015;47:a1–46.
20. Gattas DJ, Dan A, Myburgh J, Billot L, Lo S, Finfer S, et al. Fluid resuscitation with 6% hydroxyethyl starch (130/0.4 and 130/0.42) in acutely ill patients: systematic review of effects on mortality and treatment with renal replacement therapy. Intensive Care Med. 2013;39:558–68.
21. Annane D, Siami S, Jaber S, Martin C, Elatrous S, Declere AD, et al. Effects of fluid resuscitation with colloids vs crystalloids on mortality in critically ill patients presenting with hypovolemic shock: the CRISTAL randomized trial. JAMA. 2013;310:1809–17.
22. Villanueva C, Colomo A, Bosch A, Concepcion M, Hernandez-Gea V, Aracil C, et al. Transfusion strategies for acute upper gastrointestinal bleeding. N Engl J Med. 2013;368:11–21.
23. D'Amico G, Pagliaro L, Bosch J. The treatment of portal hypertension: a meta-analytic review. Hepatology. 1995;22:332–54.
24. Ioannou G, Doust J, Rockey DC. Terlipressin for acute esophageal variceal hemorrhage. Cochrane Database Syst Rev. 2003;(1):CD002147.
25. Seo YS, Park SY, Kim MY, Kim JH, Park JY, Yim HJ, et al. Lack of difference among terlipressin, somatostatin, and octreotide in the control of acute gastroesophageal variceal hemorrhage. Hepatology. 2014;60:954–63.
26. Chavez-Tapia NC, Barrientos-Gutierrez T, Tellez-Avila F, Soares-Weiser K, Mendez-Sanchez N, Gluud C, et al. Meta-analysis: antibiotic prophylaxis for cirrhotic patients with upper gastrointestinal bleeding – an updated Cochrane review. Aliment Pharmacol Ther. 2011;34:509–18.
27. Theivanayagam S, Lim RG, Cobell WJ, Gowda JT, Matteson ML, Choudhary A, et al. Administration of erythromycin before endoscopy in upper gastrointestinal bleeding: a meta-analysis of randomized controlled trials. Saudi J Gastroenterol. 2013;19:205–10.
28. Barkun AN, Bardou M, Kuipers EJ, Sung J, Hunt RH, Martel M, et al. International consensus recommendations on the management of patients with nonvariceal upper gastrointestinal bleeding. Ann Intern Med. 2010;152:101–13.
29. Min YW, Lim KS, Min BH, Gwak GY, Paik YH, Choi MS, et al. Proton pump inhibitor use significantly increases the risk of spontaneous bacterial peritonitis in 1965 patients with cirrhosis and ascites: a propensity score matched cohort study. Aliment Pharmacol Ther. 2014;40:695–704.
30. Hayat U, Lee PJ, Ullah H, Sarvepalli S, Lopez R, Vargo JJ. Association of prophylactic endotracheal intubation in critically ill patients with upper GI bleeding and cardiopulmonary unplanned events. Gastrointest Endosc. 2017;86:500–9.e1.
31. Banares R, Albillos A, Rincon D, Alonso S, Gonzalez M, Ruiz-del-Arbol L, et al. Endoscopic treatment versus endoscopic plus pharmacologic treatment for acute variceal bleeding: a meta-analysis. Hepatology. 2002;35:609–15.
32. Laine L, Cook D. Endoscopic ligation compared with sclerotherapy for treatment of esophageal variceal bleeding. A meta-analysis. Ann Intern Med. 1995;123:280–7.
33. Kang EJ, Jeong SW, Jang JY, Cho JY, Lee SH, Kim HG, et al. Long-term result of endoscopic Histoacryl (N-butyl-2-cyanoacrylate) injection for treatment of gastric varices. World J Gastroenterol. 2011;17:1494–500.
34. Ljubicic N, Biscanin A, Nikolic M, Supanc V, Hrabar D, Pavic T, et al. A randomized-controlled trial of endoscopic treatment of acute esophageal variceal hemorrhage: N-butyl-2-cyanoacrylate injection vs. variceal ligation. Hepato-Gastroenterology. 2011;58:438–43.
35. Ibrahim M, El-Mikkawy A, Abdalla H, Mostafa I, Deviere J. Management of acute variceal bleeding using hemostatic powder. United European Gastroenterol J. 2015;3:277–83.
36. Escorsell A, Pavel O, Cardenas A, Morillas R, Llop E, Villanueva C, et al. Esophageal balloon tamponade versus esophageal stent in controlling acute refractory variceal bleeding: a multicenter randomized, controlled trial. Hepatology. 2016;63:1957–67.
37. McCarty TR, Njei B. Self-expanding metal stents for acute refractory esophageal variceal bleeding: a systematic review and meta-analysis. Dig Endosc. 2016;28:539–47.

38. Vangeli M, Patch D, Burroughs AK. Salvage tips for uncontrolled variceal bleeding. J Hepatol. 2002;37:703–4.
39. Bari K, Garcia-Tsao G. Treatment of portal hypertension. World J Gastroenterol. 2012;18:1166–75.
40. D'Amico G, Pagliaro L, Bosch J. Pharmacological treatment of portal hypertension: an evidence-based approach. Semin Liver Dis. 1999;19:475–505.
41. Gournay J, Masliah C, Martin T, Perrin D, Galmiche JP. Isosorbide mononitrate and propranolol compared with propranolol alone for the prevention of variceal rebleeding. Hepatology. 2000;31:1239–45.
42. Thiele M, Krag A, Rohde U, Gluud LL. Meta-analysis: banding ligation and medical interventions for the prevention of rebleeding from oesophageal varices. Aliment Pharmacol Ther. 2012;35:1155–65.
43. Villanueva C, Graupera I, Aracil C, Alvarado E, Minana J, Puente A, et al. A randomized trial to assess whether portal pressure guided therapy to prevent variceal rebleeding improves survival in cirrhosis. Hepatology. 2017;65:1693–707.
44. Serste T, Melot C, Francoz C, Durand F, Rautou PE, Valla D, et al. Deleterious effects of beta-blockers on survival in patients with cirrhosis and refractory ascites. Hepatology. 2010;52:1017–22.
45. Leithead JA, Rajoriya N, Tehami N, Hodson J, Gunson BK, Tripathi D, et al. Non-selective beta-blockers are associated with improved survival in patients with ascites listed for liver transplantation. Gut. 2015;64:1111–9.
46. Monescillo A, Martinez-Lagares F, Ruiz-del-Arbol L, Sierra A, Guevara C, Jimenez E, et al. Influence of portal hypertension and its early decompression by TIPS placement on the outcome of variceal bleeding. Hepatology. 2004;40:793–801.
47. Garcia-Pagan JC, Caca K, Bureau C, Laleman W, Appenrodt B, Luca A, et al. Early use of TIPS in patients with cirrhosis and variceal bleeding. N Engl J Med. 2010;362:2370–9.
48. Halabi SA, Sawas T, Sadat B, Jandali A, Halabi HA, Halabi FA, et al. Early TIPS versus endoscopic therapy for secondary prophylaxis after management of acute esophageal variceal bleeding in cirrhotic patients: a meta-analysis of randomized controlled trials. J Gastroenterol Hepatol. 2016;31:1519–26.
49. Zheng M, Chen Y, Bai J, Zeng Q, You J, Jin R, et al. Transjugular intrahepatic portosystemic shunt versus endoscopic therapy in the secondary prophylaxis of variceal rebleeding in cirrhotic patients: meta-analysis update. J Clin Gastroenterol. 2008;42:507–16.
50. Wang Q, Lv Y, Bai M, Wang Z, Liu H, He C, et al. Eight millimetre covered TIPS does not compromise shunt function but reduces hepatic encephalopathy in preventing variceal rebleeding. J Hepatol. 2017;67:508–16.
51. Chen S, Li X, Wei B, Tong H, Zhang MG, Huang ZY, et al. Recurrent variceal bleeding and shunt patency: prospective randomized controlled trial of transjugular intrahepatic portosystemic shunt alone or combined with coronary vein embolization. Radiology. 2013;268:900–6.
52. Buechter M, Kahraman A, Manka P, Gerken G, Dechene A, Canbay A, et al. Partial spleen embolization reduces the risk of portal hypertension-induced upper gastrointestinal bleeding in patients not eligible for TIPS implantation. PLoS One. 2017;12:e0177401.
53. Riemenschneider T, Bermel RE, Hirner A. Results of devascularization surgery of the gastroesophageal junction in recurrent hemorrhage of esophageal and fundus varices. Zentralbl Chir. 1994;119:291–7.
54. Thomas PG, D'Cruz AJ. Distal splenorenal shunting for bleeding gastric varices. Br J Surg. 1994;81:241–4.
55. Merli M, Nicolini G, Angeloni S, Gentili F, Attili AF, Riggio O. The natural history of portal hypertensive gastropathy in patients with liver cirrhosis and mild portal hypertension. Am J Gastroenterol. 2004;99:1959–65.
56. Kim MY, Choi H, Baik SK, Yea CJ, Won CS, Byun JW, et al. Portal hypertensive gastropathy: correlation with portal hypertension and prognosis in cirrhosis. Dig Dis Sci. 2010;55:3561–7.

57. Primignani M, Carpinelli L, Preatoni P, Battaglia G, Carta A, Prada A, et al. Natural history of portal hypertensive gastropathy in patients with liver cirrhosis. The New Italian Endoscopic Club for the study and treatment of esophageal varices (NIEC). Gastroenterology. 2000;119:181–7.
58. Kouroumalis EA, Koutroubakis IE, Manousos ON. Somatostatin for acute severe bleeding from portal hypertensive gastropathy. Eur J Gastroenterol Hepatol. 1998;10:509–12.
59. Bruha R, Marecek Z, Spicak J, Hulek P, Lata J, Petrtyl J, et al. Double-blind randomized, comparative multicenter study of the effect of terlipressin in the treatment of acute esophageal variceal and/or hypertensive gastropathy bleeding. Hepato-Gastroenterology. 2002;49:1161–6.
60. Herrera S, Bordas JM, Llach J, Gines A, Pellise M, Fernandez-Esparrach G, et al. The beneficial effects of argon plasma coagulation in the management of different types of gastric vascular ectasia lesions in patients admitted for GI hemorrhage. Gastrointest Endosc. 2008;68:440–6.
61. Smith LA, Morris AJ, Stanley AJ. The use of hemospray in portal hypertensive bleeding; a case series. J Hepatol. 2014;60:457–60.

Chapter 11
Acute-On-Chronic Liver Failure

Miriam Maschmeier, Anna Hüsing-Kabar, and Hartmut H. Schmidt

Definitions

Acute-on-chronic liver failure (ACLF) describes an acute deterioration of a pre-existing chronic liver disease that results in organ failure. It is associated with a high short-term mortality rate [1]. Within the past few years, ACLF has been recognized as an important clinical entity. ACLF clearly distinguishes itself from acute liver failure (ALF) by the presence of a pre-existing liver disease. It is different from acute decompensation, as it is accompanied by multi-system organ failure and is associated with a higher mortality rate [1–3].

There is no universally accepted definition of ACLF. In fact, there are more than ten different definitions of the condition developed primarily on a theoretical basis. This hinders the identification of the subgroup of patients requiring special attention in order to decrease the high risk of mortality [4, 5].

Working independently, the Asian Pacific Association for the Study of the Liver (APASL) the European Association for the Study of the Liver (EASL), and the American Association for the Study of Liver Diseases (AASLD) have each developed a working definition of ACLF [2].

The APASL has defined ACLF as an acute hepatic insult occurring in a patient with an underlying chronic liver disease manifesting as jaundice (serum bilirubin $\geq$ 5 mg/dl (85 μmol/l)), coagulopathy (INR $\geq$ 1.5 or prothrombin activity < 40%), ascites, and/or encephalopathy within 4 weeks of onset [6]. The

M. Maschmeier (✉) · A. Hüsing-Kabar · H. H. Schmidt
Department of Transplant Medicine, University Hospital of Münster, Münster, Germany
e-mail: miriam.maschmeier@ukmuenster.de

D. Bezinover, F. Saner (eds.), *Critical Care for Potential Liver Transplant Candidates*,
https://doi.org/10.1007/978-3-319-92934-7_11

EASL and AASLD, on the other hand, describe ACLF as "an acute deterioration of a pre-existing chronic liver disease usually related to a precipitating event and associated with an increased mortality at 3 months due to multisystem organ failure" [3].

These definitions have significant differences. The APASL definition includes both patients without cirrhosis and those with compensated cirrhosis, whereas the EASL/AASLD definition includes only those with compensated and decompensated cirrhosis. The APASL definition focuses on liver failure where sepsis is not considered a precipitating event. In the EASL/AASLD definitions, extrahepatic multi-organ failure is an essential feature, and infection is considered an important trigger of ACLF [1–3, 6, 7].

These disparities can be explained by the differences in the leading causes of ACLF in the Asia-Pacific region compared to Europe and North America. In Western countries, most patients with pre-existing cirrhosis develop ACLF due to nonviral causes (e.g., bacterial infection); patients in the Asia-Pacific region, where cirrhosis is not seen as frequently, develop ACLF mainly due to viral insults (e.g., hepatitis B flares). Alcohol abuse, however, seems to be a universal problem [7]. Differences in the definitions of ACLF lead to the diagnosis of ACLF in noncomparable groups of patients, which results in different study outcomes [8].

Further insight into ACLF has been provided by two large, prospective, observational investigations performed in Europe and North America: the EASL-CLIF Acute-on-Chronic Liver Failure in Cirrhosis (CANONIC), and the North American Consortium for the Study of End-Stage Liver Disease (NACSELD). Whereas the NACSELD study focused on the mortality of infected patients with cirrhosis (leaving out other triggers), the CANONIC study included only patients with cirrhosis admitted for any acute decompensation (acute development of large amounts of ascites, hepatic encephalopathy (HE), gastrointestinal hemorrhage, bacterial infection, or any combination of these). In the CANONIC study, it was found that the mortality of cirrhotic patients with ACLF correlated with the number of organ failures. This was confirmed for cirrhotic patients with bacterial infection in the NACSELD study [5, 7]. Based on the results of the CANONIC study, the first evidence-based diagnostic criteria and prognostic scores for ACLF in cirrhotic patients have been proposed and will be discussed in this chapter.

To overcome differences and to find common ground for further research, the World Congress of Gastroenterology proposed a consensus definition in 2014. It combines features from both Eastern and Western understanding of ACLF (Table 11.1) and defines ACLF as "a syndrome in patients with chronic liver disease, with or without previously diagnosed cirrhosis, characterized by acute hepatic decompensation resulting in liver failure (jaundice and prolongation of the INR [International Normalized Ratio]) and one or more extrahepatic organ failures that is associated with increased mortality within a period of 28 days and up to 3 months from onset" [2].

Table 11.1 Alternative definitions of acute-on-chronic liver failure

APASL 2009/2014 [6]	AASLD/EASL 2011 [3]	World Congress of Gastroenterology 2014 [2]
"An acute hepatic insult manifesting as jaundice (serum bilirubin ≥ 5 mg/dl (85 μmol/l)) and coagulopathy (INR ≥ 1.5 or prothrombin activity < 40%) complicated within 4 weeks by clinical ascites and/or encephalopathy in a patient with previously diagnosed or undiagnosed chronic liver disease/cirrhosis and is associated with a high 28-day mortality"	"An acute deterioration of pre-existing chronic liver disease, usually related to a precipitating event and associated with increased mortality at 3 months due to multisystem organ failure"	"A syndrome in patients with chronic liver disease with or without previously diagnosed cirrhosis which is characterized by acute hepatic decompensation resulting in liver failure (jaundice and prolongation of the INR [International Normalized Ratio]) and one or more extrahepatic organ failures that is associated with increased mortality within a period of 28 days and up to 3 months from onset"

APASL Asian Pacific Association for the Study of the Liver, *AASLD* American Association for the Study of Liver Diseases, *EASL* European Association for the Study of the Liver

Epidemiology

Based on the results of the CANONIC und NACSELD studies, as well as data from Chinese studies using CANONIC criteria, the prevalence of ACLF in hospitalized patients with cirrhosis is between 24 and 34% [5, 7, 9, 10]. In the CANONIC study, ACLF was present in about 20% of patients at enrollment and developed in another 10% while they were hospitalized [5].

Classification and Diagnosis of ACLF in Cirrhotic Patients

ACLF Types A–C

According to the World Congress of Gastroenterology definition, acute-on-chronic liver failure can develop in patients with chronic liver disease without cirrhosis as well as in patients with compensated or decompensated cirrhosis.

Rather than one disease, ACLF is a syndrome characterized by acute decompensation, single- or multiple-organ failure, and high short-term mortality [5]. Depending on the underlying liver disease and the clinical, pathophysiologic, and prognostic features, three subtypes of ACLF have been identified (Fig. 11.1). Patients without cirrhosis who develop ACLF are Type A. A liver biopsy demonstrating signs of chronicity is necessary for confirmation and differentiation from ALF. Patients with compensated cirrhosis who develop ACLF are Type B, and those with decompensated cirrhosis are Type C [2].

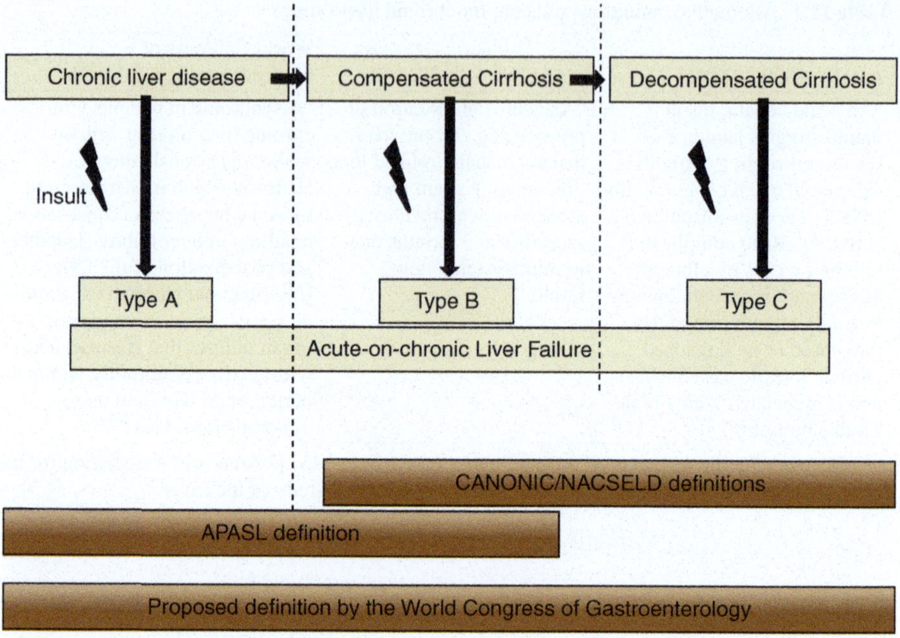

Fig. 11.1 Proposed classification of acute-on-chronic liver failure with regard to the severity of the underlying liver disease and applicable definitions (Modified from Jalan et al. (2014) [2])

Only the APASL definition (Table 11.1) applies to patients with Type A ACLF (does not include Type C ACLF). However, the ACLF scores definition of ACLF based on the CANONIC and NACSELD studies apply to patients with ACLF Types B and C.

The CANONIC Definition and ACLF Grades in Patients with Cirrhosis

The CANONIC group evaluated 1,343 patients at liver units in 29 university hospitals in Europe. Patients with either compensated or decompensated cirrhosis with or without organ failure were recruited for the study. The severity of illness was assessed by a modified CLIF-SOFA score derived from the SOFA score (sepsis-related organ failure assessment score). This score was developed to predict mortality related to sepsis [11] and is used to evaluate six organ systems: respiratory (Horovitz index), cardiovascular (hypotension and/or use of vasopressors), cerebral function (GCS), coagulation (platelet count), hepatic (bilirubin), and renal (creatinine). Depending on the assessed values for each organ system, a specific score is assigned. The sum of the subscores for all the assessed organs ranges from 0 to 24.

A SOFA score of 10 predicts a mortality of around 40%, whereas a SOFA $\geq$ 15 predicts a mortality rate of > 90%. In order to take into account specific aspects of cirrhotic patients, SOFA scores have been adjusted. To assess cerebral function, the CANONIC group replaced GCS with hepatic encephalopathy (HE) according to the West Haven criteria. The use of terlipressin, a new vasoconstrictor, has been added to the circulatory system assessment of the CLIF-SOFA score. INR is included in the assessment of the coagulation system (Table 11.2).

Based on these assessments, the authors stratified the patients into four groups:

1. No ACLF: This group comprises three subgroups:
   (a) Patients without organ failure
   (b) Patients with single non-kidney organ failure (e.g., coagulation, liver, circulatory or respiratory, serum creatinine (SCrea) <1.5 mg/dl, and no HE)
   (c) Patients with single cerebral failure and SCrea <1.5 mg/dl
   Among the recruited patients, 77.4% had no ACLF at enrollment. The 28- and 90-day mortality rates were 4.7 and 14%, respectively.
2. ACLF grade 1: This group comprises three subgroups:
   (a) Patients with single kidney failure (SCrea $\geq$2 mg/dl or dialysis)
   (b) Patients with one organ failure, SCrea ranging from 1.5 to 1.9 mg/dl and/or H.E. I°/II°
   (c) Patients with HE $\geq$ III° and SCrea ranging from 1.5 to 1.9 mg/dl

   At the time of enrollment, 11% of the patients suffered from ACLF grade 1. The 28- and 90-day mortality rates were 22.1 and 40%, respectively
3. ACLF grade 2: This group comprises patients with two organ failures. At the time of enrollment, 8% of the cohort suffered from ACLF grade 2. The 28- and 90-day mortality rates were 32 and 52.3%, respectively.
4. ACLF grade 3: This cohort comprises patients with three or more organ failures. Among the recruited patients, 3.5% suffered from ACLF grade 3. The 28- and 90-day mortality rates were 76.7 and 79.1%, respectively.

   ACLF grades and organ failures are presented in Table 11.3.

Organ failure definitions are based on specific values:

Pulmonary: Horovitz index < 200 mmHg
Renal: Creatinine $\geq$ 2 mg/dl or requirement for dialysis
Central nervous system (CNS): Hepatic encephalopathy (H.E.) $\geq$ III° Hepatic: Bilirubin $\geq$ 12 mg/dl
Circulatory: Use of any vasopressor
Coagulation: INR $\geq$ 2.5

A follow-up study aimed at developing a new score predicting the prognosis of patients with ACLF more accurately than ACLF grade 0–3 has been reported [12]. The authors created a simpler organ failure score (CLIF-C-OF). For each organ system, new cutoff points were defined to stratify organ failure into three different severity categories (Table 11.4).

Table 11.2 CLIF-SOFA score

System	Parameter	CLIF-SOFA points			
		1	2	3	4
Pulmonary	paO_2/FiO_2 mmHg SpO_2/FiO_2	≤ 400 to 300 ≤ 512 to 358	≤ 300 to 200 ≤ 357 to 215	≤ 200 to 100 ≤ 214 to 90	≤ 100 ≤ 89
Renal	SCr (mg/dL)	1.2–1.9	2.0–3.4	3.5–4.9	> 5 or dialysis
Liver	Bilirubin (mg/dl)	1.2–1.9	2.0–5.9	6.0–11.9	> 12
Circulatory	Blood pressure in mmHg/ Vasopressor in /μg/kg/min	MAP < 70	Dopamine ≤ 5 or dobutamine or terlipressin	Dopamine > 5, or adrenaline or noradrenaline ≤ 0.1	Adrenaline or noradrenaline > 0.1
Coagulation	INR	1.1 to < 1.25	1.25 ≤ INR < 1.5	1.5 ≤ INR < 2.5	2.5 ≤ INR or PLT ≤ 20 × 10^3/nl
CNS	Hepatic encephalopathy	I	II	III	IV

Table 11.3 ACLF grades

No ACLF	ACLF Grade 1	ACLF Grade 2	ACLF Grade 3
No organ failure Single organ failure and SCrea <1.5 mg/dl and no H.E. Single cerebral failure (H.E. ≥ III°-IV°) and SCrea <1.5 mg/dl	Single kidney failure Single organ failure and 1.5 ≤ SCrea ≤ 1.9 mg/dl and/or -H.E. I°-II° Single cerebral failure (H.E. III°-IV°) and 1.5 ≤ SCrea ≤ 1.9 mg/dl	Two organ failures	Three or more organ failures

According to Moreau et al. [5]
ACLF acute on chronic liver failure, *AD* acute decompensation, *HE* hepatic encephalopathy

Table 11.4 CLIF-C-OF score

Organ or System	1	2	3
Liver	Bilirubin < 6mg/dl	Bilirubin ≥ 6mg/dl and < 12 mg/dl	Bilirubin ≥ 12mg/dl
Kidney	Creatinine < 1.5mg/l 1.5-1.9mg/l	Creatinine ≥ 2mg/dl and < 3.5mg/dl	Creatinine ≥ 3.5mg/dl or RRT
Brain (West Haven Criteria for HE)	Grade 0	Grade I-II	Grade III-IV
Coagulation	INR < 2.0	INR ≥ 2.0 and < 2.5	INR ≥ 2.5
Circulation	MAP ≥ 70mmHg	MAP < 700mmHg	Use of vasopressors
Respiration PaO_2/FiO_2 or SpO_2/FiO_2	> 300 or > 357	≤ 300 and > 200 or ≤ 357 and > 214	≤ 200 or ≤ 214 or MV (unless due to HE)

Adapted from Jalan et al. [12]
Gray fields indicate organ failure
RRT renal replacement therapy, *HE* hepatic encephalopathy, *INR* international normalized ratio, *MAP* mean arterial pressure, PaO_2 arterial oxygen partial pressure, FiO_2 fraction of inspired oxygen, SpO_2 oxygen saturation, *MV* mechanical ventilation

Together with CLIF-C-OF, age and white blood cell (WBC) count were shown to be the best predictors of 28-day mortality. The CLIF-C-ACLF score can be assessed by the following equation:

$$\text{CLIF-C-ACLF} = 10 \times \left(0.33 \times \text{CLIF-OF} + 0.04 \times \text{age} + 0.63 \times \left(\text{Ln}\left(\text{WBC}\right)\right) - 2\right)$$

The score ranges between 0 and 100. The higher the score, the higher the mortality. An online application to calculate the CLIF-C-ACLF score and estimate mortality is available at the CLIF Consortium website: http://www.clifconsortium.com/.

Depending on the 28-day mortality, patients can be stratified into three categories:

1. CLIF-C-ACLF < 45 = > 28-day mortality approximately 10%
2. 45 ≤ CLIF-C-ACLF ≤ 64 = > 28-day mortality between 20 and 70%
3. CLIF-C-ACLF ≥ 65 = > 28-day mortality > 90%

The PIRO Concept in ACLF

It has been proposed that the PIRO concept (predisposition, injury, response, and organ system) be adapted to describe the complex pathophysiology of ACLF (Table 11.5) [1, 13]. In 2001, a consensus conference of intensive care societies (SCCM/ESICM/ACCP/ATS/SIS) developed a classification scheme for sepsis called PIRO, which stratifies patients on the basis of their predisposing conditions, the nature and extent of the insult (in the case of sepsis, infection), the nature and magnitude of the host response, and the degree of concomitant organ dysfunction [14].

The authors have stated that the PIRO concept is rudimentary and that extensive testing and further refinement are required before it can be presented in its final form for routine application. At present, a clinical application of PIRO is lacking for patients with sepsis.

Predisposition

Different studies have found a range of variations in the predisposition to ACLF. In the CANONIC study, patients with ACLF were significantly younger than those who did not develop ACLF. The main etiologies of cirrhosis were alcoholic liver disease (most frequent) followed by hepatitis C [5]. In patients without prior episodes of acute decompensation (ACLF type B), the course of the disease was more severe and associated with a higher mortality rate [9, 15]. In the NACSELD study, the MELD score was a significant risk factor for the development of ACLF [7].

Table 11.5 The PIRO concept in acute-on-chronic liver failure

Predisposition	Injury (=precipitating event)	Response	Organ failure
Etiology Severity of cirrhosis Age Genetic	Alcohol Drug Virus Bacterial infection Surgery	Inflammation Immune failure	CLIF-C-OF

Modified from Jalan et al. [1]

Injury (Precipitating Event)

ACLF may be triggered by precipitating hepatic or extrahepatic insults. Hepatic insults include the hepatotoxic effects of alcohol and/or drugs and viral hepatitis. Extrahepatic insults can be caused by bacterial infection, surgery, TIPS insertion, large-volume paracentesis without albumin administration, trauma, and others [1, 15]. The frequency of these triggers varies depending on the region. The CANONIC study identified bacterial infection in 33% of patients (spontaneous bacterial peritonitis, pneumonia, urinary tract and skin infections) and active alcoholism (23% of patients) to be the most frequent predisposing events [5, 16]. In Eastern countries, however, hepatotropic viral infections are more common [6]. Gastrointestinal hemorrhage was observed more often in patients with acute decompensation of cirrhosis than in patients with ACLF in the CANONIC study. The roles of different precipitating events as ACLF triggers need to be verified [15, 16].

In the CANONIC study, precipitating events were found in less than 60% of cases [5].

In some studies, including the CANONIC study, the presence and type of precipitating event were found to have no influence on mortality. Data from a Chinese population, however, suggest that the type of injury does influence the outcome of patients with ACLF. Yet, the mortality after 28 days was similar between patients with hepatic and extrahepatic insults and mortality after 3 and 12 months was significantly higher in patients with extrahepatic insults [10].

Response (Systemic Inflammation in ACLF)

The mechanisms leading to organ failure in ACLF are not completely understood. However, it is likely that inflammation plays an important role.

Inflammation may be induced by exogenic or endogenic stimuli. Exogenic stimuli include infection, mostly due to bacterial pathogens [17]. Bacterial infections are frequent in cirrhotic patients and associated with a high mortality rate [1, 5, 18]. In response to either the bacteria or molecular structures expressed by bacteria (pathogen-associated molecular patterns (PAMPs) being detected by pattern recognition receptors (PRRs, e.g., TLR, NLR, RIG, RLR) of cells of the innate immune system), a signaling cascade activates transcriptional factors (NFKB) with subsequent induction of genes responsible for the production of inflammatory cytokines. This results in collateral tissue damage, which leads to organ failure (OF). This effect is called *immunopathology* [15, 17, 19].

Data suggest that an increased innate immune response in cirrhotic patients is responsible for the development of organ failure and the development of ACLF [15].

Cirrhotic patients also have increased levels of pro- and anti-inflammatory cytokines [8, 15]. In an animal model, cirrhotic rats had significantly higher TNF-α levels than those without cirrhosis after being exposed to lipopolysaccharide (LPS, a PAMP)

[15]. Accordingly, freshly isolated monocytes, or peripheral blood mononuclear cells of cirrhotic patients, produced higher pro-inflammatory cytokine levels after ex vivo exposure to LPS. Increased production of those cytokines is associated with increased mortality [15]. Patients with spontaneous bacterial peritonitis have high levels of pro-inflammatory cytokines and, thus, have an increased risk of renal failure [15].

Inflammation might be caused by exogenous ligands such as structural elements of bacteria, e.g., PAMPs, or nonviable bacteria not detected by standard diagnostic measures. Endogenous ligands released by dying or damaged cells (e.g., danger-associated molecular patterns (DAMPs), extracellular matrix, heat-shock proteins, or nucleic acids) can also trigger excessive (sterile) inflammation [17]. This might be relevant in patients with acute alcoholic hepatitis, HBV-related hepatitis flares, or liver injury induced by drugs [17].

Tissue damage can be caused directly by bacteria via toxins or virulence factors. The impact of direct tissue damage as a mechanism for organ failure in cirrhosis is unknown [15, 19].

Another factor that can lead to tissue damage is failed tolerance [20]. When immunopathology causes an excessive inflammatory response, anti-inflammatory treatment might be beneficial. If tissue homeostasis or tissue damage is mediated by the pathogen itself, anti-inflammatory therapy might harm the patient further [15]. If an immune suppressed state (sepsis-like immune paralysis) develops with decreased production of inflammatory cytokines, patients are at risk of developing secondary infections and have increased mortality [18, 21]. Similar to patients with sepsis, lower levels of ex vivo TNF-α and HLA DR expression were found after an LPS challenge in patients with ACLF [21].

Organ Failure

Please see Tables 11.2 and 11.4.

Management of ACLF

It is beyond the scope of this chapter to discuss in detail the treatment of each failing organ.

The main insight is that there is currently no specific treatment for ACLF. The principle of treatment is the early identification of the syndrome and the factors that trigger ACLF [15]. Given that infections (e.g., spontaneous bacterial peritonitis, urinary tract infection, and pneumonia) are the most frequent precipitating events, they should always be screened for and – if detected – therapy should be initiated immediately.

Data from the CANONIC study clearly demonstrate that the first 7 days after initiation of specific treatment are important and ACLF patients should be treated in an intensive care environment. ACLF is a dynamic syndrome, where 50% of the patients improve their clinical condition, 30% remain unchanged, and 20% worsen. Some patients will qualify for transplantation. Every patient should initially receive supportive organ therapy and be re-evaluated after 3 days. This applies even to those patients with a CLIF-C-OF $\geq$ 65 and predicted mortality of > 90%.

Key Points

1. ACLF is a specific syndrome characterized by acute deterioration of a pre-existing liver disease, organ failure, and high short-term mortality. A 28-day-mortality rate correlates with the grade of ACLF, ranging from 22% (grade 1) to 73% (grade 3).
2. One of the most important precipitating factors in patients with ACLF is infection. Bacteria release PAMPs, which are recognized by PRR. Tissue damage related to pathogens is increased by an altered cell function.
3. A substantial number of ACLF cases are not related to bacterial infections. Tissue damage and OF are probably related to excessive host response, activating the same PRR, either by PAMPs released by already killed bacteria or DAMPs, which are proteins released from dying cells.
4. The CLIF-SOFA score and the simplified version, the CLIF-C-OF score, are based on an assessment of six organ systems. The CLIF-C-OF score together with age and WBC allows the calculation of the CLIF-C-ACLF score, which specifically predicts short-term mortality.
5. The general management of ACLF requires rapid identification and treatment of potential triggers.

References

1. Jalan R, Gines P, Olson JC, Mookerjee RP, Moreau R, Garcia-Tsao G, et al. Acute-on chronic liver failure. J Hepatol. 2012;57(6):1336–48.
2. Jalan R, Yurdaydin C, Bajaj JS, Acharya SK, Arroyo V, Lin HC, et al. Toward an improved definition of acute-on-chronic liver failure. Gastroenterology. 2014;147(1):4–10.
3. Olson JC, Kamath PS. Acute-on-chronic liver failure: concept, natural history, and prognosis. Curr Opin Crit Care. 2011;17(2):165–9.
4. Wlodzimirow KA, Eslami S, Abu-Hanna A, Nieuwoudt M, Chamuleau RA. A systematic review on prognostic indicators of acute on chronic liver failure and their predictive value for mortality. Liver Int. 2013;33(1):40–52.
5. Moreau R, Jalan R, Gines P, Pavesi M, Angeli P, Cordoba J, et al. Acute-on-chronic liver failure is a distinct syndrome that develops in patients with acute decompensation of cirrhosis. Gastroenterology. 2013;144(7):1426–37, 1437 e1421–1429.
6. Sarin SK, Kedarisetty CK, Abbas Z, Amarapurkar D, Bihari C, Chan AC, et al. Acute-on-chronic liver failure: consensus recommendations of the Asian Pacific Association for the Study of the Liver (APASL) 2014. Hepatol Int. 2014;8(4):453–71.
7. Bajaj JS. Defining acute-on-chronic liver failure: will east and west ever meet? Gastroenterology. 2013;144(7):1337–9.

8. Zhang J, Gao S, Duan Z, Hu KQ. Overview on acute-on-chronic liver failure. Front Med. 2016;10(1):1–17.
9. Li H, Chen LY, Zhang NN, Li ST, Zeng B, Pavesi M, et al. Characteristics, diagnosis and prognosis of acute-on-chronic liver failure in cirrhosis associated to hepatitis B. Sci Rep. 2016;6:25487.
10. Shi Y, Zheng MH, Yang Y, Wei W, Yang Q, Hu A, et al. Increased delayed mortality in patients with acute-on-chronic liver failure who have prior decompensation. J Gastroenterol Hepatol. 2015;30(4):712–8.
11. Vincent JL, Moreno R, Takala J, Willatts S, De Mendonca A, Bruining H, et al. The SOFA (Sepsis-related Organ Failure Assessment) score to describe organ dysfunction/failure. On behalf of the Working Group on Sepsis-Related Problems of the European Society of Intensive Care Medicine. Intensive Care Med. 1996;22(7):707–10.
12. Jalan R, Saliba F, Pavesi M, Amoros A, Moreau R, Gines P, et al. Development and validation of a prognostic score to predict mortality in patients with acute-on-chronic liver failure. J Hepatol. 2014;61(5):1038–47.
13. Jalan R, Stadlbauer V, Sen S, Cheshire L, Chang YM, Mookerjee RP. Role of predisposition, injury, response and organ failure in the prognosis of patients with acute-on-chronic liver failure: a prospective cohort study. Crit Care. 2012;16(6):R227.
14. Levy MM, Fink MP, Marshall JC, Abraham E, Angus D, Cook D, et al. 2001 SCCM/ESICM/ACCP/ATS/SIS international sepsis definitions conference. Crit Care Med. 2003;31(4):1250–6.
15. Arroyo V, Moreau R, Jalan R, Gines P, E-CCC S. Acute-on-chronic liver failure: a new syndrome that will re-classify cirrhosis. J Hepatol. 2015;62(1 Suppl):S131–43.
16. Moreau R, Jalan R, Arroyo V. Acute-on-chronic liver failure: recent concepts. J Clin Exp Hepatol. 2015;5(1):81–5.
17. Moreau R. The pathogenesis of ACLF: the inflammatory response and immune function. Semin Liver Dis. 2016;36(2):133–40.
18. Bernal W, Jalan R, Quaglia A, Simpson K, Wendon J, Burroughs A. Acute-on-chronic liver failure. Lancet. 2015;386(10003):1576–87.
19. Hernaez R, Sola E, Moreau R, Gines P. Acute-on-chronic liver failure: an update. Gut. 2017;66(3):541–53.
20. Medzhitov R, Schneider DS, Soares MP. Disease tolerance as a defense strategy. Science. 2012;335(6071):936–41.
21. Wasmuth HE, Kunz D, Yagmur E, Timmer-Stranghoner A, Vidacek D, Siewert E, et al. Patients with acute on chronic liver failure display "sepsis-like" immune paralysis. J Hepatol. 2005;42(2):195–201.

Chapter 12
Critical Care of the Acute Liver Failure Patient

Thomas A. Verbeek, Geraldine C. Diaz, and John F. Renz

Introduction

Acute liver failure (ALF) is the abrupt deterioration of hepatic function in an individual with no previous history of liver disease. A rare life-threatening condition with an annual incidence of approximately 2,000 cases in the United States, ALF requires expert, multidisciplinary care to achieve optimal outcomes.

The severity of ALF is characterized by hepatic synthetic dysfunction, abnormal liver biochemistry, an elevated international normalized ratio (INR), and encephalopathy [1, 2]. Survival rates for patients with ALF have improved significantly in developed countries thanks to earlier recognition, critical care advances, antiviral therapy, and triage to specialized centers offering highly specific therapy and orthotopic liver transplantation (OLT) when necessary [3].

Definition

Acute liver failure is defined by the onset of hepatic encephalopathy and coagulopathy within 26 weeks of jaundice in a patient without preexisting liver disease [4]. In the adult population, the presence of encephalopathy distinguishes ALF from acute

T. A. Verbeek
Department of Anesthesiology, Penn State College of Medicine, Hershey, PA, USA

G. C. Diaz (✉)
Department of Anesthesiology, University of Illinois at Chicago, Chicago, IL, USA
e-mail: gdiaz@uic.edu

J. F. Renz
Department of Surgery, University of Chicago, Chicago, IL, USA

D. Bezinover, F. Saner (eds.), *Critical Care for Potential Liver Transplant Candidates*,
https://doi.org/10.1007/978-3-319-92934-7_12

liver injury (ALI) and forms the basis for a temporal ALF classification. ALF is classified into hyperacute, acute, and subacute phenotypes depending on the time from jaundice to encephalopathy [5, 6]. Hyperacute ALF has an interval of jaundice to encephalopathy of 7 days or less; acute liver failure occurs with a jaundice to encephalopathy interval of 8–28 days; and subacute liver failure is classified as a jaundice to encephalopathy interval of greater than 28 days [6, 7].

Acute liver failure has replaced the classic term "fulminant hepatic failure," which was defined as severe liver injury with the onset of hepatic encephalopathy within 8 weeks of initial symptoms in the absence of preexisting liver disease [8]. Changes in the definition of ALF over time reflect clinical experience recognizing etiology, time from jaundice to onset of encephalopathy, patient age, and underlying physiology as principal contributors to outcomes [1, 2].

The time interval from jaundice to encephalopathy may suggest etiology, potential complications, and the prognosis of supportive medical therapy. Typically, hyperacute liver failure is the result of intentional acetaminophen-induced ALF (AIALF) or viral exposure [1, 2]. It is characterized by a marked coagulopathy, increased transaminases, and severe encephalopathy, with only a minority of cases needing OLT.

Subacute liver failure is typically associated with idiosyncratic drug-induced liver injury, autoimmune hepatitis, unintentional AIALF, or an idiopathic virus/toxin and has a very low incidence of spontaneous recovery. Coagulopathy and encephalopathy are not as pronounced in the early phase of disease but persistently deteriorate despite medical therapy. Encephalopathy is often very subtle and difficult to diagnose. The response to medical therapy is consistently poor in this group compared to that of patients with hyperacute liver failure. Subacute liver failure is associated with a low incidence of cerebral edema [1, 2].

The temporal classification of ALF is not universally accepted, and the 2011 American Association for the Study of Liver Diseases (AASLD) position paper on the management of acute liver failure cautions against the use of the terms hyperacute, acute, and subacute, as they have limited prognostic significance, which should be interpreted within the context of the etiology and the patient's clinical condition [9, 10].

Incidence and Etiology

The incidence of ALF varies geographically. In developed countries, the incidence of ALF is relatively rare, fewer than 10 cases/million. The incidence, however, is probably higher in Asia and developing nations where the prevalence of hepatitis A, B, and E is markedly higher [11].

ALF can be caused by many conditions, and etiology has a significant impact on the anticipated clinical course (Table 12.1). Worldwide, viral infections are the most common causes of ALF. In addition to hepatitis A, B, and E, other DNA viruses including the herpes virus family (cytomegalovirus, Epstein-Barr virus, herpes

Table 12.1 Etiologies of acute liver failure [1, 2, 9, 11–14]

Drug-induced	Acetaminophen	
	Non-acetaminophen	Isoniazid
		Phenytoin
		Valproate
		Propylthiouracil
		Nitrofurantoin
	Recreational	Cocaine
		Ecstasy (3,4-methylenedioxy-N-methylamphetamine)
Viruses	Hepatitis (A, B, D, and E)	
	Herpes	Cytomegalovirus
		Epstein-Barr
		Herpes simplex
		Varicella zoster
	Adenovirus	
	Parvovirus B19	
Autoimmune hepatitis		
Metabolic disorders	Wilson's disease	
	Heatstroke	
Pregnancy	Acute fatty liver of pregnancy	
	HELLP syndrome	
Budd-Chiari syndrome		
Amanita phalloides		
Indeterminate		

simplex, varicella zoster), adenovirus, and parvovirus may cause acute liver injury and, in rare cases, ALF. Hepatitis A and E are the principal contributors to global mortality due to the rapidity of clinical progression in areas where OLT is restricted or unavailable [1].

Etiologies of ALF have evolved over time. In developed nations, drug-induced liver injury is the leading cause of ALF, as opposed to hepatitis B in the past [2]. AIALF is the most common cause of ALF in the United States and the United Kingdom, whereas idiosyncratic drug-induced liver injury is the leading cause in Europe [9, 11–14]. Acetaminophen overdose in the United Kingdom is typically intentional, whereas in the United States, it is often secondary to unintentional, chronic ingestion of analgesic products [3, 15]. Chronic ingestion of acetaminophen over a period of days to weeks is associated with a greater risk of progression to OLT than is a single deliberate overdose [1, 2]. Hepatotoxicity from acetaminophen is dose-dependent and predictable but may be confounded by the presence of other substances such as aspirin and alcohol [16]. Intentional acetaminophen ingestion resulting in ALF typically exceeds 10 grams with unintentional daily doses exceeding 4 grams per day [5]. Notably, acetaminophen-related toxicity is exacerbated by conditions resulting in glutathione depletion, such as alcoholism and malnutrition [17]. Idiosyncratic drug-induced ALF is less common than AIALF but exhibits a greater progression to encephalopathy and OLT [1, 2].

Autoimmune hepatitis, Budd-Chiari syndrome, *Amanita phalloides* ingestion, Wilson's disease, fatty liver of pregnancy, and HELLP (hemolysis, elevated liver enzymes, low platelets) syndrome remain infrequent etiologies. ALF during pregnancy typically mandates delivery of the fetus and should be triaged to a referral center where specialized neonatal care as well as intensive management including potential liver transplantation exists [18].

Acute hepatic ischemic injury and malignant infiltration are secondary etiologies of ALF where recovery depends on treatment of the initiating condition. Acute hepatic ischemia is typically due to cardiopulmonary collapse from sepsis; however, reactive vasoconstriction secondary to the recreational use of cocaine or MDMA (3,4-methylenedioxy-N-methylamphetamine, also known as ecstasy) can prompt a similar syndrome. A variation of ALF with a particularly poor prognosis is reactivation of hepatitis B from a latent subclinical infection without established chronic liver disease. This condition classically presents in patients who are immunocompromised from treatment, such as chemotherapy, of a systemic disease [1].

A meticulous search for the cause of ALF as early as possible following clinical presentation is essential to optimizing therapy and formulating a prognosis. Transplant-free survival is up to 90% among patients with acetaminophen, hepatitis A, or pregnancy-related ALF, whereas other etiologies require liver transplantation more frequently. Increased age, elevated transaminase and bilirubin levels, and coagulopathy are associated with an increased risk of death [1, 2]. Despite extensive investigation, the cause of liver injury with acute liver failure remains indeterminate in one fifth of patients. ALF of indeterminate cause is associated with poor survival without OLT [3].

Diagnosis, Initial Management, and Triage

Early management focuses on investigating the etiology and assessing the extent of the patient's hepatic impairment. Most patients on initial presentation are suffering from acute liver injury with constitutional complaints of fatigue, malaise, and loss of appetite with or without new-onset jaundice. Alternatively, the patient may have been found unconscious following an intentional acetaminophen ingestion. Recognition of hyperacute ALF can be difficult, as jaundice may be subtle or the patient may be mistakenly diagnosed with chronic liver disease [1]. In all cases, a thorough history including diet, travel, illicit drug use, duration of symptoms, and sexual history is paramount and may require referencing additional sources such as an accompanying relative or friend or the patient's general practitioner as the patient may be impaired. Typically, obtaining the psychosocial and medical histories requires considerable effort. The diagnostic evaluation is summarized in Table 12.2.

Table 12.2 Investigations and specific therapies for initial management of acute liver failure [1, 2, 19, 20]

Etiology			Diagnostic evaluation	Specific therapy
Drug-induced			Clinical history, prescriptions, over-the-counter medication and supplements, herbal medications, diet	
	Acetaminophen		Acetaminophen level	NAC
	Recreational (cocaine, MDMA)		Urine and serum toxicology	
Viral infection	Hepatitis	HAV	IgM anti-HAV	
		HBV	HBsAG IgM anti-HBc HBV DNA RT-PCR	Entecavir
		HDV	IgM, IgG anti-HDV, HDV RNA	
		HEV	IgM, IgG anti-HEV, HEV RNA PCR	
	Other viruses	Cytomegalovirus	CMV IgM	
		Epstein-Barr	EBV IgM	
		Herpes simplex	HSV IgM	Acyclovir
		Varicella zoster	VZV IgM	
Autoimmune			ANA SMA	Steroids
Wilson's disease			Ceruloplasmin Serum copper Urine copper Kayser-Fleischer rings	Chelation Dialysis
Budd-Chiari syndrome			Ultrasound, CT, MRI Hematology consult	Anticoagulation TIPS
Pregnancy	Acute fatty liver		β-HCG	Delivery
	HELLP syndrome			
Indeterminate			Liver biopsy	

ANA antinuclear antibody, *β-HCG* beta human chorionic gonadotrophin, *CMV* cytomegalovirus, *EBV* Epstein-Barr virus, *EKG* electrocardiogram, *HAV* hepatitis A virus, *HBV* hepatitis B virus, *HBsAG* hepatitis B surface antigen, *HDV* hepatitis D virus, *HEV* hepatitis E virus, *HSV* herpes simplex virus, *IgG* immunoglobulin G, *IgM* immunoglobulin M, *MDMA* 3,4-methylenedioxy-N-methylamphetamine, *NAC* N-acetyl cysteine, *PCR* polymerase chain reaction, *RT-PCR* reverse transcription polymerase chain reaction, *SMA* anti-smooth muscle antibody, *TIPS* transjugular intrahepatic portosystemic shunt, *VZV* varicella zoster virus

Intensive care management is required for this patient population. The main goal is to provide optimal conditions for hepatocyte regeneration while preventing further hepatic or additional organ system injury [4, 21]. Early treatment or removal of the inciting agent while maintaining homeostasis and preventing complications associated with hepatic impairment facilitates regeneration. Specific therapies may be an antiviral agent, a chelating agent, steroids, or glutathione repletion depending on the etiology (see Table 12.2).

The Rumack-Matthew acetaminophen toxicity nomogram is useful in determining the likelihood of serious liver damage due to acetaminophen ingestion, but it is unreliable in the setting of unintentional acetaminophen ingestion over an extended period of time, acetaminophen ingestion in combination with additional toxins, malnutrition, alcoholism, or glutathione depletion [16, 22]. AIALF is mediated by the production of N-acetyl-p-benzoquinone imine (NAPQI). The majority of ingested acetaminophen is conjugated to form nontoxic metabolites; however, a minority is shunted to the cytochrome P450 system where NAPQI is produced. NAPQI is neutralized by glutathione, which is rapidly depleted within hepatocytes. Once glutathione is depleted, NAPQI initiates hepatocyte necrosis [16, 22]. Cytochrome P450 activity may be significantly increased following induction by phenytoin, carbamazepine, or alcohol, resulting in accelerated NAPQI production and hepatic injury. Conversely, glutathione depletion secondary to malnutrition, eating disorders, alcoholism, or chronic acetaminophen ingestion facilitates hepatotoxicity. N-acetylcysteine (NAC) replenishes glutathione to inactivate NAPQI. For acetaminophen ingestion, the time interval from ingestion to initiation of NAC corresponds to the outcome [1]. When administered within 24 h of a single ingestion, NAC can minimize toxicity from massive acetaminophen doses with very low mortality [1, 2]. NAC should be administered even if there is doubt concerning the timing, dose, or plasma concentration of acetaminophen [21].

NAC improves systemic hemodynamics and tissue oxygen delivery and demonstrates antioxidant and immunologic effects [21]. It is a well-tolerated drug with only minor side effects such as nausea, vomiting, diarrhea, and constipation frequently reported. In rare cases, intravenous NAC has been associated with bronchospasm. Administration is easy and does not require monitoring. The length of administration is variable secondary to clinical improvement, death, or OLT rather than time or serum acetaminophen levels [4, 21].

NAC has not demonstrated clear efficacy in the setting of non-acetaminophen-induced acute liver failure (NAIALF). In a prospective, randomized trial comparing NAC and placebo among NAIALF patients demonstrating various grades of encephalopathy, Lee et al. reported improved transplant-free survival with NAC in patients exhibiting grade I/II encephalopathy but no benefit in the presence of grade III/IV encephalopathy [23, 24]. Although the role of NAC in the treatment of NAIALF is not as clearly defined, initiation of NAC therapy remains indicated in all ALF cases, as the morbidity averted by early therapy prior to confirmation of AIALF exceeds the small risk of a NAC-associated complication should the etiology not be acetaminophen-related.

Table 12.3 King's College Criteria for urgent liver transplant indication [25, 28]

Acetaminophen-induced acute liver failure (AIALF)	Arterial pH < 7.3 following adequate volume resuscitation	
	OR Grade III or IV encephalopathy *PLUS* INR > 6.5 or PT >100 s *PLUS* Creatinine > 3.4 mg/dl (300 μmol/l) (acute kidney injury)	
Non-acetaminophen-induced acute liver failure (NAIALF)	INR > 6.7, PT > 100 s	
	OR Three (3) of the following:	
		Unfavorable etiology: drug-induced, Wilson's disease, indeterminate
		Age < 10 years or > 40 years
		Onset of encephalopathy > 7 days after onset of jaundice
		INR > 4, PT > 50 s
		Bilirubin > 17.5 (300 μmol/l) mg/dl

Multiple prognostic scoring systems exist that predict recovery from ALF. While each has unique advantages and disadvantages, the AASLD does not recommend relying entirely on a single prognostic system. Rather, integration of multiple systems within the clinical context is required [10]. Initially reported in 1989, the King's College Criteria (KCC) is the most widely applied prognostic system (Table 12.3) [25]. It was the first system to distinguish between AIALF and NAIALF etiologies. The sensitivity and specificity of KCC for AIALF have historically been higher than for NAIALF [26]. McPhail et al. recently reported a meta-analysis demonstrating a sensitivity and specificity of 58 and 89%, respectively, for AIALF versus 58 and 74%, respectively, for NAIALF [27]. Sensitivity and specificity improve with the inclusion of serum lactate when used during patient care [28, 29].

The Clichy criteria were developed from a cohort of acute hepatitis B patients and incorporate serum factor V levels as a prognostic indicator [5]. In an analysis, factor V levels below 20% in patients ≤ 30 years or < 30% in older patients strongly predicted mortality. The Eurotransplant International Foundation is a nonprofit organization responsible for coordinating organ transplants in Austria, Belgium, Croatia, Germany, Hungary, Luxembourg, the Netherlands, and Slovenia. Eurotransplant uses the Clichy criteria for high-urgency liver transplantation listing in patients with ALF associated with viral hepatitis. The criteria are factor V activity < 20 or 30% depending on age and HE ≥ grade III. However, as the ALF population has changed, subsequent studies have demonstrated the Clichy criteria to be less efficacious than KCC [10, 30, 31].

The Model for End-Stage Liver Disease (MELD) score, the Acute Liver Failure Study Group index, and the APACHE III scoring system have all been proposed as alternative prognostic systems [32–34]. Each has shown promise; yet, no prognostic system has demonstrated sufficiently consistent accuracy to warrant recognition as the standard [10].

Table 12.4 West Haven encephalopathy grading system [35]

Grade	Clinical description
I	Trivial lack of awareness, euphoria or anxiety, shortened attention span, impaired performance of addition or subtraction
II	Lethargy or apathy, minimal disorientation to time or place, subtle personality change, inappropriate behavior
III	Somnolence to semi-stupor, responsive to verbal stimuli, confusion, gross disorientation
IV	Coma

Table 12.5 Clinical indicators for immediate transfer to a quaternary care center

Any etiology except single-episode acetaminophen ingestion
Progression from acute liver injury to acute liver failure
Encephalopathy or altered mental status attributable to hepatic insufficiency
Additional organ system involvement
Acetaminophen ingestion that has not responded to N-acetylcysteine therapy after a 12-h observation window
Jaundice

After initial evaluation and early therapy, the mental status assessment should be repeated regularly to distinguish acute liver injury from ALF. A commonly used index of hepatic encephalopathy is the West Haven criteria (Table 12.4) [35]. Although this is a semiquantitative scale with high interobserver variability, the degree of encephalopathy does approximate the presence of cerebral edema [1, 2, 21]. For West Haven grade I or II encephalopathy, the risk of cerebral edema is low. However, the risk of cerebral edema exponentially increases with grade III and IV encephalopathy [36]. Any unexplained mental status changes observed establishes a diagnosis of ALF, and an immediate non-contrast CT of the brain to evaluate for cerebral edema is indicated. Any sign of intracranial hypertension such as seizures, decerebrate posturing, altered pupil reactivity, or abnormal oculovestibular reflexes warrants immediate investigation and referral to a facility that can offer liver transplantation. A non-contrast CT of the brain when acetaminophen has been excluded as the etiology is recommended.

The clinical indicators for immediate triage to a facility with the capacity for OLT are summarized in Table 12.5. Immediate triage indicators include (1) any etiology except single-episode acetaminophen ingestion, (2) encephalopathy or any altered mental status that cannot be explained, (3) any other organ system involvement (renal insufficiency/failure, fever, hypertension, cerebral edema, and seizures), (4) acetaminophen ingestion that has not responded to N-acetylcysteine therapy after a 12-h observation window, and (5) jaundice. Pending transfer, patients require intensive care monitoring as their condition may deteriorate rapidly.

Management of Acute Liver Failure at a Quaternary Care Facility

Evaluation for OLT is indicated in patients who meet the definition of ALF. Patients should be transferred to an intensive care unit, as they may deteriorate rapidly. Ideally, NAC therapy should be initiated prior to the patient being transferred to a quaternary care center where subspecialty medical care is available. At this time, the goals of care are to confirm the initial diagnostic evaluation and initiate appropriate etiology-directed therapy, to monitor for further hepatic decompensation, to support homeostasis to facilitate hepatic regeneration, and to prevent complications. Among ALF patients, the most common causes of death are sepsis and cerebral herniation [1, 2].

ALF is characterized by low systemic vascular resistance and increased cardiac output [1, 2, 37]. ALF patients are typically hypovolemic from poor oral intake secondary to malaise, nausea and vomiting, as well as diarrhea. Hemodynamic support to maintain systemic perfusion is essential, as hypotension is associated with increased encephalopathy and mortality [38, 39]. Intravascular volume expansion with balanced salt solutions or fresh frozen plasma is initiated according to the patient's acid-base, electrolyte, and coagulation status [1]. The goals of circulatory support depend on the presence or absence of encephalopathy. In the absence of encephalopathy, a mean arterial pressure (MAP) of $\geq$ 65 mmHg is sufficient; however, this should be increased to a MAP of $\geq$ 75 mmHg when encephalopathy is present. Cerebral perfusion pressure, when available, should be targeted to 60–80 mmHg. Hyperchloremic acidosis should be avoided due to its deleterious effects on cerebral perfusion [19, 21, 40].

Fluid resuscitation should be carefully monitored by physical examination, pulse pressure variation, or echocardiography, as volume overload may worsen the patient's respiratory status and cerebral edema [41]. An arterial catheter is very helpful for the assessment of blood gases, pH, and lactate, frequent blood sampling, and verification of systemic perfusion. Central venous and pulmonary arterial catheters subject the patient to a risk of infection, and benefits should outweigh the risks. Every effort must be made to protect renal function by facilitating adequate hemodynamics and avoiding nephrotoxic drugs [42–44].

Hypotension in the presence of effective circulating volume requires initiation of vasopressors and is a significant milestone in the disease progression of ALF [4, 19]. Initiating vasopressors mandates an arterial catheter for systemic blood pressure and acid-base monitoring. The transplant service should be made aware of the patient's requirement for vasopressors [21]. Norepinephrine is the initial vasopressor of choice for raising MAP while minimizing tachycardia and preserving splanchnic and cerebral blood flow [45, 46]. Maintenance of systemic vascular tone and acid-base balance is observed in most ALF patients on low-dose norepinephrine. However, routine pH and lactate monitoring is essential, as a small subset of patients will require escalating vasopressors and demonstrate increasing hyperlactatemia despite adequate volume resuscitation. Persistently increasing vasopressor requirements, acidosis, renal failure, seizures, or loss of consciousness signal an impending terminal stage of disease, which should prompt immediate discussion with the transplant service as to the expected poor outcome after OLT [47].

If a second vasopressor is required, vasopressin is preferred as it potentiates norepinephrine's alpha-receptor vasoactive response. Because of its potential to increase intracranial pressure (ICP), vasopressin should be restricted to use as a second-line therapy for hemodynamic support and limited to a dose of 0.04 U/min [45]. Epinephrine is not indicated, as it may compromise hepatic blood flow in patients with ALF [48]. Patients with persistent hypotension without metabolic acidosis should be evaluated for adrenal insufficiency [49].

Early endotracheal intubation should be considered in the setting of seizure, agitation, or progressive encephalopathy to minimize the risk of aspiration, which could defer or exclude OLT [4]. ALF patients should receive sedation for laryngoscopy, as this procedure may transiently increase ICP. Cisatracurium, a non-depolarizing neuromuscular blocker, is the preferred muscle relaxant, as its metabolism is independent of renal and hepatic function. Succinylcholine should be avoided, as it may increase ICP [45].

ALF patients often spontaneously hyperventilate, which does not require treatment [50]. Endotracheal intubation marks another ominous clinical milestone, which should prompt discussions between the various clinical teams to reevaluate current management and the role of OLT. Goals are partial carbon dioxide pressures at the lower end of normal (30–35 mmHg) with low tidal volumes (6 ml/kg predicted body weight) to reduce the risk of acute respiratory distress syndrome [19]. Plateau pressure should be kept at < 30 cmH_2O along with the lowest level of positive end-expiratory pressure that achieves adequate oxygenation in order to limit increases in ICP and decreased hepatic blood flow [4, 48]. Sustained hyperventilation to $PaCO_2$ levels below 30 mmHg may require increased sedation and mandatory modes of ventilation. The patient's head should be elevated to 30° and maintained in a neutral position, orotracheal suctioning and other noxious stimuli should be minimized [4]. Forced hyperventilation should be instituted for impending brain stem herniation [45]. Intubated ALF patients require sedation. Although propofol potentiates γ-aminobutyric acid-related neurotransmission modulation that may worsen encephalopathy, it is preferred over short-acting benzodiazepines whose metabolism can be widely variable. Propofol infusion should be minimized to avoid propofol infusion syndrome. It is unusual for ALF patients to have pain. If necessary, short-acting opioids such as fentanyl are recommended over morphine and meperidine [4]. Following endotracheal intubation, the patient should receive non-contrast head computed tomography (CT) to reevaluate for evidence of cerebral edema and to assess the need for cerebral pressure monitoring.

Cerebral edema resulting in intracranial hypertension and cerebral herniation is a leading cause of ALF-associated mortality in patients with grades III and IV encephalopathy. Intracranial hypertension is defined as an intracranial pressure of > 25 mmHg and is associated with mortality exceeding 50% [3]. In an autopsy

Table 12.6 Management of cerebral edema in acute liver failure [1, 2, 4, 19, 21, 30]

Endotracheal intubation	
Sedation	
Head elevation to 30°	
Hemodynamics	MAP ≥ 75 mmHg
	CPP ≥ 60 mmHg
Cerebral monitoring	Intracranial pressure monitor
	Transcranial Doppler
Osmotic therapy	Mannitol
	Hypertonic saline
Hypothermia	33–36 °C
Hyperammonemia	Continuous renal replacement therapy
Salvage therapies	Hyperventilation
	Indomethacin
	Plasma exchange
	Hepatectomy with portocaval shunt

series, a majority of patients who expired from ALF had demonstrated histological evidence of cerebral edema [51]. The pathophysiology is multifactorial and involves inflammatory mediators, acute osmotic disturbances, altered glutamine-dependent neurotransmitter activity, neuronal oxidative stress, impaired mitochondrial function, and elevated circulating ammonia concentrations, resulting in astrocyte swelling.

Early recognition of neurologic impairment with proactive intensive management has reduced the incidence of neurological death (Table 12.6) [21]. ICP monitoring should be considered in patients listed for OLT who are intubated or demonstrate advanced (stage III/IV) encephalopathy; however, ICP monitoring has not been demonstrated to improve survival, and its role in the management of ALF remains controversial [52]. In a retrospective study of NAIALF patients by Karvellas et al., mortality was higher among those with ICP monitoring and was associated with a more than 5% incidence of intracranial hemorrhage [53].

The time to discuss placement of an ICP monitor is not when a patient is in the intensive care unit. Rather, the development of a protocol through discussions with the transplant team, neurosurgery, anesthesiology, and critical care is the preferred way to avoid ambiguity. Important topics for discussion include the type of catheter and the coagulation parameters necessary for ICP monitor placement. Epidural ICP monitors are safer but may overestimate ICP, whereas intraventricular ICP monitors are associated with a high incidence of intracranial hemorrhage and should be avoided. Another point of contention is the conditions necessary for ICP monitor insertion. ALF-associated coagulopathies and thrombocytopenia are exceedingly difficult to correct through transfusion. Prospective, randomized trials are necessary to define the benefit of ICP monitoring.

The use of ICP monitoring has declined as alternative modalities have become available. Transcranial Doppler sonography (TCD) is a noninvasive alternative to direct ICP monitoring that has been validated for the measurement of cerebral blood flow [54]. Several acoustic windows facilitate evaluation of the cerebral vasculature [55]. The transtemporal window evaluates the middle cerebral artery, the anterior cerebral artery, the posterior cerebral artery, and the terminal portion of the internal carotid artery prior to bifurcation. It is the benchmark view for cerebral blood flow assessment in ALF patients. Some patients may not demonstrate an adequate acoustic window, and false positives may occur in patients who are hyperventilated or demonstrate diffuse intravascular disease, severe cardiac regurgitation, or hyperdynamic circulatory physiology. Near-infrared spectroscopy (NIRS) is a noninvasive technique for measuring regional cerebral oxygen saturation. NIRS may be valuable in monitoring critical changes in cerebral oxygenation and blood volume [56].

Initial therapy for intracranial hypertension is volume and electrolyte repletion. Astute management of the ALF patient's volume status is essential, particularly as the disease progresses. Mannitol should be administered provided serum osmolality remains below 320 mosm/l. Elevated serum sodium may prevent the progression of intracranial hypertension. Thus, serum sodium should be targeted to between 145 and 155 meq/l [10]. Infusion of hypertonic saline presents the body with a high sodium load and should be limited [57]. Osmotic demyelination in these patients is extremely rare due to the short duration of changes in serum sodium concentration, and prophylactic therapy for intracranial hypertension is not recommended. Corticosteroids have not demonstrated a benefit in ALF except in the treatment of adrenal insufficiency [48, 58]. Indomethacin at a dose of 25 mg or 0.5 mg/kg intravenously over 1 min acutely decreases ICP by causing cerebral vasoconstriction. Its nephrotoxic effects limit its application to salvage therapy in patients with refractory ICH [4]. Some patients may be volume-overloaded and hyponatremic. In these situations, administration of mannitol or dialysis to remove excess volume and correct the hyponatremia is recommended.

As hyperammonemia is central to the pathophysiology of cerebral edema, arterial ammonia concentration should be closely monitored. Lowering ammonia levels theoretically reduces astrocyte swelling and dysfunction. Bernal et al. identified high ammonia concentrations as an independent risk factor for the development of intracranial hypertension with a low incidence observed below 150 μmol/l [3]. Risk factors for the development of intracranial hypertension related to hyperammonemia include an arterial ammonia concentration exceeding 200 μmol/l, a sustained level of at least 150 μmol/l despite treatment, an age $\leq$ 35 years, and concurrent renal or cardiovascular failure [1, 2, 42].

Hyperammonemia should be treated aggressively with continuous renal replacement therapy (CRRT) utilizing high-filtration volume (90 ml/kg/h) for arterial ammonia concentrations exceeding 200 μmol/l [1, 40, 59]. Renal dysfunction is common among ALF patients and may result from direct nephrotoxicity or systemic circulatory dysfunction [37, 40]. Hypokalemia and metabolic acidosis increase renal ammonia production. Early initiation of CRRT lowers circulating ammonia, promotes metabolic consistency, facilitates hemodynamic stability, and corrects disturbances before hemodynamic collapse and intracranial hypertension occur [40, 44].

Lactulose, neomycin, rifaximin, and L-ornithine-L-aspartate are used to attenuate hepatic encephalopathy in patients with chronic liver disease. Unfortunately, these agents have not demonstrated a clear benefit in the treatment of ALF, and lactulose may actually be deleterious [21]. Lactulose may result in dehydration, hyponatremia, and abdominal distention, which can increase intra-abdominal pressure, decrease cerebral perfusion, and interfere with surgery. Rifaximin is a nonabsorbable antibiotic with few side effects, which is frequently prescribed in conjunction with lactulose. Use of rifaximin has also not demonstrated a clear benefit [53, 60]. L-ornithine-L-aspartate has demonstrated efficacy in reducing ammonia levels in patients with ESLD. However, prospective, randomized studies in ALF have failed to show a benefit in terms of a reduction of encephalopathy, disease severity, or mortality.

Therapeutic hypothermia has been utilized for decades as a late-stage option to reduce cerebral edema in progressing ALF. Hypothermia has wide-ranging effects on cerebral blood flow and brain metabolism, including by altering lactate production and glucose, ammonia, and glutamate metabolism [10, 61, 62]. Systemic hemodynamics often improve with the initiation of therapy. Unfortunately, some trials utilizing moderate hypothermia as prophylaxis against intracranial hypertension failed to delay the onset or severity of disease [63, 64]. In addition, hypothermia is not without adverse effects, which include coagulopathy, enhanced susceptibility to infection, and cardiac arrhythmia. The decision to employ therapeutic hypothermia is largely an empiric one. If the patient is a relatively good candidate for OLT, i.e., is hemodynamically stable, and there is no immediate donor availability, therapeutic hypothermia as a late option to potentially bridge to OLT can be considered. However, in the setting of an excellent donor readily available, hemodynamic instability, potentially septic physiology, deteriorating hemodynamics, or additional organ system failure(s), therapeutic hypothermia can be deferred. The goal core temperature would be 33–36 °C with daily surveillance cultures [1].

Fever must be treated aggressively by pharmacologic (acetaminophen, indomethacin, non-steroidal anti-inflammatory drugs) as well as non-pharmacological means including cooling blankets or fans [4]. Shivering should be alleviated by sedation or small doses of meperidine.

Seizure activity in ALF patients may present atypically, and a high index of suspicion must be maintained. Seizure activity should be treated immediately. Electroencephalography (EEG) is a noninvasive monitoring modality that can be performed at the bedside. While hepatic encephalopathy does not demonstrate specific EEG changes, there is a correlation between EEG findings and the level of encephalopathy. EEG can be very useful in diagnosing and treating seizure activity that may be difficult to diagnose otherwise [65]. Prophylactic administration of phenytoin to avert seizures has not demonstrated a benefit [66].

Barbiturate coma is an anecdotal therapy now rarely considered except in the presence of continuing seizure activity. Barbiturate metabolism is reduced in ALF and neurological assessment becomes impossible. Furthermore, systemic hypotension is common, and seizures may occur on cessation of the drug. While propofol sedation has largely replaced barbiturate coma, the necessity for such interventions signals an extremely grave condition requiring continuous intense monitoring, as progression to herniation is frequent [10].

When therapies are deployed to control ICP, attention to slow de-escalation of therapy post-OLT or with spontaneous recovery is essential, as intracranial pressure normalization lags behind liver recovery [40]. Normalization of sodium levels by no more than 10 meq/l/day and gradual rewarming are essential to optimize neurologic recovery; however, despite optimal therapy, patients who demonstrate cerebral edema often demonstrate permanent cognitive impairment [67, 68].

Multi-system organ failure secondary to sepsis is a major risk factor for developing cerebral edema and the most common cause of death among ALF patients [38, 39]. ALF patients are naturally immunodeficient due to a compensatory anti-inflammatory response that follows the initial systemic inflammatory response syndrome (SIRS) triggered by massive hepatocellular necrosis [69, 70]. Hepatocellular necrosis and profound endotoxemia increase the potential for translocation of bacteria and fungi, exposing the ALF patient to potential infections that may preclude liver transplantation [10, 71]. Thus, meticulous attention to infection control, including surveillance cultures, handwashing, and minimizing central venous access are essential [21]. Central venous catheters placed at an outside hospital should preferably be removed or replaced [48]. Progression from ALF to sepsis can be subtle and may manifest without fever or leukocytosis. C-reactive protein is produced exclusively by hepatocytes and is an unreliable marker of infection in ALF [71]. Hemodynamic compromise, hypoxia, seizures, and progressive encephalopathy are often the presenting symptoms that should trigger an exhaustive search for a source of infection [72]. There are insufficient data to recommend routine antibiotic prophylaxis in all patients with ALF [73].

Appropriate management of hemostasis is an essential aspect of care that is frequently poorly understood. An elevated INR is a universal finding and a component of the definition of ALF. Reduced INR reflects impaired hepatic synthetic function but does not indicate a bleeding diathesis. The liver is responsible for the production of procoagulant as well as anticoagulant factors. A reduction in anticoagulant proteins such as proteins C and S, as well as antithrombin, may occur concomitantly with a decrease in procoagulant factors synthesized by the liver, but the INR test will reflect only the procoagulant activity [74–76]. Fibrinolysis can be activated or impaired via endothelial cell injury, increased circulating factor VIII, or altered von Willebrand factor activity. Thus, the ALF patient may be in a balanced hemostatic state or a hyper- or hypo-coagulable state depending on local factors.

Hemostasis in the ALF patient should be approached as a very fluid situation depending on bacterial translocation, transfusion of blood products, thrombosis, fibrinolysis, or cytokine-mediated inflammation. Paradoxically, overt bleeding is observed in only a minority of ALF patients with most hemostatic morbidity associated with thrombotic complications [4]. Hemorrhage is typically gastrointestinal in origin with hemostatic complications usually associated with poor medical management or disease progression to SIRS and multi-system organ failure [74, 75].

Transfusion is dictated by clinical evaluation, viscoelastic thromboelastometry (VET), and the need to perform procedures. VET provides near real-time assessment of hemostasis and should be utilized often to confirm a clinical finding or guide the type and amount of product to be transfused [1, 4, 21]. A VET may be normal, suggesting a balanced hemostatic state [76]. In this situation, transfusion should be deferred, as there are no data to support correction of abnormal routine coagulation tests in the absence of clinically significant hemorrhage [40]. If a procedure is necessary, a decision regarding possible platelet administration should be based on assessments of clot strength (VETs) or on significant thrombocytopenia $< 50 \times 10^9/\mu l$ [75, 77]. An exception to this practice is the placement of an ICP monitor in the setting of an elevated INR. In this situation, more aggressive coagulation management can be considered. Recombinant factor VII utilization has been associated with thrombotic complications and cannot be currently recommended [78]. VET-guided use of four factor prothrombin complex concentrate in cirrhotic patients undergoing OLT appears to be safe [79], but data on its use in ALF are lacking.

Prophylaxis against bleeding and thrombotic complications is a critical element of care. ALF patients should receive proton pump inhibitors, parenteral vitamin K, and intermittent leg compression devices [10]. In the absence of ICP monitoring, Lisman et al. have reported the use of low molecular weight heparin in select patients [74]. Utilization of heparin to prevent or treat thrombosis of renal replacement catheters and circuits has also been reported [10, 80].

Proper transfusion practice in patients with ALF is essential. Protocol-based transfusion practices involving all engaged disciplines should be developed preemptively to deliver consistent high-quality care.

Nutritional support optimizes hepatic regeneration. ALF patients demonstrate increased energy expenditure with protein catabolism requiring nutritional support to preserve muscle mass and augment immune function [1, 2, 4, 21]. Glucose, potassium, magnesium, and phosphate require frequent monitoring. Hypoglycemia exacerbates cerebral metabolic injury and must be prevented by preemptive intravenous dextrose infusion [40]. Hypophosphatemia due to hepatocyte regeneration should be managed aggressively. Nutrition should be enteral to facilitate immune function, enterocyte health, and enterohepatic circulation [10]. Enteral nutrition also avoids the need for central venous access and reduces the risk of sepsis. Daily enteral administration of 1.0–1.5 g protein per kilogram body weight is recommended with frequent monitoring of arterial ammonia and adjustment for progressive hyperammonemia or evidence of ICH [1, 4, 21].

Toxic liver syndrome is a preterminal phase of ALF characterized by complete liver necrosis with critical multi-organ dysfunction and SIRS. These patients become profoundly acidotic and hemodynamically unstable despite escalating therapy. The recognition of progressive acidosis and escalating vasopressor requirements is an emergency that requires the complete care team to assess the possibility of OLT. In these situations, the performance of an urgent hepatectomy with creation of a temporary portocaval shunt is typically the final option as a bridge to OLT. The goal is to remove the necrotic liver tissue to dampen the SIRS response. Transplantation for toxic liver syndrome as a two-stage procedure was initially reported by Ringe et al., who noted hemodynamic and metabolic stabilization in patients waiting for an allograft [81]. Use of this technique has subsequently been reported for liver trauma, spontaneous hepatic rupture, HELLP syndrome, and acute deterioration of chronic liver disease [82–84]. Sanabria Mateos et al. reported a series of six patients over a 22-year period with anhepatic times ranging from 330 to 2,640 min [84]. While anhepatic, patients received hemofiltration with plasma separation. Variable periods of hemodynamic stability and control of acidosis were observed, but overall survival was excellent with five of six recipients surviving urgent OLT. The longest anhepatic period reported is 66 h in a child with primary nonfunction following OLT [82]. Urgent hepatectomy with temporary portocaval shunt may be useful in two distinct clinical situations. The first and most likely to result in a successful outcome is when a donor has been identified but the ALF patient is demonstrating worsening SIRS. In this situation, it is reasonable to transport the patient to the operating room with the expectation that he/she will remain there until OLT is performed. In the second situation, an urgent hepatectomy with temporary portocaval shunt is performed as a final bridge to OLT when a donor has yet to be identified. Hemodynamic stability can be expected for a variable period of time followed by cardiac and cerebral collapse. In this situation, the patient may be returned to the intensive care unit but must be monitored intensively to verify candidacy, as the development of contraindications to OLT can be subtle [47].

Artificial Liver Support

Extracorporeal liver assist devices are rapidly emerging technologies designed to support the ALF patient as a bridge to recovery or OLT. These systems facilitate hemodynamic stability through detoxification and possible production of trophic factors [85, 86]. The molecular adsorbent recirculating system (MARS) utilizes an albumin-impregnated high-flux dialysis membrane with albumin or fresh frozen plasma dialysate [2, 85]. The extracorporeal liver assist device (ELAD) incorporates porcine or human hepatocyte cell lines, which are attached to dialysis cartridges and utilized for hemofiltration [85, 86]. High-volume plasma exchange (HVP) utilizing fresh frozen plasma has demonstrated a potential survival benefit [87, 88].

Conclusion

ALF is a rapidly evolving condition characterized by hepatic synthetic dysfunction, abnormal liver function tests, an elevated INR, and encephalopathy. Early medical management focuses on identifying an etiology and determining the time period from jaundice to encephalopathy. The identification of encephalopathy or unexplained altered mental status is a sentinel event that signals progression of acute liver injury to ALF. ALF requires intensive care hospitalization in a quaternary care center capable of orthotopic liver transplantation. The goals of care are (1) to confirm the initial diagnostic evaluation and initiate appropriate etiology-directed therapy, (2) to monitor for further hepatic decompensation, (3) to render homeostasis support to facilitate hepatic regeneration and minimize extrahepatic organ dysfunction, and (4) to prevent iatrogenic complications. Outcomes have continually improved through the creation of protocol-driven, specialized, multidisciplinary care. Most patients will recover without OLT. However, OLT remains a life-saving option.

Key Points

1. Acute liver failure (ALF) is a life-threatening disease that requires multidisciplinary care for optimal outcomes.
2. Most cases of ALF in the United States and the United Kingdom are due to acetaminophen ingestion and are self-limiting, not requiring liver transplantation.
3. All ALF patients should receive N-acetyl cysteine.
4. Early management of ALF focuses on finding the cause and assessing the degree of hepatic impairment.
5. The most common causes of death in ALF are sepsis and cerebral herniation.
6. Management of ALF in a quaternary care facility consists of supportive measures to assist hepatic regeneration, measures to avoid complications, and liver transplantation when indicated.

References

1. Bernal W, Wendon J. Acute liver failure. N Engl J Med. 2013;369(26):2525–34.
2. Cardoso FS, Marcelino P, Bagulho L, Karvellas CJ. Acute liver failure: an up-to-date approach. J Crit Care. 2017;39:25–30.
3. Bernal W, Hyyrylainen A, Gera A, Audimoolam VK, McPhail MJ, Auzinger G, et al. Lessons from look-back in acute liver failure? A single centre experience of 3300 patients. J Hepatol. 2013;59(1):74–80.
4. Stravitz RT, Kramer AH, Davern T, Shaikh AO, Caldwell SH, Mehta RL, et al. Intensive care of patients with acute liver failure: recommendations of the U.S. Acute Liver Failure Study Group. Crit Care Med. 2007;35(11):2498–508.
5. Bernuau J, Rueff B, Benhamou JP. Fulminant and subfulminant liver failure: definitions and causes. Semin Liver Dis. 1986;6(2):97–106.
6. O'Grady JG, Williams R. Classification of acute liver failure. Lancet. 1993;342(8873):743.
7. O'Grady JG, Schalm SW, Williams R. Acute liver failure: redefining the syndromes. Lancet. 1993;342(8866):273–5.
8. Trey C, Davidson CS. The management of fulminant hepatic failure. Prog Liver Dis. 1970;3:282–98.
9. Ostapowicz G, Fontana RJ, Schiødt FV, Larson A, Davern TJ, Han SH, et al. Results of a prospective study of acute liver failure at 17 tertiary care centers in the United States. Ann Intern Med. 2002;137(12):947–54.

10. Lee WM, Stravitz RT, Larson AM. Introduction to the revised American Association for the Study of Liver Diseases Position Paper on acute liver failure 2011. Hepatology. 2012;55(3):965–7.
11. Acharya SK, Batra Y, Hazari S, Choudhury V, Panda SK, Dattagupta S. Etiopathogenesis of acute hepatic failure: Eastern versus Western countries. J Gastroenterol Hepatol. 2002;17(Suppl 3):S268–73.
12. Gulmez SE, Larrey D, Pageaux GP, Bernuau J, Bissoli F, Horsmans Y, et al. Liver transplant associated with paracetamol overdose: results from the seven-country SALT study. Br J Clin Pharmacol. 2015;80(3):599–606.
13. Hadem J, Tacke F, Bruns T, Langgartner J, Strnad P, Denk GU, et al. Etiologies and outcomes of acute liver failure in Germany. Clin Gastroenterol Hepatol. 2012;10(6):664–9.e2.
14. Areia M, Romãozinho JM, Ferreira M, Amaro P, Leitão MC. Fulminant hepatic failure: a Portuguese experience. Eur J Gastroenterol Hepatol. 2007;19(8):665–9.
15. Bernal W, Auzinger G, Dhawan A, Wendon J. Acute liver failure. Lancet. 2010;376(9736):190–201.
16. Rumack BH, Matthew H. Acetaminophen poisoning and toxicity. Pediatrics. 1975;55(6):871–6.
17. Myers RP, Shaheen AA, Li B, Dean S, Quan H. Impact of liver disease, alcohol abuse, and unintentional ingestions on the outcomes of acetaminophen overdose. Clin Gastroenterol Hepatol. 2008;6(8):918–25; quiz 837
18. Mikolajczyk AE, Renz J, Diaz G, Alpert L, Hart J, Te HS. Massive hepatic infarction caused by HELLP syndrome. ACG Case Rep J. 2017;4:e81.
19. Stravitz RT. Critical management decisions in patients with acute liver failure. Chest. 2008;134(5):1092–102.
20. Manka P, Verheyen J, Gerken G, Canbay A. Liver failure due to acute viral hepatitis (A-E). Visc Med. 2016;32(2):80–5.
21. Willars C. Update in intensive care medicine: acute liver failure. Initial management, supportive treatment and who to transplant. Curr Opin Crit Care. 2014;20(2):202–9.
22. Lee WM. Drug-induced hepatotoxicity. N Engl J Med. 2003;349(5):474–85.
23. Lee WM, Hynan LS, Rossaro L, Fontana RJ, Stravitz RT, Larson AM, et al. Intravenous N-acetylcysteine improves transplant-free survival in early stage non-acetaminophen acute liver failure. Gastroenterology. 2009;137(3):856–64, 864.e1.
24. Singh S, Hynan LS, Lee WM, Acute Liver Failure Study Group. Improvements in hepatic serological biomarkers are associated with clinical benefit of intravenous N-acetylcysteine in early stage non-acetaminophen acute liver failure. Dig Dis Sci. 2013;58(5):1397–402.
25. O'Grady JG, Alexander GJ, Hayllar KM, Williams R. Early indicators of prognosis in fulminant hepatic failure. Gastroenterology. 1989;97(2):439–45.
26. McPhail MJ, Wendon JA, Bernal W. Meta-analysis of performance of Kings's College Hospital Criteria in prediction of outcome in non-paracetamol-induced acute liver failure. J Hepatol. 2010;53(3):492–9.
27. McPhail MJ, Farne H, Senvar N, Wendon JA, Bernal W. Ability of King's college criteria and model for end-stage liver disease scores to predict mortality of patients with acute liver failure: a meta-analysis. Clin Gastroenterol Hepatol. 2016;14(4):516–25.e5; quiz e43–e45
28. Bernal W, Donaldson N, Wyncoll D, Wendon J. Blood lactate as an early predictor of outcome in paracetamol-induced acute liver failure: a cohort study. Lancet. 2002;359(9306):558–63.
29. Mendizabal M, Silva MO. Liver transplantation in acute liver failure: a challenging scenario. World J Gastroenterol. 2016;22(4):1523–31.
30. Rabinowich L, Wendon J, Bernal W, Shibolet O. Clinical management of acute liver failure: results of an international multi-center survey. World J Gastroenterol. 2016;22(33):7595–603.
31. Pauwels A, Mostefa-Kara N, Florent C, Lévy VG. Emergency liver transplantation for acute liver failure. Evaluation of London and Clichy criteria. J Hepatol. 1993;17(1):124–7.
32. Yantorno SE, Kremers WK, Ruf AE, Trentadue JJ, Podesta LG, Villamil FG. MELD is superior to King's college and Clichy's criteria to assess prognosis in fulminant hepatic failure. Liver Transpl. 2007;13(6):822–8.

33. Rutherford A, King LY, Hynan LS, Vedvyas C, Lin W, Lee WM, et al. Development of an accurate index for predicting outcomes of patients with acute liver failure. Gastroenterology. 2012;143(5):1237–43.
34. Fikatas P, Lee JE, Sauer IM, Schmidt SC, Seehofer D, Puhl G, et al. APACHE III score is superior to King's College Hospital criteria, MELD score and APACHE II score to predict outcomes after liver transplantation for acute liver failure. Transplant Proc. 2013;45(6):2295–301.
35. Conn HO, Leevy CM, Vlahcevic ZR, Rodgers JB, Maddrey WC, Seeff L, et al. Comparison of lactulose and neomycin in the treatment of chronic portal-systemic encephalopathy. A double blind controlled trial. Gastroenterology. 1977;72(4 Pt 1):573–83.
36. Muñoz SJ. Difficult management problems in fulminant hepatic failure. Semin Liver Dis. 1993;13(4):395–413.
37. Tsai MH, Chen YC, Lien JM, Tian YC, Peng YS, Fang JT, et al. Hemodynamics and metabolic studies on septic shock in patients with acute liver failure. J Crit Care. 2008;23(4):468–72.
38. Vaquero J, Polson J, Chung C, Helenowski I, Schiodt FV, Reisch J, et al. Infection and the progression of hepatic encephalopathy in acute liver failure. Gastroenterology. 2003;125(3):755–64.
39. Karvellas CJ, Pink F, McPhail M, Cross T, Auzinger G, Bernal W, et al. Predictors of bacteraemia and mortality in patients with acute liver failure. Intensive Care Med. 2009;35(8):1390–6.
40. Kandiah PA, Olson JC, Subramanian RM. Emerging strategies for the treatment of patients with acute hepatic failure. Curr Opin Crit Care. 2016;22(2):142–51.
41. Audimoolam VK, McPhail MJ, Willars C, Bernal W, Wendon JA, Cecconi M, et al. Predicting fluid responsiveness in acute liver failure: a prospective study. Anesth Analg. 2017;124(2):480–6.
42. Lee WM. Acute liver failure. N Engl J Med. 1993;329(25):1862–72.
43. Leithead JA, Ferguson JW, Bates CM, Davidson JS, Lee A, Bathgate AJ, et al. The systemic inflammatory response syndrome is predictive of renal dysfunction in patients with non-paracetamol-induced acute liver failure. Gut. 2009;58(3):443–9.
44. Davenport A. Continuous renal replacement therapies in patients with liver disease. Semin Dial. 2009;22(2):169–72.
45. Stravitz RT, Kramer DJ. Management of acute liver failure. Nat Rev Gastroenterol Hepatol. 2009;6(9):542–53.
46. Steiner LA, Johnston AJ, Czosnyka M, Chatfield DA, Salvador R, Coles JP, et al. Direct comparison of cerebrovascular effects of norepinephrine and dopamine in head-injured patients. Crit Care Med. 2004;32(4):1049–54.
47. O'Grady J. Timing and benefit of liver transplantation in acute liver failure. J Hepatol. 2014;60(3):663–70.
48. Patton H, Misel M, Gish RG. Acute liver failure in adults: an evidence-based management protocol for clinicians. Gastroenterol Hepatol (N Y). 2012;8(3):161–212.
49. Harry R, Auzinger G, Wendon J. The clinical importance of adrenal insufficiency in acute hepatic dysfunction. Hepatology. 2002;36(2):395–402.
50. Warrillow SJ, Bellomo R. Preventing cerebral oedema in acute liver failure: the case for quadruple-H therapy. Anaesth Intensive Care. 2014;42(1):78–88.
51. Scott TR, Kronsten VT, Hughes RD, Shawcross DL. Pathophysiology of cerebral oedema in acute liver failure. World J Gastroenterol. 2013;19(48):9240–55.
52. Smith M. Monitoring intracranial pressure in traumatic brain injury. Anesth Analg. 2008;106(1):240–8.
53. Karvellas CJ, Fix OK, Battenhouse H, Durkalski V, Sanders C, Lee WM, et al. Outcomes and complications of intracranial pressure monitoring in acute liver failure: a retrospective cohort study. Crit Care Med. 2014;42(5):1157–67.
54. Kawakami M, Koda M, Murawaki Y. Cerebral pulsatility index by transcranial Doppler sonography predicts the prognosis of patients with fulminant hepatic failure. Clin Imaging. 2010;34(5):327–31.
55. Kassab MY, Majid A, Farooq MU, Azhary H, Hershey LA, Bednarczyk EM, et al. Transcranial Doppler: an introduction for primary care physicians. J Am Board Fam Med. 2007;20(1):65–71.

56. Paschoal FM, Nogueira RC, Ronconi KA, de Lima Oliveira M, Teixeira MJ, Bor-Seng-Shu E. Multimodal brain monitoring in fulminant hepatic failure. World J Hepatol. 2016;8(22):915–23.
57. Murphy N, Auzinger G, Bernel W, Wendon J. The effect of hypertonic sodium chloride on intracranial pressure in patients with acute liver failure. Hepatology. 2004;39(2):464–70.
58. Karkhanis J, Verna EC, Chang MS, Stravitz RT, Schilsky M, Lee WM, et al. Steroid use in acute liver failure. Hepatology. 2014;59(2):612–21.
59. Bernal W, Hall C, Karvellas CJ, Auzinger G, Sizer E, Wendon J. Arterial ammonia and clinical risk factors for encephalopathy and intracranial hypertension in acute liver failure. Hepatology. 2007;46(6):1844–52.
60. Mohsenin V. Assessment and management of cerebral edema and intracranial hypertension in acute liver failure. J Crit Care. 2013;28(5):783–91.
61. Vaquero J. Therapeutic hypothermia in the management of acute liver failure. Neurochem Int. 2012;60(7):723–35.
62. Jalan R, Olde Damink SW, Deutz NE, Hayes PC, Lee A. Moderate hypothermia in patients with acute liver failure and uncontrolled intracranial hypertension. Gastroenterology. 2004;127(5):1338–46.
63. Bernal W, Murphy N, Brown S, Whitehouse T, Bjerring PN, Hauerberg J, et al. A multicentre randomized controlled trial of moderate hypothermia to prevent intracranial hypertension in acute liver failure. J Hepatol. 2016;65(2):273–9.
64. Karvellas CJ, Todd Stravitz R, Battenhouse H, Lee WM, Schilsky ML, Group UALFS. Therapeutic hypothermia in acute liver failure: a multicenter retrospective cohort analysis. Liver Transpl. 2015;21(1):4–12.
65. Ellis AJ, Wendon JA, Williams R. Subclinical seizure activity and prophylactic phenytoin infusion in acute liver failure: a controlled clinical trial. Hepatology. 2000;32(3):536–41.
66. Bhatia V, Batra Y, Acharya SK. Prophylactic phenytoin does not improve cerebral edema or survival in acute liver failure – a controlled clinical trial. J Hepatol. 2004;41(1):89–96.
67. Porcher R, Vaquero J. Hypothermia in acute liver failure: what got lost in translation? J Hepatol. 2016;65(2):240–2.
68. Lee WM. Recent developments in acute liver failure. Best Pract Res Clin Gastroenterol. 2012;26(1):3–16.
69. Bernsmeier C, Antoniades CG, Wendon J. What's new in acute liver failure? Intensive Care Med. 2014;40(10):1545–8.
70. Singanayagam A, Bernal W. Update on acute liver failure. Curr Opin Crit Care. 2015;21(2):134–41.
71. Donnelly MC, Hayes PC, Simpson KJ. Role of inflammation and infection in the pathogenesis of human acute liver failure: clinical implications for monitoring and therapy. World J Gastroenterol. 2016;22(26):5958–70.
72. Singh T, Gupta N, Alkhouri N, Carey WD, Hanouneh IA. A guide to managing acute liver failure. Cleve Clin J Med. 2016;83(6):453–62.
73. Karvellas CJ, Cavazos J, Battenhouse H, Durkalski V, Balko J, Sanders C, et al. Effects of antimicrobial prophylaxis and blood stream infections in patients with acute liver failure: a retrospective cohort study. Clin Gastroenterol Hepatol. 2014;12(11):1942–9.e1.
74. Lisman T, Stravitz RT. Rebalanced hemostasis in patients with acute liver failure. Semin Thromb Hemost. 2015;41(5):468–73.
75. Stravitz RT, Lisman T, Luketic VA, Sterling RK, Puri P, Fuchs M, et al. Minimal effects of acute liver injury/acute liver failure on hemostasis as assessed by thromboelastography. J Hepatol. 2012;56(1):129–36.
76. Lisman T, Porte RJ. Rebalanced hemostasis in patients with liver disease: evidence and clinical consequences. Blood. 2010;116(6):878–85.
77. British Committee for Standards in H, Blood Transfusion Task Force. Guidelines for the use of platelet transfusions. Br J Haematol. 2003;122(1):10–23.

78. Pavese P, Bonadona A, Beaubien J, Labrecque P, Pernod G, Letoublon C, et al. FVIIa corrects the coagulopathy of fulminant hepatic failure but may be associated with thrombosis: a report of four cases. Can J Anaesth. 2005;52(1):26–9.
79. Kirchner C, Dirkmann D, Treckmann JW, Paul A, Hartmann M, Saner FH, et al. Coagulation management with factor concentrates in liver transplantation: a single-center experience. Transfusion. 2014;54(10 Pt 2):2760–8.
80. Agarwal B, Shaw S, Hari MS, Burroughs AK, Davenport A. Continuous renal replacement therapy (CRRT) in patients with liver disease: is circuit life different? J Hepatol. 2009;51(3):504–9.
81. Ringe B, Pichlmayr R, Lübbe N, Bornscheuer A, Kuse E. Total hepatectomy as temporary approach to acute hepatic or primary graft failure. Transplant Proc. 1988;20(1 Suppl 1):552–7.
82. Hammer GB, So SK, Al-Uzri A, Conley SB, Concepcion W, Cox KL, et al. Continuous venovenous hemofiltration with dialysis in combination with total hepatectomy and portocaval shunting. Bridge to liver transplantation. Transplantation. 1996;62(1):130–2.
83. Domínguez Fernández E, Lange K, Lange R, Eigler FW. Relevance of two-stage total hepatectomy and liver transplantation in acute liver failure and severe liver trauma. Transpl Int. 2001;14(3):184–90.
84. Sanabria Mateos R, Hogan NM, Dorcaratto D, Heneghan H, Udupa V, Maguire D, et al. Total hepatectomy and liver transplantation as a two-stage procedure for fulminant hepatic failure: a safe procedure in exceptional circumstances. World J Hepatol. 2016;8(4):226–30.
85. Karvellas CJ, Subramanian RM. Current evidence for extracorporeal liver support systems in acute liver failure and acute-on-chronic liver failure. Crit Care Clin. 2016;32(3):439–51.
86. Karvellas CJ, Gibney N, Kutsogiannis D, Wendon J, Bain VG. Bench-to-bedside review: current evidence for extracorporeal albumin dialysis systems in liver failure. Crit Care. 2007;11(3):215.
87. Karvellas CJ, Stravitz RT. High volume plasma exchange in acute liver failure: dampening the inflammatory cascade? J Hepatol. 2016;64(1):10–2.
88. Larsen FS, Schmidt LE, Bernsmeier C, Rasmussen A, Isoniemi H, Patel VC, et al. High-volume plasma exchange in patients with acute liver failure: an open randomised controlled trial. J Hepatol. 2016;64(1):69–78.

Chapter 13
Liver Assist Systems for Bridging to Transplantation: Devices and Concepts

Nathanael Raschzok, Karl Herbert Hillebrandt, and Igor M. Sauer

Introduction

Liver transplantation (LT) is the gold standard for treating patients with acute liver failure and chronic liver diseases (CLDs), as well as those in the early stages of hepatocellular carcinoma [1]. During LT, the diseased organ is replaced by a healthy graft, which provides the body with all the functions of the liver, including detoxification and synthesis as well as direct and indirect regulation of the acid-base status and electrolytes. The removal of the diseased organ from circulation resolves the portal hypertension that is responsible for dramatic changes in the patient's hemodynamics.

Organ Shortage

The success of liver transplantation is increasingly limited by the lack of suitable donor organs. In 2016, 1,450 patients were listed for liver transplantation in Germany; yet, only 888 liver transplantations could be performed [2]. In the UNOS region, 14,134 patients were on the waiting list for LT, although only 7,841 liver transplantations could be performed [3]. This significant organ shortage for liver transplantation is due to the success of intensive care medicine and to the increasing

N. Raschzok (✉) · K. H. Hillebrandt · I. M. Sauer
Department of Surgery, Campus Charité Mitte | Campus Virchow-Klinikum, Experimental Surgery and Regenerative Medicine, Charité – Universitätsmedizin Berlin, Berlin, Germany
e-mail: nathanael.raschzok@charite.de

D. Bezinover, F. Saner (eds.), *Critical Care for Potential Liver Transplant Candidates*,
https://doi.org/10.1007/978-3-319-92934-7_13

number of patients who are too sick to serve as donors for liver transplantation. The problem is not only the insufficient number of donations, but also the quality of the potentially available grafts. For example, about 20% of liver grafts must be rejected from transplantation due to fatty liver disease. Based on the actual trends in the prevalence of diabetes and obesity, it has been estimated that the overall use of liver grafts will fall from 78% to 44% by 2030 [4]. According to the 2017 publication, "Study on the Uptake and Impact of the EU Action Plan on Organ Donation and Transplantation (2009–2015) in the EU Member States," nearly 33,000 transplants were performed in the 28 EU member states in 2015 [5, 6]. Nevertheless, 56,000 patients still remained on waiting lists, irrespective of the type of organ needed, and over 3,800 died while waiting for a new organ by the end of the same year [6]. The demand for organs in the EU exceeds the supply by far. This phenomenon is observed in every member state, although to varying degrees, and it is currently one of the main issues in the field of organ transplantation, alongside other major issues such as organ trafficking and transplant tourism [7].

The allocation system based on the Model for End-Stage Liver Disease (MELD) is designed to ensure that the candidates who most urgently need a transplant are most likely to receive one [11]. Certainly, MELD-based allocation has led to a significant reduction in the mortality of exactly those candidates. On the other hand, the waiting time for patients with chronic liver disease has increased dramatically. In Germany, this situation has led to a decrease in the number of patients on the waiting list for liver transplantation [9]. Moreover, in patients with HCC within the Milan criteria who would have been treated by LT in the past, currently performed liver resection is not a definitive treatment for this condition. In parallel, at least in Germany, the mortality rate after a liver transplantation is rising because of the protocol whereby the sickest patients are first to receive a transplant [10].

MELD-based allocation has led to a reduction in the mortality rate of patients with advanced liver disease. However, not all patients with acute liver failure can be treated by liver transplantation. For example, patients are rendered ineligible for transplantation due to various causes, including sepsis, the unavailability of a suitable graft, and conditions associated with potential liver regeneration. In addition, patients who continue to consume alcohol even as they are experiencing acute deterioration are ineligible for a liver transplant.

Clinical Needs

The idea of extracorporeal liver support was developed in order to solve these problems by providing temporary support for the failing liver. Liver assist devices should, from a conceptual point of view, help to either bridge the time until a suitable liver graft becomes available (bridging to transplantation) or give the patient's liver a chance to regenerate (bridging to regeneration). Liver assist devices should, therefore, be designed to provide all the functions of the liver, i.e., detoxification, regulation, and synthesis.

Artificial and Bioartificial Liver Support: Concepts and Clinical Results

As the accumulation of toxins not cleared by the failing liver is the most critical problem in liver failure, the removal of these substances can significantly improve the patient's condition. This led to the development of artificial filtration and adsorption devices – referred to as artificial liver support devices. The complex tasks of the liver's synthetic function, however, have to be addressed by bioartificial liver support systems.

Artificial Liver Support Systems

Artificial liver support systems are designed to clear the blood of albumin-bound, hydrophobic substances. Additional adsorbers or acceptors of substances are necessary to enhance mass exchange. Artificial liver support devices are usually based on membrane separation and use sorbents including charcoal and anion or cation exchangers. Albumin, which is the predominant carrier of toxins in the patient's blood, serves as an acceptor substance.

Based on this idea, the Molecular Adsorbent Recirculating System (MARS) was developed. This system consists of a dialysis circuit, a blood circuit, and an albumin circuit. It is based on a hemodialysis system, where dialysate is modified using albumin (Fig. 13.1a). A high-flux hemodialysis filter separates the albumin solution from the patient's blood. Human albumin is used in the albumin circuit as dialysate. Albumin acts as the acceptor substance for albumin-bound toxins and is partly regenerated by passing an anion exchanger and a charcoal adsorber in a closed circuit [11].

Even simpler, a single pass albumin dialysis (SPAD) uses standard renal replacement therapy machines without an additional perfusion pump system. The patient's blood flows through a circuit with a high-flux hollow fiber filter during hemodiafiltration. The other side of this membrane is cleaned, in counter-directional flow, with an albumin solution, which is simply discarded after passing through the filter (Fig. 13.1c) [12].

The Prometheus System (FPSA, Prometheus, Fresenius Medical Care, Bad Homburg, Germany) uses membranes with larger pores, which separate a certain fraction of plasma proteins, including the toxin-loaded albumin, from the patient's blood (Fig. 13.1b). Fractionated plasma separation and adsorption allow the patient's own albumin to be regenerated via passage through two adsorption matrices in a secondary circuit. An albumin-permeable polysulfone membrane is used to filter the patient's albumin fraction into the secondary circuit [13]. The Hepa Wash procedure (Hepa Wash GmbH, Munich, Germany) is a further variation of albumin dialysis. Instead of regenerating the albumin with adsorbers or discarding it, this procedure is based on changes in pH and temperature that allow the albumin to be regenerated (Fig. 13.1d) [14].

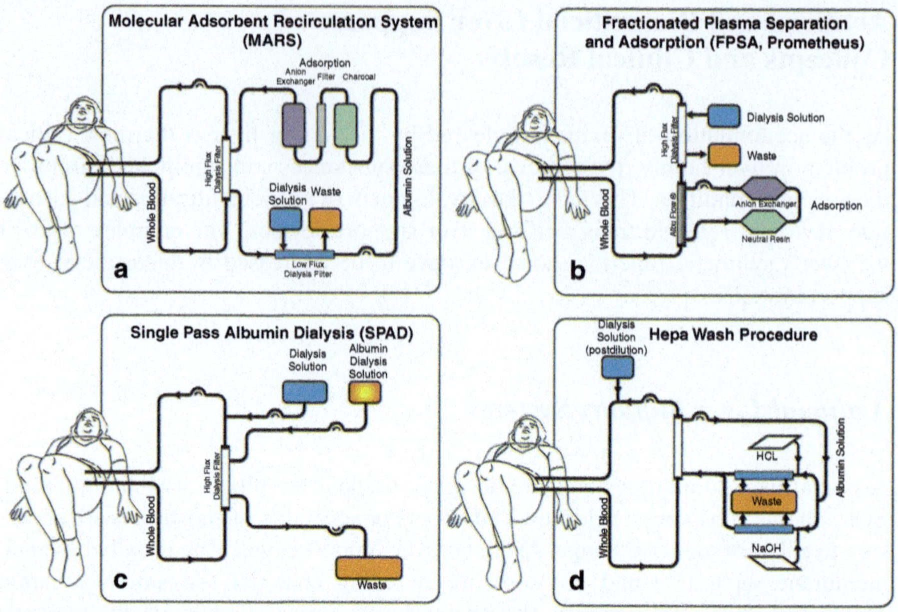

Fig. 13.1 Schematic representation of current artificial liver support systems: (**a**) Molecular Adsorbent Recirculation System (MARS). (**b**) Fractionated plasma separation and adsorption (FPSA, Prometheus). (**c**) Single-pass albumin dialysis (SPAD). (**d**) Albumin dialysis and targeted manipulation of dialysis fluid pH (HepaWash Advanced Organ Support, ADVOS)

Bioartificial Liver Support Systems

Bioartificial liver support devices were developed to not only support the failing detoxification function of the diseased liver but also to address the failing regulatory (e.g., acid-base status, amino acids) and synthetic function (e.g., albumin, glucose, lipids, coagulation factors, even unknown substances). These functions can be enabled only by the use of hepatic cells. As extracorporeal liver perfusion requires complex logistics and depends on intact liver grafts, several different liver support bioreactors have been developed, which enable the cultivation of isolated liver cells in a more suitable mode for integration into clinical perfusion systems and for prolonged cell culture function.

The HepatAssist system developed by Demetriou et al. is based on cryopreserved porcine hepatocytes within the intercapillary space of a device resembling a modified dialysis cartridge (Fig. 13.2a). The patient's plasma ultrafiltrates directly through the cartridges via an activated charcoal adsorber and an oxygenator [15].

The extracorporeal liver assist device (ELAD) uses approximately 200 g of cell line originating from human hepatoblastoma (C3A, derived from HepG2) in a similar setting (Fig. 13.2b). The cells are separated from the patient's plasma by hollow fiber membranes and an integrated charcoal adsorber as well as a membrane oxygenator. This is necessary to support detoxification and maintain the oxygen supply of the cells [16].

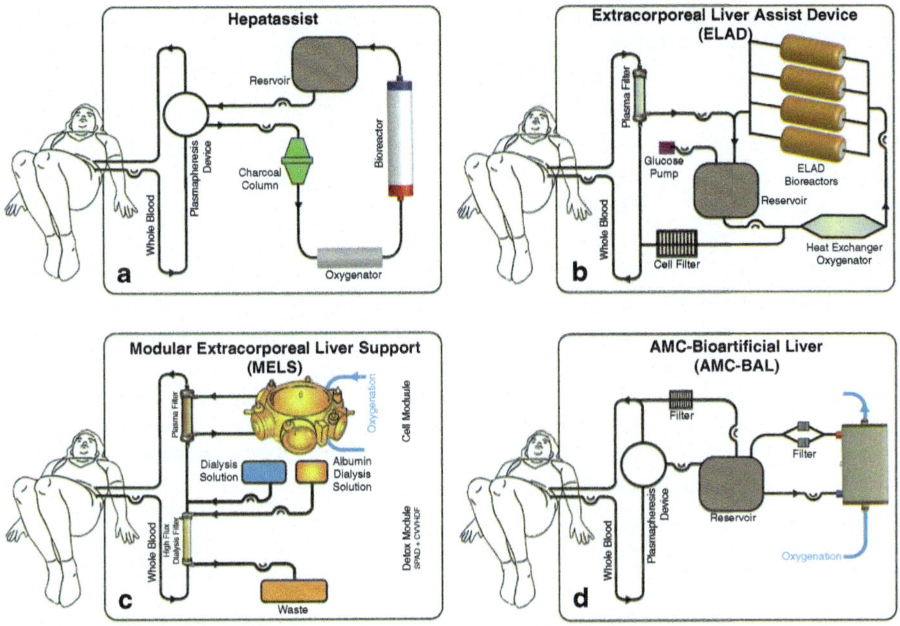

Fig. 13.2 Bioartificial liver support systems (schematic images). (**a**) HepatAssist. (**b**) Extracorporeal liver assist device (ELAD). (**c**) Modular extracorporeal liver support (MELS). (**d**) AMC-bioartificial liver

The modular extracorporeal liver support (MELS) systems combine a bioreactor with CVVHDF and SPAD for the removal of water-soluble and albumin-bound toxins. The bioreactor is based on two hydrophilic polyethersulfone membrane bundles and a hydrophobic multilayer hollow fiber bundle for oxygenation and was charged with primary porcine [17] or human liver cells [18] (Fig. 13.2c).

The Academisch Medisch Centrum Bioartificial Liver (AMC-BAL) differs from other systems in one major respect: instead of separating the patient's plasma from the extracorporeally applied liver cells by a membrane, the plasma is in direct contact with the cells. A non-woven polyester matrix is used for this approach to offer a large surface area for the inoculated primary porcine cells to attach and form aggregates between the fibers [19] (Fig. 13.2d).

Clinical Evaluation of Extracorporeal Liver Support

In general, randomized, controlled, and adequately powered studies evaluating artificial and bioartificial liver support are rare. A summary of key ECLS trials is provided in Table 13.1 (modified from Olson and Karvellas [20]). Five prospective randomized control trials (RCTs) have been used as a basis for

Table 13.1 Studies demonstrating biochemical improvements by extracorporeal liver support in patients with acute liver failure

Nr.	Author/year	Device	Survival
1	Mitzner, 2000	MARS	Yes (38% vs. 0% at 7 days)
2	Heemann, 2002	MARS	Yes (90% vs. 55% at 30 days)
3	Sen, 2004	MARS	No (45% in both)
4	Laleman, 2006	MARS/Prometheus	N/A
5	Hassinien, 2007	MARS	N/A
6	Kribben, 2012	Prometheus	No effect on 28/90-day survival
7	Banares, 2013	MARS	No effect on 28-day survival
8	Lake, 2016	ELAD	(90-day 59% vs. 62%, $p = 0.74$)
9	Sauer, unpublished	MELS	
10	Larsen, 2016	High-Volume Plasma Exchange Versus Standard Medical Treatment in Patients With Acute Liver Failure	Significant 90-day survival benefit in patients receiving plasma exchange

Adapted from Olson and Karvellas [20]

evaluating MARS [21–25]. Prometheus was evaluated in one RCT regarding the survival of patients with acute-on-chronic liver failure (ACLF). The use of MARS and Prometheus in patients with ACLF has been evaluated in two studies [25, 26]. Although both studies demonstrated an acceptable safety profile, no increase in the probability of survival was found. Clinical data on SPAD are limited to case reports and small series. Bioartificial liver support concepts have also been evaluated in small studies only, with the exception of the HepatAssist system. In an RCT with 171 patients with acute liver failure or primary graft non-function after LT, the 30-day survival rates were 71% versus 62%, respectively, for the HepatAssist device compared with standard care ($p = 0.26$). However, survival in the subgroup of patients with fulminant/subfulminant hepatic failure was significantly higher in the BAL group compared with the control group ($p = 0.048$) [27]. Artificial and bioartificial support systems did not appear to affect mortality in acute liver failure. Stutchfield et al., in a meta-analysis of RCTs, evaluated the role of contemporary extracorporeal liver support concepts related to patients with acute liver failure or ACLF [28]. They concluded that these systems appeared to improve survival in acute liver failure.

In conclusion, artificial and bioartificial liver support devices have demonstrated biochemical improvement in patients with acute liver failure and patients with hepatic encephalopathy, but their effects have failed to correlate with the survival benefit in larger methodologically robust studies. Thus, the use of extracorporeal liver support systems is currently not recommended as standard care in patients with acute liver failure or ACLF [20]. Four studies are currently recruiting patients with the purpose of evaluating the effect of artificial liver support systems, although there are currently no studies underway to address bioartificial liver support (Table 13.2).

Table 13.2 Active studies listed on ClinicalTrials.gov addressing liver support systems for treatment of liver failure

Nr.	Study title	Status
1	Safety and Efficacy of hiHep Bioartificial Liver Support System to Treat Acute Liver Failure	Not yet recruiting
2	Early Postoperative Extracorporeal Liver Support Therapy as a Tool to Manage Post-Hepatectomy Liver Failure	Recruiting
3	Comparison of Two Liver Dialysis Systems: MARS versus SPAD in Severe Liver Failure	Recruiting
4	High-Volume Plasma Exchange Versus Standard Medical Treatment in Patients with Acute Liver Failure	Recruiting
5	Molecular Adsorbent Recirculating System (MARS®) in Hypoxic Hepatitis	Recruiting

Limitations of Extracorporeal Liver Support Systems

There are a number of problems associated with the use of artificial and bioartificial liver support systems.

1. Lack of a reliable, safe, highly metabolically active, and easily expandable human cell source. Human tumor cell lines (e.g., hepatoblastoma cells) are characterized by an impaired metabolic function and a certain risk of metastatic cells spreading via leaking hollow fibers. Primary porcine cells have limited metabolic biocompatibility, and the suitability of these types of cells as sources for clinical application is open to question due to their immunogenicity (anti-pig IgG and IgM were seen after clinical application) and the risk for xenozoonoses.
2. The membrane of bioartificial liver support systems is a major technical problem of this system. Mass exchange is limited due to the artificial separation by membranes in the patient's blood from plasma and – in most systems – plasma from hepatic cells. In addition, owing to the resistance of the bundles of hollow fibers, flow rates within the bioreactors are low (100–200 ml/min) compared to those of in vivo perfusion (~1500 ml/min).

Hepatocyte Transplantation

Hepatocyte transplantation was initially developed as an alternative therapeutic approach to the solid organ transplantation approach for various liver conditions [29]. Hepatocyte transplantation is based on the administration of liver cells in suspension, which implies several potential advantages over whole-organ transplantation. Preparation includes the isolation of hepatocytes from donor livers or liver segments that were unused for whole-organ transplantation or rejected from transplantation. Hepatocyte transplantation could expand the donor pool for liver grafts and theoretically allow the treatment of multiple patients with cells from one donor organ. Hepatocytes can be cryopreserved, which enables the pooling of cells and on-demand applications. Cells can then be either infused into the liver or into an ectopic implantation site such as the spleen or the peritoneal cavity. This method is also less invasive than whole-organ transplantation and offers the chance to treat critically ill or very young patients who are not suitable for whole-organ transplantation. Transplanted hepatocytes engrafted in the recipient liver or at the ectopic implantation site provide metabolic activity without the need to remove the diseased liver. Thus, the native liver can be left in place and may have a chance of recovery [30, 31].

Hepatocyte transplantation has been clinically evaluated for the same major indications if LT is required [29] (Table 13.1). However, hepatocyte transplantation has not yet achieved sustainable benefits for patients with acute liver failure or chronic liver disease [29]. The reasons for this deficit are (1) the inability to transplant a sufficient number of cells in order to provide hepatic capacity similar to that afforded by a full liver graft and according to the patient's need and (2) the inability of hepatocytes to engraft in the cirrhotic or severely damaged liver. Clinical studies on hepatocyte transplantation in acute liver failure have been stopped, and currently there is no study listed on ClinicalTrials.gov addressing hepatocyte transplantation for this application.

However, clinical data from a small series suggest that hepatocyte transplantation can be an effective bridging strategy for patients suffering from inborn metabolic liver disorders. Especially in cases with a single deficient enzyme such as urea cycle defects [32–38] or glycogen storage disease [39], transplanted hepatocytes can fulfill the missing function such that it is not necessary to replace the organ. According to the current literature, approximately 40 children and adults have received hepatocyte transplantation for liver-based metabolic disease [29]. Hepatocyte transplantation is proven to be feasible and safe, and a majority of the cases demonstrated temporal clinical improvements, e.g., bilirubin or urea reduction or the presence of soluble factors synthesized by transplanted cells. However, almost all the patients had to undergo LT a few months after hepatocyte transplantation due to a recurrence or further aggravation of the disease.

Thus, there are several issues to consider regarding successfully treating liver disease by hepatocyte transplantation [40]. First, evidence for the long-term engraftment and function of transplanted cells in humans is still lacking. Possible reasons for the unsustainable long-term outcome of hepatocyte transplantation include insufficient cell translocation through the endothelial cell barrier [41], insufficient cell engraftment [42], and destruction of the engrafted cells by the immune system [43, 44]. In order to address this issue, Jorns et al. recently investigated the concept of preconditioning by partial hepatectomy prior to hepatocyte transplantation in two patients with Crigler-Najjar syndrome type I [45]. Their data suggest that this procedure provided a regenerative stimulus to the transplanted cells. However, the grafts were lost early after transplantation, presumably due to humoral rejection. Soltys et al. investigated preparative hepatic irradiation as another concept for preconditioning prior to hepatocyte transplantation [46]. Again, their concept was initially successful, but the recipient had to undergo LT shortly thereafter. Another major challenge is that primary human hepatocytes are currently the only source for clinical hepatocyte transplantation. With the continually decreasing number of available organs for hepatocyte isolation, there is a critical scarcity of hepatocytes for transplantation. Strategies to overcome this issue include the use of stem cells or induced pluripotent stem cells to generate hepatocytes. However, the safety of such cells has not yet been proven [47, 48].

In conclusion, hepatocyte transplantation is still an experimental approach that has some potential to become a clinically routine method for liver support prior to liver transplantation, especially in newborns and children with genetic metabolic liver diseases. Whether or not hepatocyte transplantation might be suitable for liver support in patients with acute liver failure or cirrhosis has yet to be established.

Future Concepts: Bioengineered Liver

The treatment of end-stage liver disease and acute liver failure remains a clinically relevant problem. Despite three decades of scientific efforts on artificial and bioartificial liver support, LT remains the gold standard. However, whole-organ transplantation is invasive and limited by the unavailability of suitable donor organs [49]. Further, whole-organ transplantation requires lifelong immunosuppression of the recipient. Although immunosuppressive regimens have improved tremendously during the last decade, unwanted effects such as high infection rates, elevated risk for cancer and lymphoproliferative diseases, and long-term graft failure are limiting factors [50, 51].

To overcome these problems, the new technique of de- and re-cellularization was developed and has been of great interest to the field of regenerative medicine and tissue engineering over the last decade. During the process of decellularization, the organ is perfused through the vascular system with different ionic, chemical, physical, or enzymatic agents to remove cells and other immunogenic molecules (e.g., DNA, alpha-Gal epitopes) from the organs, in order to obtain the extracellular matrix (ECM) [52]. The ECM, in general, preserves the complex, three-dimensional microanatomy of an organ, including its "vascular framework," and, on the liver specifically, it also preserves the framework of the biliary system [53].

These natural liver scaffolds can then be used for repopulation with parenchymal (e.g., hepatocytes) as well as non-parenchymal liver (e.g., sinusoidal endothelial) cells to generate vascularized (and thus perfusable with whole blood) and metabolic functional bioengineered livers. These elegant techniques could be used to create human-scale bioengineered liver grafts (Fig. 13.3).

As they are highly conserved across species, ECM proteins are unlikely to induce immunogenic reactions, even in allogenic or xenogenic host organisms [54, 55]. Due to this knowledge, human-scale xenogenic liver scaffolds (e.g., porcine) may be used as a foundation for repopulation in a clinical setting [49, 52]. To achieve a clinically relevant metabolic liver function, there is a tremendous need for highly

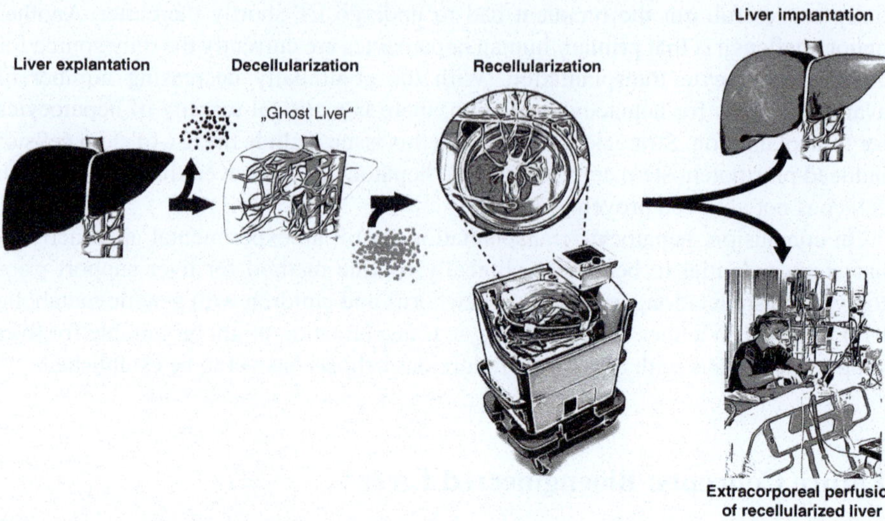

Fig. 13.3 Concept of liver de- and re-cellularization as well as the potential clinical applications (schematic image)

active liver cells. Liver cell isolation from discharged liver grafts has been described but has not yet reached an adequate cell yield [52, 56]. Nevertheless, the use of isolated liver cells for repopulation would again require immunosuppressive therapy. Since the introduction of human-induced pluripotent stem cells (hiPSC), there has been great interest in the field of recellularization [52].

With the use of patient-derived iPSC for the recellularization of human-size liver scaffolds, the engineering of a personalized liver graft, which requires no or only slight immunosuppression, would be possible. However, the induction of human pluripotent stem cells, their differentiation, and finally their expansion to clinically relevant masses require novel, enhanced, and optimized protocols for all the stated steps.

After a period of maturation and in the case of iPSC-derived hepatocytes, cell differentiation in a bioreactor, this autologous graft could be used for extracorporeal perfusion (bridging to regeneration or bridging to transplantation) or – in the future – could even be implanted.

Since the first description of whole-liver de- and re-cellularization in 2010 [53], the field has quickly expanded. Over the years, various whole-organ decellularization protocols for the livers of mice, rats, ferrets, pigs, and sheep, as well as human livers, have been developed [53, 57–64]. Furthermore, over the last several years, numerous protocols for the recellularization of rodent- and human-scale liver scaffolds demonstrating metabolic function and cell survival in vitro have been published [53, 59, 60, 62, 65–67]. Nevertheless, none of these experiments reached a relevant cell mass with respect to the model. As mentioned before, iPSC may offer such an approach.

Another problem is the blood coagulation within the vascular system after the implantation or in vitro whole blood perfusion of decellularized or only parenchymatous recellularized liver grafts [68]. This problem occurs due to the fact that the vascular network in the decellularized matrix consists of uncovered collagen fibers, which induce clotting. Therefore, at present, most groups address the repopulation of the vascular network as "re-endothelialization." Thus, the challenge is to cover all parts of the vascular network of ECM from the main branches of the portal vein down to the sinusoidal structures with endothelium or another appropriate structure.

So far, a few studies have shown partial re-endothelialization in vitro, covering the big vessel branches with an endothelial cell monolayer [53, 60, 69–71]. Other approaches to overcoming the issue of blood coagulation are to cross-link the collagen surface or to cover the vascular ECM with immobilized heparin layers [66, 72, 73].

However, in only some of these studies did researchers implant the re-endothelialized or heparinized liver grafts in vivo for up to 72 h [53, 62, 66, 70]. None of these studies show long-term metabolic function or graft survival.

Another area for which many questions remain is the reconstruction of the biliary tract [68]. The presence of cholangiocytes after recellularization with fetal or neonatal cell mixtures has been investigated in only a handful of studies [60, 67]. For these bioengineered livers to be used successfully in the setting of bridging to transplantation or bridging to regeneration, effective bile excretion will be essential.

Another underrepresented topic is the immunogenicity of decellularized liver tissue. Up to now, there is no universal definition for which properties an "optimal" decellularized matrix should have [74]. Based on earlier works, it is stated that decellularized tissue is not immunogenic, and the following three criteria are fulfilled: (1) < 50 ng dsDNA/mg ECM dry weight, (2) < 200 bp DNA fragment length, and (3) lack of visible nuclear material [30]. However, the immunogenicity of decellularized liver tissue has not been investigated in a systematic way. In several studies, decellularized liver tissue has been implanted even in xenogenic models with no adverse effects [64, 75]. Moreover, they demonstrated an infiltration of host cells into the decellularized matrix, which proves the biocompatibility of the tissue [64, 75]. However, systematic investigations are needed to address this issue.

In conclusion, the technique of de- and re-cellularization has the potential for a clinical translation to a personalized bioengineered liver graft. Alternatively, in the future these systems may be suitable as bridging systems. Nevertheless, some major obstacles must be addressed: (1) the need for sufficient cell expansion of iPSC-derived hepatocytes, (2) a patent vasculature as a basis for bioengineering perfusable liver grafts. Therefore, the re-endothelialization must be optimized and may be combined with a biochemical surface sealing.

If it is possible to address these major issues, as well as the problem of bile excretion, de- and re-cellularization may prove capable of overcoming the hurdles faced in using other bioartificial livers. However, the next decade will show us whether this technique can actually deliver in practice.

Key Points

1. The aim of bioartificial liver support systems is to provide all the functions of the liver for patients with liver failure by either bridging to transplantation or bridging to regeneration.
2. Artificial liver support systems have been developed to filter albumin-bound toxins. Although a handful of devices have been tested and used in clinical settings, none is recommended for routine intensive care.
3. Hepatocyte transplantation has been evaluated as an alternative treatment approach to solid organ transplantation or bridging to transplantation. However, the benefit of this approach has been demonstrated only for infants with metabolic diseases.
4. Bioengineered liver manufacturing using the technique of de- and re-cellularization is a promising approach. However, several problems such as cell source or adequate vascular perfusion are currently limiting factors in terms of transitioning these techniques to the clinic.

References

1. Alqahtani SA. Update in liver transplantation. Curr Opin Gastroenterol. 2012;28(3):230–8.
2. Jahresbericht Organspende und Transplantation in Deutschland 2016. Deutsche Stiftung Organtransplantation. p. 82.
3. www.unos.org.
4. Pais R, Barritt AS 4th, Calmus Y, Scatton O, Runge T, Lebray P, Poynard T, Ratziu V, Conti FJ. NAFLD and liver transplantation: current burden and expected challenges. J Hepatol. 2016;65(6):1245–57. https://doi.org/10.1016/j.jhep.2016.07.033. Epub 2016 Jul 30.
5. Study on the uptake and impact of the EU Action Plan on organ donation and transplantation (2009–2015) in the EU Member States. European Commission. 2017. pp. 5–7.
6. Council of Europe. Newsletter Transplant. International figures on donation and transplantation 2015. 2016. p. 16, pp. 43–45.
7. Council of Europe. Trafficking in organs, tissues and cells and trafficking in human beings for the purpose of the removal of organs. 2009.
8. Kamath PS1, Kim WR, Advanced Liver Disease Study Group. The model for end-stage liver disease (MELD). Hepatology. 2007;45(3):797–805.
9. Tacke F, Kroy DC, Barreiros AP, Neumann UP. Liver transplantation in Germany. Liver Transpl. 2016;22(8):1136–42. https://doi.org/10.1002/lt.24461.
10. Otto G. Liver transplantation: an appraisal of the present situation. Dig Dis. 2013;31(1):164–9. https://doi.org/10.1159/000347213. Epub 2013 Jun 17.
11. Mitzner SR. Extracorporeal liver support-albumin dialysis with the Molecular Adsorbent Recirculating System (MARS). Ann Hepatol. 2011;10:21–8.
12. Sauer IM, Goetz M, Steffen I, et al. In vitro comparison of the molecular adsorbent recirculation system (MARS) and single-pass albumin dialysis (SPAD). Hepatology. 2004;39:1408–144.
13. Rifai K. Fractionated plasma separation and adsorption: current practice and future options. Liver Int. 2011;31:13–5.
14. Al-Chalabi A, et al. Evaluation of the Hepa Wash(R) treatment in pigs with acute liver failure. BMC Gastroenterol. 2013;13:83.

15. Demetriou AA, Brown RS Jr, Busuttil RW, et al. Prospective, randomized, multicenter, controlled trial of a bioartificial liver in treating acute liver failure. Ann Surg. 2004;239:660–70.
16. Sussman NL, Gislason GT, Conlin CA, et al. The Hepatix extracorporeal liver assist device: initial clinical experience. Artif Organs. 1994;18:390–6.
17. Sauer IM, Kardassis D, Zeillinger K, Pascher A, Gruenwald A, Pless G, Irgang M, Kraemer M, Puhl G, Frank J, Müller AR, Steinmüller T, Denner J, Neuhaus P, Gerlach JC. Clinical extracorporeal hybrid liver support–phase I study with primary porcine liver cells. Xenotransplantation. 2003;10(5):460–9.
18. Sauer IM, Zeilinger K, Pless G, et al. Extracorporeal liver support based on primary human liver cells and albumin dialysis – treatment of a patient with primary graft non-function. J Hepatol. 2003;39:649–53.
19. van de Kerkhove MP, Di Florio E, Scuderi V, et al. Phase I clinical trial with the AMC-bioartificial liver. Int J Artif Organs. 2002;25:950–9.
20. Olson JC, Karvellas CJ. Critical care management of the cirrhotic patient awaiting liver transplant in the intensive care unit. Liver Transpl. 2017;23:1465.
21. Mitzner SR, et al. Improvement of hepatorenal syndrome with extracorporeal albumin dialysis MARS: results of a prospective, randomized, controlled clinical trial. Liver Transpl Off Publ Am Assoc Study Liver Dis Int Liver Transpl Soc. 2000;6:277–86.
22. Heemann U, et al. Albumin dialysis in cirrhosis with superimposed acute liver injury: a prospective, controlled study. Hepatology. 2002;36:949–58.
23. Sen S, et al. Pathophysiological effects of albumin dialysis in acute-on-chronic liver failure: a randomized controlled study. Liver Transpl Off Publ Am Assoc Study Liver Dis Int Liver Transpl Soc. 2004;10:1109–19.
24. Hassanein TI, et al. Randomized controlled study of extracorporeal albumin dialysis for hepatic encephalopathy in advanced cirrhosis. Hepatology. 2007;46:1853–62.
25. Banares R, et al. Extracorporeal albumin dialysis with the molecular adsorbent recirculating system in acute-on-chronic liver failure: the RELIEF trial. Hepatology. 2013;57:1153–62.
26. Kribben A, et al. Effects of fractionated plasma separation and adsorption on survival in patients with acute-on-chronic liver failure. Gastroenterology. 2012;142:782–789.e783.
27. Demetriou AA, et al. Prospective, randomized, multicenter, controlled trial of a bioartificial liver in treating acute liver failure. Ann Surg. 2004;239:660–7. ; discussion 667–70.
28. Stutchfield BM, Simpson K, Wigmore SJ. Systematic review and meta-analysis of survival following extracorporeal liver support. Br J Surg. 2011;98:623–31.
29. Dhawan A, Puppi J, Hughes RD, Mitry RR. Human hepatocyte transplantation: current experience and future challenges. Nat Rev Gastroenterol Hepatol. 2010;7(5):288–98. ** of considerable interest, as this article reviews the current state of clinical LCT.
30. Dhawan A, Strom SC, Sokal E, Fox IJ. Human hepatocyte transplantation. Methods Mol Biol. 2010;640:525–34.
31. Hughes RD, Mitry RR, Dhawan A. Current status of hepatocyte transplantation. Transplantation. 2012;93(4):342–7.
32. Strom SC, Fisher RA, Rubinstein WS, et al. Transplantation of human hepatocytes. Transplant Proc. 1997;29(4):2103–6.
33. Horslen SP, McCowan TC, Goertzen TC, et al. Isolated hepatocyte transplantation in an infant with a severe urea cycle disorder. Pediatrics. 2003;111(6 Pt 1):1262–7.
34. Stéphenne X, Najimi M, Smets F, Reding R, de Ville de Goyet J, Sokal EM. Cryopreserved liver cell transplantation controls ornithine transcarbamylase deficient patient while awaiting liver transplantation. Am J Transplant. 2005;5(8):2058–61.
35. Puppi J, Tan N, Mitry RR, et al. Hepatocyte transplantation followed by auxiliary liver transplantation – a novel treatment for ornithine transcarbamylase deficiency. Am J Transplant. 2008;8(2):452–7.
36. Meyburg J, Das AM, Hoerster F, et al. One liver for four children: first clinical series of liver cell transplantation for severe neonatal urea cycle defects. Transplantation. 2009;87(5):636–41.

37. Stéphenne X, Najimi M, Sibille C, Nassogne MC, Smets F, Sokal EM. Sustained engraftment and tissue enzyme activity after liver cell transplantation for argininosuccinate lyase deficiency. Gastroenterology. 2006;130(4):1317–23.
38. Dhawan A, Mitry RR, Hughes RD. Hepatocyte transplantation for liver-based metabolic disorders. J Inherit Metab Dis. 2006;29(2–3):431–5.
39. Allen KJ, Mifsud NA, Williamson R, Bertolino P, Hardikar W. Cell-mediated rejection results in allograft loss after liver cell transplantation. Liver Transpl. 2008;14(5):688–94.
40. Soltys KA, Soto-Gutiérrez A, Nagaya M, et al. Barriers to the successful treatment of liver disease by hepatocyte transplantation. J Hepatol. 2010;53(4):769–74.
41. Schneider A, Attaran M, Meier PN, et al. Hepatocyte transplantation in an acute liver failure due to mushroom poisoning. Transplantation. 2006;82(8):1115–6.
42. Khan AA, Habeeb A, Parveen N, et al. Peritoneal transplantation of human fetal hepatocytes for the treatment of acute fatty liver of pregnancy: a case report. Trop Gastroenterol. 2004;25(3):141–3.
43. Baccarani U, Adani GL, Sanna A, et al. Portal vein thrombosis after intraportal hepatocytes transplantation in a liver transplant recipient. Transpl Int. 2005;18(6):750–4.
44. Strom SC, Fisher RA, Thompson MT, et al. Hepatocyte transplantation as a bridge to orthotopic liver transplantation in terminal liver failure. Transplantation. 1997;63(4):559–69.
45. Jorns C, Nowak G, Nemeth A, Zemack H, Mörk LM, Johansson H, Gramignoli R, Watanabe M, Karadagi A, Alheim M, Hauzenberger D, van Dijk R, Bosma PJ, Ebbesen F, Szakos A, Fischler B, Strom S, Ellis E, Ericzon BG. De novo donor-specific HLA antibody formation in two patients with Crigler-Najjar syndrome type I following human hepatocyte transplantation with partial hepatectomy preconditioning. Am J Transplant. 2016;16(3):1021–30.
46. Soltys KA, Setoyama K, Tafaleng EN, Soto Gutiérrez A, Fong J, Fukumitsu K, Nishikawa T, Nagaya M, Sada R, Haberman K, Gramignoli R, Dorko K, Tahan V, Dreyzin A, Baskin K, Crowley JJ, Quader MA, Deutsch M, Ashokkumar C, Shneider BL, Squires RH, Ranganathan S, Reyes-Mugica M, Dobrowolski SF, Mazariegos G, Elango R, Stolz DB, Strom SC, Vockley G, Roy-Chowdhury J, Cascalho M, Guha C, Sindhi R, Platt JL, Fox IJ. Host conditioning and rejection monitoring in hepatocyte transplantation in humans. J Hepatol. 2017;66(5):987–1000.
47. Touboul T, Hannan NR, Corbineau S, et al. Generation of functional hepatocytes from human embryonic stem cells under chemically defined conditions that recapitulate liver development. Hepatology. 2010;51(5):1754–65.
48. Espejel S, Roll GR, McLaughlin KJ, et al. Induced pluripotent stem cell-derived hepatocytes have the functional and proliferative capabilities needed for liver regeneration in mice. J Clin Invest. 2010;120(9):3120–6.
49. Struecker B, Raschzok N, Sauer IM. Liver support strategies: cutting-edge technologies. Nat Rev Gastroenterol Hepatol. 2014;11(3):166–76.
50. Yee ML, Tan HH. Use of everolimus in liver transplantation. World J Hepatol. 2017;9(23):990–1000.
51. Zhou J, Hu Z, Zhang Q, Li Z, Xiang J, Yan S, Wu J, Zhang M, Zheng S. Spectrum of De novo cancers and predictors in liver transplantation: analysis of the scientific registry of transplant recipients database. PLoS One. 2016;11(5):e0155179. https://doi.org/10.1371/journal.pone.0155179. eCollection 2016.
52. Faulk DM, Wildemann JD, Badylak SF. Decellularization and cell seeding of whole liver biologic scaffolds composed of extracellular matrix. J Clin Exp Hepatol. 2015;5(1):69–80.
53. Uygun BE, Soto-Gutierrez A, Yagi H, Izamis ML, Guzzardi MA, Shulman C, Milwid J, Kobayashi N, Tilles A, Berthiaume F, Hertl M, Nahmias Y, Yarmush ML, Uygun K. Organ reengineering through development of a transplantable recellularized liver graft using decellularized liver matrix. Nat Med. 2010;16(7):814–20.
54. Londono R, Badylak SF. Biologic scaffolds for regenerative medicine: mechanisms of in vivo remodeling. Ann Biomed Eng. 2015;43(3):577–92.
55. Badylak SF. Decellularized allogeneic and xenogeneic tissue as a bioscaffold for regenerative medicine: factors that influence the host response. Ann Biomed Eng. 2014;42(7):1517–27.

56. Alexandrova K, Griesel C, Barthold M, Heuft HG, Ott M, Winkler M, Schrem H, Manns MP, Bredehornsp T, Net M, MMI V, Kafert-Kasting S, Arseniev L. Large-scale isolation of human hepatocytes for therapeutic application. Cell Transplant. 2005;14(10):845–53.
57. Zhou P, Lessa N, Estrada DC. Decellularized liver matrix as a carrier for the transplantation of human fetal and primary hepatocytes in mice. Liver Transpl. 2011;17(4):418–27.
58. Struecker B, Butter A, Hillebrandt K, Polenz D, Reutzel-Selke A, Tang P, Lippert S, Leder A, Rohn S, Geisel D, Denecke T, Aliyev K, Jöhrens K, Raschzok N, Neuhaus P, Pratschke J, Sauer IM. Improved rat liver decellularization by arterial perfusion under oscillating pressure conditions. J Tissue Eng Regen Med. 2017;11(2):531–41.
59. Soto-Gutierrez A, Zhang L, Medberry C, Fukumitsu K, Faulk D, Jiang H, Reing J, Gramignoli R, Komori J, Ross M, Nagaya M, Lagasse E, Stolz D, Strom SC, Fox IJ, Badylak SF. A whole-organ regenerative medicine approach for liver replacement. Tissue Eng Part C Methods. 2011;17(6):677–86. Epub 2011 Apr 20.
60. Baptista PM, Siddiqui MM, Lozier G, Rodriguez SR, Atala A, Soker S. The use of whole organ decellularization for the generation of a vascularized liver organoid. Hepatology. 2011;53(2):604–17.
61. Struecker B, Hillebrandt KH, Voitl R, Butter A, Schmuck RB, Reutzel-Selke A, Geisel D, Joehrens K, Pickerodt PA, Raschzok N, Puhl G, Neuhaus P, Pratschke J, Sauer IM. Porcine liver decellularization under oscillating pressure conditions: a technical refinement to improve the homogeneity of the decellularization process. Tissue Eng Part C Methods. 2015;21(3):303–13.
62. Barakat O, Abbasi S, Rodriguez G, Rios J, Wood RP, Ozaki C, Holley LS, Gauthier PK. Use of decellularized porcine liver for engineering humanized liver organ. J Surg Res. 2012;173(1):e11–25.
63. Verstegen MMA, Willemse J, van den Hoek S, Kremers GJ, Luider TM, van Huizen NA, Willemssen FEJA, Metselaar HJ, IJzermans JNM, van der Laan LJW, de Jonge J. Decellularization of whole human liver grafts using controlled perfusion for transplantable organ bioscaffolds. Stem Cells Dev. 2017;26(18):1304–15. https://doi.org/10.1089/scd.2017.0095. Epub 2017 Jul 31.
64. Mazza G, Rombouts K, Rennie Hall A, Urbani L, Vinh Luong T, Al-Akkad W, Longato L, Brown D, Maghsoudlou P, Dhillon AP, Fuller B, Davidson B, Moore K, Dhar D, De Coppi P, Malago M, Pinzani M. Decellularized human liver as a natural 3D-scaffold for liver bioengineering and transplantation. Sci Rep. 2015;5:13079.
65. Butter A, Aliyev K, Hillebrandt KH, Raschzok N, Kluge M, Seiffert N, Tang P, Napierala H, Muhamma AI, Reutzel-Selke A, Andreou A, Pratschke J, Sauer IM, Struecker B. Evolution of graft morphology and function after recellularization of decellularized rat livers. J Tissue Eng Regen Med. 2018;12(2):e807–16.
66. Bao J, Shi Y, Sun H, Yin X, Yang R, Li L, Chen X, Bu H. Construction of a portal implantable functional tissue-engineered liver using perfusion-decellularized matrix and hepatocytes in rats. Cell Transplant. 2011;20(5):753–66.
67. Hassanein W, Uluer MC, Langford J, Woodall JD, Cimeno A, Dhru U, Werdesheim A, Harrison J, Rivera-Pratt C, Klepfer S, Khalifeh A, Buckingham B, Brazio PS, Parsell D, Klassen C, Drachenberg C, Barth RN, JC LM. Recellularization via the bile duct supports functional allogenic and xenogenic cell growth on a decellularized rat liver scaffold. Organogenesis. 2017;13(1):16–27.
68. Collin de l'Hortet A, Takeishi K, Guzman-Lepe J, Handa K, Matsubara K, Fukumitsu K, Dorko K, Presnell SC, Yagi H, Soto-Gutierrez A. Liver-regenerative transplantation: regrow and reset. Am J Transplant. 2016;16(6):1688–96.
69. Hussein KH, Park KM, Kang KS, Woo HM. Heparin-gelatin mixture improves vascular reconstruction efficiency and hepatic function in bioengineered livers. Acta Biomater. 2016;38:82–93.

70. Ko IK, Peng L, Peloso A, Smith CJ, Dhal A, Deegan DB, Zimmerman C, Clouse C, Zhao W, Shupe TD, Soker S, Yoo JJ, Atala A. Bioengineered transplantable porcine livers with re-endothelialized vasculature. Biomaterials. 2015;40:72–9.
71. Zhou P, Huang Y, Guo Y, Wang L, Ling C, Guo Q, Wang Y, Zhu S, Fan X, Zhu M, Huang H, Lu Y, Wang Z. Decellularization and Recellularization of rat livers with hepatocytes and endothelial progenitor cells. Artif Organs. 2016;40(3):E25–38.
72. Wang Y, Bao J, Wu X, Wu Q, Li Y, Zhou Y, Li L, Bu H. Genipin crosslinking reduced the immunogenicity of xenogeneic decellularized porcine whole-liver matrices through regulation of immune cell proliferation and polarization. Sci Rep. 2016;6:24779.
73. Bao J, Wu Q, Sun J, Zhou Y, Wang Y, Jiang X, Li L, Shi Y, Bu H. Hemocompatibility improvement of perfusion-decellularized clinical-scale liver scaffold through heparin immobilization. Sci Rep. 2015;5:10756.
74. Crapo PM, Gilbert TW, Badylak SF. An overview of tissue and whole organ decellularization processes. Biomaterials. 2011;32(12):3233–43.
75. Mirmalek-Sani SH, Sullivan DC, Zimmerman C, Shupe TD, Petersen BE, Am J. Immunogenicity of decellularized porcine liver for bioengineered hepatic tissue. Am J Pathol. 2013;183(2):558–65.

Index

D. Bezinover, F. Saner (eds.), *Critical Care for Potential Liver Transplant Candidates*,
https://doi.org/10.1007/978-3-319-92934-7

The manufacturer's authorised representative in the EU is Springer Nature Customer Service Centre GmbH, Europaplatz 3, 69115 Heidelberg, Germany. If you have any concerns regarding our products, please contact ProductSafety@springernature.com

Printed and bound by CPI Group (UK) Ltd, Croydon, CR0 4YY

22/09/2026

02221065-0001